Reconstructive Surgery of the Esophagus

Mark K. Ferguson, MD
Professor, Department of Surgery
The University of Chicago

Futura Publishing Company, Inc.
Armonk, NY
www.futuraco.com

Library of Congress Cataloging-in-Publication Data

Ferguson, Mark K.
Reconstructive surgery of the esophagus / by Mark K. Ferguson.
p. ; cm.
Includes bibliographical references and index.
ISBN 0-87993-494-8 (hardcover : alk. paper)
1. Esophagus—Surgery. I. Title.
[DNLM: 1. Esophagus—surgery. 2. Esophageal Diseases—surgery.
WI 250 F353r 2001]
RD539.5 .F47 2001
617.5'48—dc21

2001040911

Futura Publishing Company, Inc.
135 Bedford Road
Armonk, New York 10504
www.futuraco.com

ISBN #:0-87993-494-8

Printed in the United States of America on acid-free paper.

Contents

Dedication

To my wife, Phyllis, whose love and support have made enjoyment of my life and my career possible.

To my son, Ben, whose dreams I hope are fulfilled and fulfilling.

To my uncle, Donald J. Ferguson, MD, PhD, who, by striving for perfection in the imperfect world of surgery, was an inspiration to two generations of physicians.

Preface

The art of esophageal surgery is now over 100 years old. Many of the problems faced by the early pioneers of esophageal surgery remain clinical issues today. During my training, I often heard the phrase "if it was easy, everyone would want to do it." This sentiment is particularly apropos of esophageal reconstructive surgery. Although the occasional esophageal surgeon will approach straightforward operations such as fundoplication and hiatal hernia repair with aplomb, contemplation of the more difficult reconstructive operations typically produces anxiety, and some surgeons experience real apprehension. The reasons for this trepidation lie in the technical complexity of the operations, the physical stamina that is often required, and the seemingly unending list of potential complications associated with such procedures. These issues were extant a century ago and remain the bane of the esophageal surgeon to this day.

Reconstructive surgery of the esophagus is not a science, but a discipline that requires knowledge of a host of different and sometimes arcane aspects of physiology and anatomy. The esophagus and related structures extend from the base of the tongue to the stomach, traversing three anatomic regions which are claimed as the province of at least that number of surgical specialties. Esophageal reconstructive surgery, perhaps more than any other discipline, has simultaneously enjoyed the respect and aversion of diverse specialists who have tasted both the frustration and the joy of its demands.

There are a number of excellent recently published books that deal with esophageal surgery in general and reconstructive surgery in particular. One might reasonably ask why another book on esophageal surgery was thought necessary. The aim of this book is different than that of the general esophageal texts. What I hope to provide is a systematic and comprehensive analysis of information on esophageal reconstruction that exists perhaps nowhere else in a single source. This text contains references to most original source material as well as to reviews of relevant subjects. Basic science information is provided whenever possible. This permits examination of current dogma and provides a basis for rational decision making with regards to esophageal reconstruction.

Using this information, I have endeavored to provide a synthesis of various aspects of esophageal reconstructive surgery that is based primarily on evidence and as little as possible on my own personal preferences. The careful reader will find evidence of my teaching and personal clinical experience in many places. However, I hope to have differentiated fact from opinion and to have indicated where my opinion diverges from the information available in the literature. The result is a text that provides the practicing surgeon with indications for and descriptions of available options for esophageal reconstruction. It also contains the information necessary to help avoid common problems associated with esophageal reconstructive surgery and to manage complications when they occur (as they most certainly will).

The text is liberally illustrated with original line drawings that depict the relevant anatomy and steps associated with each procedure. Even the least astute viewer will immediately recognize the lack of artistic value in these renderings. They are designed to be functional and to convey the necessary information that will provide a guide to each procedure and permit most surgeons to steer clear of common pitfalls.

I have many people to thank for the impact they have had on my career and on the writing of this book. My uncle, Dr. Donald Ferguson, was the first individual who inspired me to pursue surgery as a discipline. He was the quintessential role model for me throughout medical school and residency training. From my medical school years on, my mentors included some giants of esophageal surgery. Dr. Tom DeMeester was among my professors who stimulated my interest in both benign and malignant esophageal diseases. Dr. David Skinner became Chairman of the Department of Surgery at the University of Chicago the year I entered medical school there. He was first my professor, then my mentor, and ultimately we became friends and colleagues on the faculty. His fearless approach to clinical problems, consummate surgical skill, and endless good cheer provided all the impetus I needed to look on the esophagus as the most fascinating field of surgical endeavor. It was through Dr. Skinner that I had an opportunity to work with Mr. Ronald Belsey, one of the pioneers of esophageal surgery. After Mr. Belsey's retirement from his position at the Bristol Royal Infirmary, he spent six months of each year on the faculty at the University of Chicago during a memorable decade. Thus, I was exposed simultaneously to the thoughts of three world-renowned esophageal surgeons. A wealth of information was exchanged at each of our Saturday morning conferences and during the many esophageal operations that took place. It was during this period that much of the basic knowledge I posses regarding esophageal surgery and physiology was accumulated.

During this period, I also had the privilege of training with a number of the next generation of accomplished esophageal surgeons, including Drs. Carlos Pellegrini, Alex Little, Keith Naunheim, and Nasser Altorki, each of whom is a good friend and each of whom has taught me much about surgery of the esophagus. My mentors attracted many visitors, and I had the opportunity to become acquainted with a number of surgeons from outside of the United States who also enjoyed international reputations. I have learned a great deal from these individuals through our discussions over the years. Finally, my association with members of the general surgery and thoracic surgery societies over the years have been very rewarding, and I am grateful to a host of individuals for their friendship and guidance. Close personal friends in the community of esophageal surgeons include Drs. Victor Trastek, Mark Orringer, Joseph Miller, Toni Lerut, Andre Duranceau, Sergio Stipa, Luigi Bonavina, Romeo Bardini, Gerald O'Sullivan, Manjit Bains, Alberto Ruol, Gilles Beauchamp, Douglas Mathisen, the late Andrea Segalin, Clemente Iascone, and Stanley Fell. Others whose counsel and friendship I value include Alberto Peracchia, J. Rudiger Siewert, Clem Hiebert, Glyn Jamieson, Nobutoshi Ando, Hiroshi Watanabe, Anthony Watson, Hiroshi Akiyama, Guo Jun Huang, the late Lucius Hill, F. Henry Ellis, Jr., Arnulf Holscher, Dorothea Liebermann-Meffert, James Maher, Philip Donahue, Attila Csendes, John Wong, Tetsuru Nishihira, Aldo Moraldi, Bruno Zilberstein, Jean-Marie Collard, and Kin-Ichi Nabeya.

The practice of esophageal surgery requires meticulous attention to detail, to the extent that successful surgery is not usually possible without the help of resident surgeons and fellows. I have been privileged to work with a large number of truly outstanding individuals during my nearly two decades of clinic practice at the University of Chicago. I am grateful for the care they provided my patients and for what I have learned from each of them.

The staff at Futura publishing has been outstanding throughout the writing of this book. Special thanks go to Mr. Steven Korn, the publisher who was instrumental in getting me to complete this project. His frequent phone calls during the eight years from the inception of this book until its publication provided the encouragement and support that allowed me finally to focus on the project and to complete the majority of the writing within the span of a single year. I also am indebted to Kirstin Bellhouse, my editor, whose knowledge, skill, and positive outlook have made even the normally mundane work of getting my writing into print a great pleasure.

My hope is that this book will permit the reader to take a fresh look at a subject that is mired in history and convention and that has not been strongly influenced by the types of advances that have occurred in other more common surgical disciplines during the last decade. Perhaps this will stimulate original ideas and the development of new approaches to these problems. The investigation of basic esophageal physiology is ongoing and may contribute to a better understanding of the pathophysiology of disease and the functional consequences of esophageal reconstruction. Molecular and genetic therapies may obviate the need for many current surgical procedures. No doubt new surgical techniques will be devised and current techniques will be modified as minimally invasive approaches. Progress in the development of cultured or artificial tissues may render harvesting of reconstructive tissues obsolete. The text provides guidance as to the areas in which most improvement is necessary.

Surgeons are blessed with the knowledge and skill to be able to restore swallowing and digestive functions to patients who, a few decades ago, were destined to live without the hope of ever eating. It is a privilege to be a part of this effort and to hopefully stimulate the future work of others in this field.

Chapter 1

History of Esophageal Reconstructive Surgery

Esophageal reconstruction, even with the benefit of a century of experience and modern surgical techniques, remains a daunting task in the hands of most physicians. That surgeons now routinely expect a successful outcome is due in large part to the efforts of a small group of intrepid individuals who were faced with seemingly insurmountable obstacles. Their operations were performed on an organ that resisted successful anastomosis, that was seemingly too long to permit replacement in a single stage, and that was located in the thorax, the opening of which meant almost certain death for the patient. They succeeded in overcoming each of these obstacles in the early part of the twentieth century, permitting the next generation of surgeons to accumulate extensive practical experience with esophageal reconstruction. Based on this work, surgeons now have available numerous options for esophageal reconstruction that allow operations to be tailored to the individual patient. The contributions of many of these historical figures have been summarized previously by Meade, on whose invaluable book much of this chapter is based.[1]

Indications for esophageal reconstruction early in the twentieth century were somewhat different than those today. Esophageal cancer was recognized in the late nineteenth century as a disease for which treatment was primarily palliative, despite Mikulicz' suggestion that carcinoma of the esophagus should have a high rate of cure after resection.[2] Treatment of esophageal cancer in the latter half of the nineteenth century was largely confined to dilation of malignant strictures. In 1877, the first resection of the esophagus was performed by Czerny in Heidelberg.[3] A summary of nine resections for cancer reported by 1885, in which no reconstruction was attempted in the four short-term survivors, further discouraged attempts at both esophageal resection and replacement.[2] In fact, in the reports by Torek and Zaaijer in 1913 of the first successful

From Ferguson MK: *Reconstructive Surgery of the Esophagus* Armonk, NY: Futura Publishing Company, Inc., © 2002.

transthoracic esophagectomies for carcinoma, no reconstruction was performed initially.[4,5] It wasn't until two decades later that successful simultaneous transthoracic esophagectomy and reconstruction was described.

In contrast to malignant esophageal strictures, benign strictures were recognized frequently and were considered appropriate for aggressive intervention. At the close of the nineteenth century most benign strictures were secondary to caustic ingestion. Corrosive substances were sold in general stores without proper labeling or warnings on the packaging, leading to many instances of accidental ingestion in addition to their frequent use in suicide attempts. Many of the resultant strictures were difficult to dilate due to their length and degree of fibrosis. Peptic strictures undoubtedly existed, but were not formally described until 1910 by Chevalier Jackson,[6] and were more easily dilated than were caustic strictures. When dilation therapy failed, few options were available to palliate dysphagia. Internal esophagotomy had been attempted during the middle and late nineteenth century with disastrous results,[7] opening the way for attempts at stricture bypass or esophageal replacement.

Proposed and Experimental Reconstructive Techniques

A variety of techniques for esophageal reconstruction were proposed in the late nineteenth and early twentieth centuries, many of which were used experimentally on cadavers or animals. The stomach was among the first organs to be proposed as a possible esophageal replacement. In 1895, Biondi suggested that the stomach could be pulled into the chest, where an anastomosis could be constructed between it and the esophagus.[8] Gosset reported results of such a transdiaphragmatic esophagogastrostomy performed in dogs in 1903.[9] An extrathoracic tube created from the greater curvature of the stomach was used for reconstruction in both cadavers and dogs by Beck and Carrell in a fashion that was to be popularized much later (Figure 1-1).[10] A similar proposal was made by Hirsch who suggested that a gastric tube could be formed from the anterior surface of the stomach.[11] In 1920, Kirschner reported experimental results of an antesternal pull-up of the whole stomach, rather than a reverse gastric tube, performed in both cadavers and dogs (Figure 1-2).[12] At this early date, despite the work that had been done, the level of enthusiasm for use of the stomach in esophageal reconstruction was quite low. The use of jejunum as an esophageal substitute was originally described by Wullstein in 1904.[13] Lexer subsequently suggested that a skin tube could be fashioned, in the manner originally described by Bircher,[14] to bridge the gap between the cervical esophagus and the proximal end of the antethoracic jejunal segment.[15]

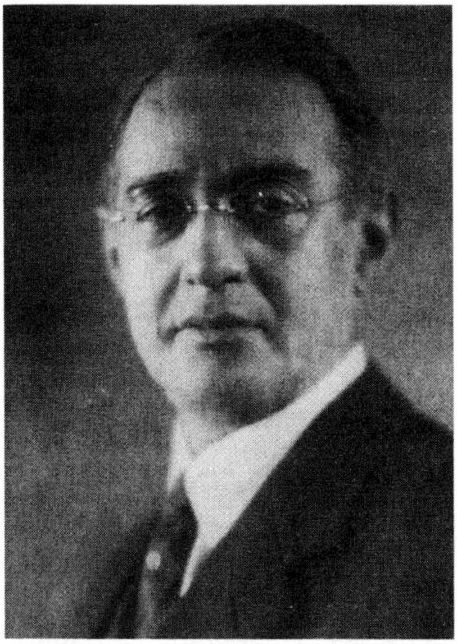

Figure 1-1. Carl Beck (1856-1911). From Meade RH, *A History of Thoracic Surgery*, 1961. Courtesy of Charles C. Thomas, Publisher, Ltd., Springfield, IL.

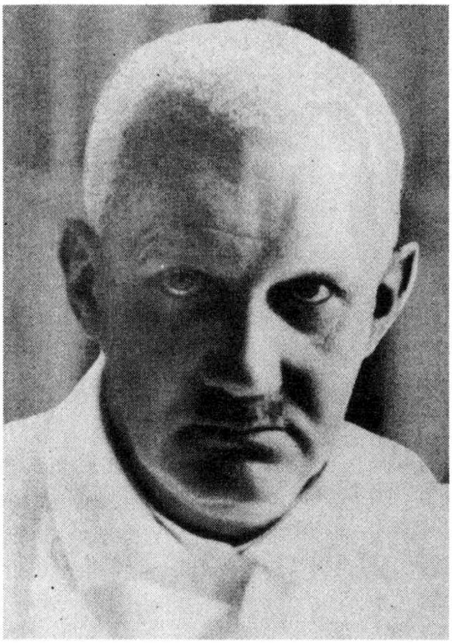

Figure 1-2. Martin B. Kirschner (1879-1942). From Meade RH, *A History of Thoracic Surgery*, 1961. Courtesy of Charles C. Thomas, Publisher, Ltd., Springfield, IL.

Early Clinical Reconstructive Efforts

Early efforts at esophageal surgery were hindered by substantial obstacles, including the lack of antiseptic techniques and antibiotics and a poor understanding of the physiology of the pleural space. Antiseptic techniques were in the arduous process of being adopted during the formative years of esophageal surgery. Wound infection was common, and healing by primary intention, especially of esophageal anastomoses, was unusual. The lack of antibiotics for perioperative use in esophageal surgery meant that the slightest intrapleural leak of esophageal contents portended a life-threatening infection. Entry into the pleural space while patients were under ether anesthesia delivered through a mask resulted in severe cardiovascular instability and a high risk of intraoperative death. If a patient was fortunate enough to survive, the lack of appropriate drainage techniques often led to postoperative empyema, a common cause of operative mortality. For these reasons, early operations for esophageal reconstruction were performed extrapleurally.

Skin Flaps

One of the first descriptions of the use of a skin tube as a replacement for a segment of the esophagus was published by Mikulicz in 1886.[2] Following resection of the cervical esophagus and creation of an external esophagostomy, the fistula subsequently was closed using the skin of the neck as a plastic substitute. The patient died some months later, having been able to ingest normal food for 3 months following reconstruction. The use of skin tubes for reconstruction of the cervical esophagus was also reported by Garre in 1898.[16] In 1894, Bircher constructed an extrathoracic skin tube for the purpose of bridging the gap between the cervical esophagus and stomach.[14] He performed a gastrostomy to connect to the distal end of the skin tube 6 weeks after construction of the tube, and demonstrated that liquids would pass through the tube and into the stomach. He never anastomosed the cervical esophagus to the tube for fear that solids would not pass. Both of his patients died in the early postoperative period. Denk performed a transhiatal esophagectomy for cancer in 1913 and reconstructed the patient using an antethoracic skin tube.[17] The Bircher technique was first successfully completed by Payr in 1917.[18] Dissatisfaction with results of these techniques prompted further investigation into the use of stomach and bowel as reconstructive tissues.

Stomach

The Hungarian Jianu reported his experience with creation of a tube from the greater curve of the stomach after the fashion of Beck (Figure 1-3).[10,19] He brought the tube subcutaneously to the neck, devising what was subsequently known as the Beck-Jianu operation. A similar operation was proposed by Halpern.[20] Willy Meyer reported its use in three pa-

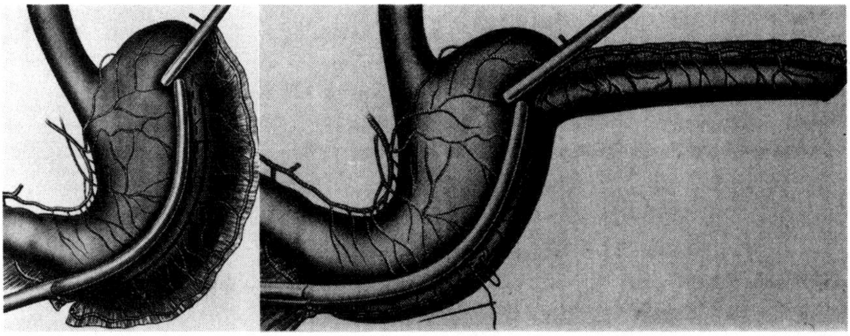

Figure 1-3. Jianu's technique of creating a reversed gastric tube from the greater curvature of the stomach. The greater curve is clamped and the line of division is indicated (left). After division, the cut edges are oversewn to create the gastric tube (right). From Meyer W: Oesophagoplasty. *Ann Surg* 1913;58:289-295.

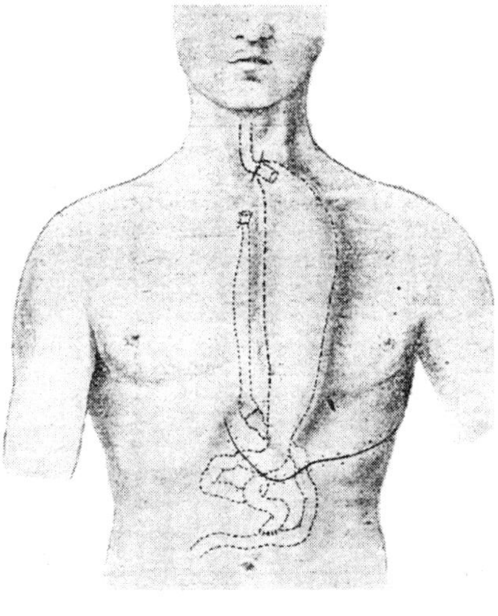

Figure 1-4. Kirschner's technique for an isoperistaltic, subcutaneous gastric pull-up. From Kirschner: Ein neues Verfahren der Oesophagoplastik. *Arch Klin Chir* 1920;114:606-663. Springer-Verlag, with permission.

tients.[21] The procedure was used by Lotheissen, who described an initial favorable experience and, a decade later, a much larger experience in 44 patients.[22-23] In contrast to use of a gastric tube, Fink divided the duodenum, mobilized the whole stomach, and brought it through a subcutaneous tunnel to the suprasternal notch in an antiperistaltic fashion. The esophagus and duodenum were subsequently connected using a skin tube.[24] Kirschner first performed an isoperistaltic gastric pull-up in 1920 for a patient with a lye stricture, using a subcutaneous tunnel for the pull-up and a direct cervical esophagogastric anastomosis (Figure 1-4).[12]

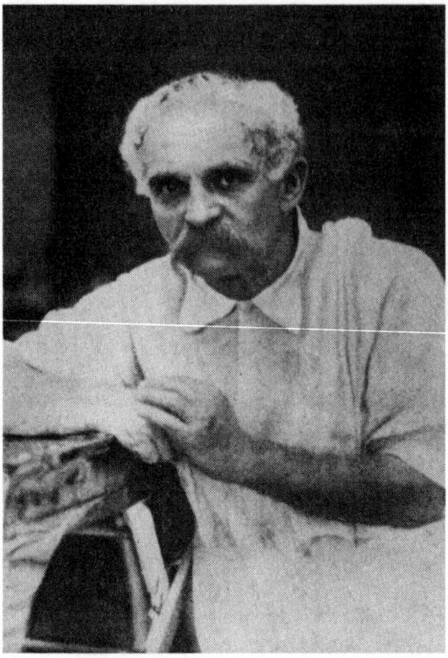

Figure 1-5. Cesar Roux (1857-1934). From Meade RH, *A History of Thoracic Surgery*, 1961. Courtesy of Charles C. Thomas, Publisher, Ltd., Springfield, IL.

Jejunum

The use of jejunum as an esophageal substitute was reported by Roux in 1907, who brought an isolated segment of jejunum through a subcutaneous tunnel for subsequent anastomosis to the stomach distally and the esophagus proximally (Figure 1-5).[25] A similar technique was used by Herzen, who performed the reconstruction in three stages.[26] In the fashion of Lexer, the Roux operation was combined with that of Bircher, and the use of an antethoracic jejuno-dermato-esophagoplasty became popular for reconstruction, particularly for corrosive strictures.[15]

Colon

Kelling first described the clinical use of colon as an esophageal substitute in 1911.[27] A segment of transverse colon was brought subcutaneously in an isoperistaltic fashion and its distal end was anastomosed to the stomach. In a subsequent stage a skin tube was created which was to be connected between the cervical esophagus and the colon. This was never completed, as the patient died of carcinoma. Subsequent modifications included the use of an antiperistaltic segment of transverse colon[28] and the use of an isoperistaltic segment of cecum and ascending colon.[29]

Summary

In 1934, Ochsner and Owens published an overview of extrathoracic esophageal reconstruction techniques in use up to that time for manage-

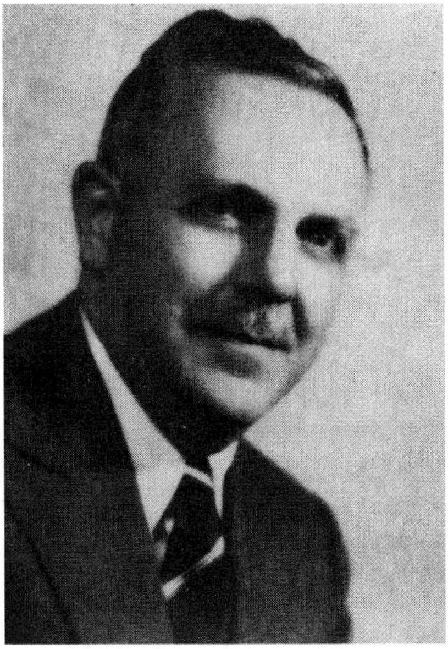

Figure 1-6. Alton Ochsner (1896-1981). From Meade RH, *A History of Thoracic Surgery,* 1961. Courtesy of Charles C. Thomas, Publisher, Ltd., Springfield, IL.

ment of esophageal obstruction (Figure 1-6).[30] It should come as no surprise that, due to the low rate of success of each of the procedures described above, a wide variety of methods were in use. A total of 242 operations in 240 patients were evaluated and were grouped according to the techniques employed. These included 1) dermato-esophagoplasty, using full thickness skin flaps or inlay grafts lining a skin tunnel (Figure 1-7); 2) jejuno-esophagoplasty; 3) jejuno-dermato-esophagoplasty; 4) colo-esophagoplasty; 5) gastro-esophagoplasty using a gastric tube or whole stomach; and 6) a variety of miscellaneous or incomplete operations (Table 1-1). Operations were performed for a benign stricture (usually secondary to caustic ingestion) in 55% of patients and for a malignant stricture in 13%. The underlying problem was unstated in 32% and was probably unknown in many of these patients.

Their review represents a watershed, albeit an unintentional one, between the largely unsuccessful reconstructive attempts of the first three decades of the twentieth century and the rapidly improving expertise developed during the subsequent several decades. To their credit, Ochsner and Owens recognized that the ideal method of replacement of an obstructed thoracic esophagus is removal of the diseased portion and reconstruction of the esophagus in the posterior mediastinum. However, they went on to state that "such operations are attended with an extremely high mortality and, therefore, are not feasible or justified." Based on its overall high rate of success, they recommended jejuno-dermato-esophagoplasty as the procedure of choice, despite the large number of operations

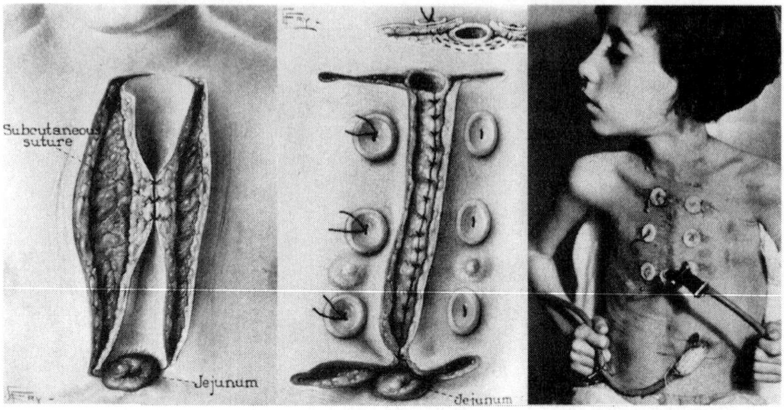

Figure 1-7. The technique for creating a dermatoesophagoplasty is illustrated (left), and its partially complete postoperative appearance is apparent (right). From Ochsner A, Owens N: Anterothoracic oesophagoplasty for impermeable stricture of the oesophagus. *Ann Surg* 1934;100:1055-1091, with permission.

Table 1-1.
Early Results of Extrathoracic Esophageal Reconstruction.

Procedure	Patients (%)	Mortality (%)	Completed (%)	Good Results (%)
Dermatoplasty	32 (13.4)	30.0	63.3	37.5
Jejunoplasty	36 (14.8)	46.7	43.3	33.3
Jejuno-dermatoplasty	100 (41.3)	22.8	66.0	46.0
Coloplasty	20 (8.2)	25.8	61.1	45.0
Gastroplasty (Tube)	24 (9.9)	27.8	11.1	8.3
Gastroplasty (Whole stomach)	22 (9.1)	66.7	45.4	27.3

*From Ochsner and Owens, 1934.[30]

Mortality is computed as deaths divided by the total number of outcomes reported.

Operations completed is calculated for the total number of cases for which an outcome was reported.

Good results are the total number of good outcomes divided by the total number of operated patients.

and inordinate length of time required to accomplish reconstruction using this technique.

Evolution of Current Techniques

In an address before the American Surgical Association in 1909, Willy Meyer summarized the current state-of-the-art regarding esophagogastrostomy following intrathoracic resection of the esophagus (Figure 1-

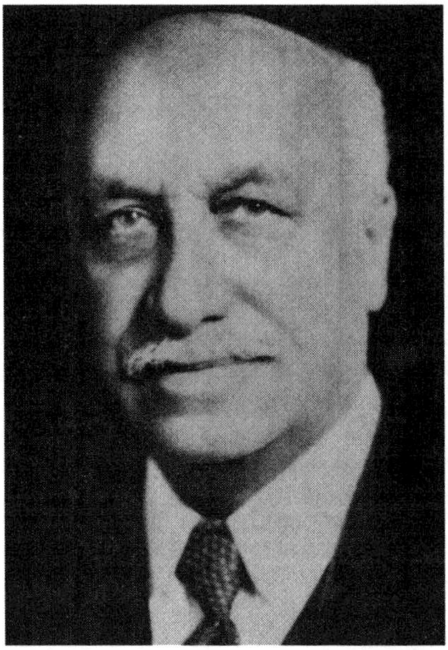

Figure 1-8. Willie Meyer (1880-1952). From Meade RH, *A History of Thoracic Surgery*, 1961. Courtesy of Charles C. Thomas, Publisher, Ltd., Springfield, IL.

8).[31] Encouraged by recent developments in operating under differential pressure, initially advanced by Sauerbruch, Meyer described his own differential pressure chamber and encouraged exploratory thoracotomy in all patients with esophageal cancer as an attempt to improve outcome through resection. Despite the fact that the efforts of six European surgeons had failed to yield a single survivor from this disease, Meyer was undaunted, stating that "even should the first 50 or 100 or 200 cases operated upon for cancer of the oesophagus die, may be [sic] the 51st, 101st, or 201st will live." Though few of his contemporaries were willing to sacrifice the requisite number of patients to achieve this goal, it is likely that many shared the belief that substantial improvement in the treatment of esophageal cancer was possible.

Ironically, improvements that eventually permitted routine esophagectomy and reconstruction were largely unrelated to surgical techniques per se. Advances in anesthetic management, a better understanding of requirements for fluid and electrolyte replacement during and after major surgical intervention, and the development of methods for safe blood transfusion all contributed to improved surgical outcomes. Arguably the most important among these was the development of techniques for positive pressure ventilation through an endotracheal tube, which ultimately permitted safe thoracotomy nearly a century after the introduction of general anesthesia.

The concept of tracheal intubation was not new in the early 1900s. Endotracheal intubation was used to resuscitate drowning victims in the

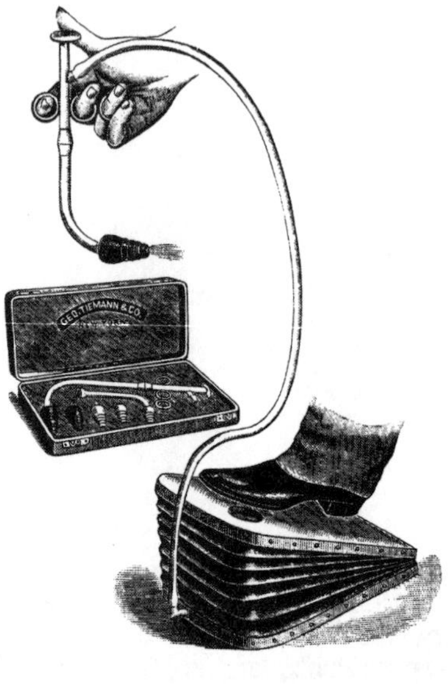

Figure 1-9. The Fell-O'Dwyer apparatus for positive pressure ventilation. From Matas R: Intralaryngeal insufflation. *JAMA* 1900;34:1371-1375, 1468-1473, copyrighted 1900, American Medical Association, with permission.

late eighteenth century, and blind orotracheal intubation was practiced by Macewen and O'Dwyer a century later.[32-34] In 1893, Fell described the use of bellows attached to the endotracheal tube to achieve positive pressure ventilation (Figure 1-9). The "Fell-O'Dwyer" apparatus was welcomed by Matas and Tuffier,[35,36] but its potential was not fully recognized, and it was never adopted for general clinical use in thoracic surgery. Based on instrumentation introduced by Kirstein and the experience of Chevalier Jackson in direct laryngoscopy,[37] techniques of intratracheal insufflation were described by Meltzer and Auer,[38] and were applied clinically using an air-ether combination by Elsberg after the turn of the century.[39] Nevertheless, during World War I the most common technique for delivering anesthetic gases was use of an air-tight mask and positive end-expiratory gas insufflation.

International conflict stimulates scientific advances in many arenas, and the practice of anesthesia following the Great War was no exception. The need for controlled ventilation to permit safe operations on patients requiring repair of maxillofacial injuries incurred during the war prompted reintroduction of the technique of endotracheal intubation by Rowbotham and Magill.[40] Intubation under direct vision was pioneered by Gale and Waters in the United States and by Magill in the United Kingdom in the early 1930s.[41,42] The introduction of specialized endotracheal tubes permitted separate ventilation of individual lungs. Intermittent positive pressure breathing using a closed anesthesia circuit and the use of the paralytic agent curare provided the final and important steps

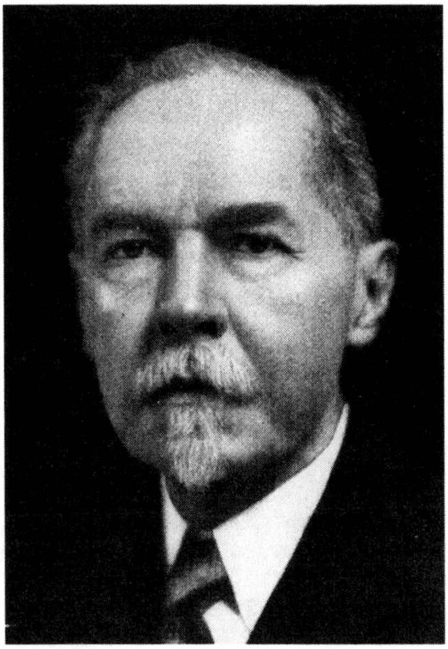

Figure 1-10. Franz Torek (1861-1938). From Meade RH, *A History of Thoracic Surgery*, 1961. Courtesy of Charles C. Thomas, Publisher, Ltd., Springfield, IL.

necessary to allow mechanically controlled ventilation in thoracic surgical patients.[43-46]

Transthoracic Esophagectomy and Reconstruction

Torek's successful transthoracic esophagectomy in 1913 was performed with the patient under an anesthetic provided by intratracheal ether insufflation (Figure 1-10).[4] That the patient survived the operation was due in part to extensive pleural adhesions that prevented the lung from collapsing. Tissue reconstruction was never performed, and the patient took liquids orally which passed from a cervical esophagostomy through a tube into a gastrostomy for 11 years thereafter (Figure 1-11). Other sporadic reports of transthoracic esophagectomy appeared,[5,47-51] but the successful use of modern techniques of reconstruction was not published until 20 years after Torek's original description.

Based on extensive experimental work in animals, the Japanese surgeon Ohsawa was the first to describe the successful performance of a transthoracic esophagectomy and intrathoracic esophagogastrostomy or esophagojejunostomy.[52] That achievement was quickly followed by similar reports from Marshall in Boston and Adams and Phemister in Chicago (Figure 1-12).[53,54] Information subsequently came to light that, during this same period, Yudin of Moscow had developed a successful experience with immediate reconstruction of the esophagus following esophagectomy,

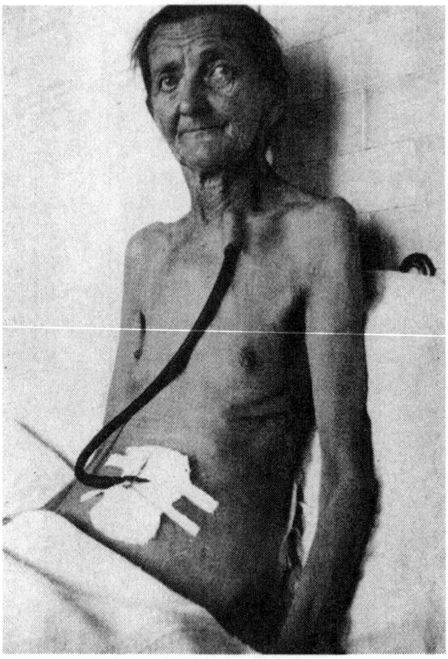

Figure 1-11. The first patient to undergo a successful transthoracic esophagectomy, performed by Torek in 1913. Reprinted with permission from the American College of Surgeons, *Surg Gynecol Obstet* 1913; 16:614-617.

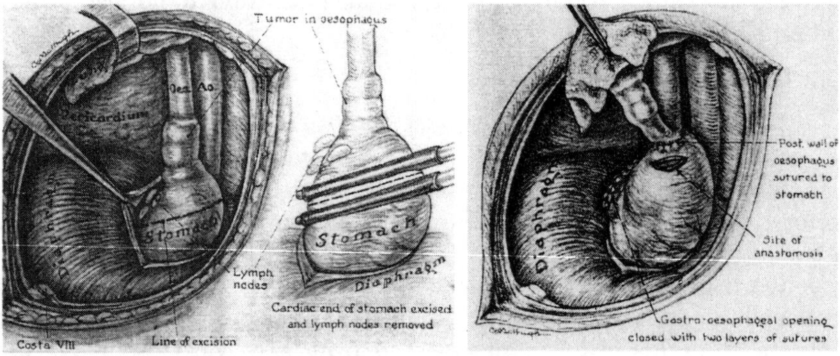

Figure 1-12. The technique for distal esophagectomy (left) and intrathoracic esophagogastrostomy (right) originally described by Adams and Phemister in 1938. From Adams WE, Phemister DB: Carcinoma of the lower thoracic esophagus. Report of a successful resection and esophagogastrostomy. *J Thorac Surg* 1938;7:621-632, with permission.

employing a segment of jejunum brought through a subcutaneous tunnel.[55] Although surgeons continued to perform esophagectomy after the manner of Torek during the 1930s and 1940s,[56-59] the benefits of immediate reconstruction were quickly apparent. These initial successes prompted intense activity directed at identifying the best organ for use in intrathoracic esophageal reconstruction.

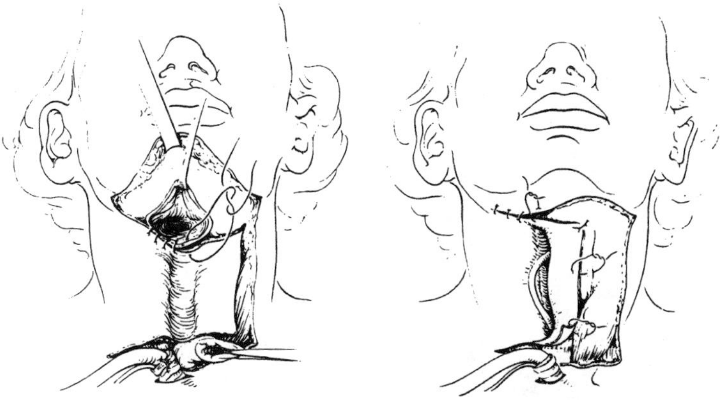

Figure 1-13. The use of a skin flap for replacement of the cervical esophagus, according to the method of Wookey. After resection of the larynx and cervical esophagus, a skin flap is used to create the posterior wall of the neo-esophagus (left) after which the skin flap is rotated to permit completion of the tube (right). Reprinted with permission from the American College of Surgeons, *Surg Gynecol Obstet* 1942;75:499-506.

Skin Flaps

Despite the necessity of performing staged operations, skin flaps continued in use as a primary means of reconstruction for many years. Wookey advocated construction of skin-lined tubes following treatment of carcinoma of the pharynx and for thoracic inlet esophageal lesions (Figure 1-13).[60,61] Ladd used skin tubes for antethoracic reconstruction in patients with esophageal atresia.[62] Watson and Converse developed a technique for radical resection of cervical esophageal cancers, performing reconstruction with skin and pedicled flaps.[63] The summary of Bricker and Burford in 1957 sounded the death knell for primary reconstrucion with skin flaps. Among 16 operated patients, there was only one good result, and only five patients survived.[64] Thereafter, the trend was away from skin flaps for reconstruction due to the need for staged operations, the high incidence of fistulas, and the generally poor results. The techniques are now reserved for use when visceral segment replacement has failed or is inadequate.

Stomach

Despite the early success with stomach pull-up for esophageal reconstruction, and the observation by Kirschner that the stomach can be used routinely for a cervical esophagogastrostomy, there was initial concern as to how far the stomach could be stretched cephalad without compromis-

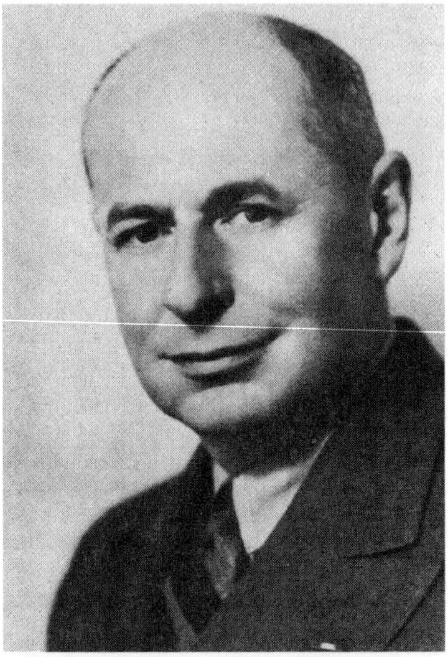

Figure 1-14. Edward Churchill (1895-1972). From Meade RH, *A History of Thoracic Surgery*, 1961. Courtesy of Charles C. Thomas, Publisher, Ltd., Springfield, IL.

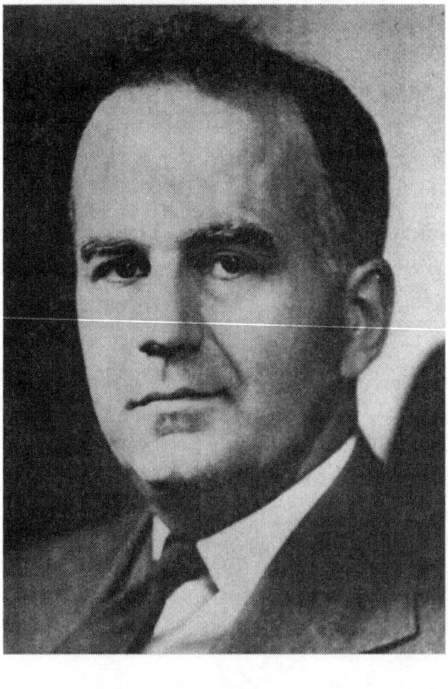

Figure 1-15. Richard Sweet (1901-1962). From Meade RH, *A History of Thoracic Surgery*, 1961. Courtesy of Charles C. Thomas, Publisher, Ltd., Springfield, IL.

ing its blood supply. In 1942, Churchill and Sweet recommended direct esophagogastrostomy only if the esophagus could be transected below the inferior pulmonary vein,[65] but additional experience led Sweet to conclude that anastomoses could be accomplished safely as high as the aortic arch (Figures 1-14, 1-15).[66] The classic reports of Lewis and Sweet in 1946

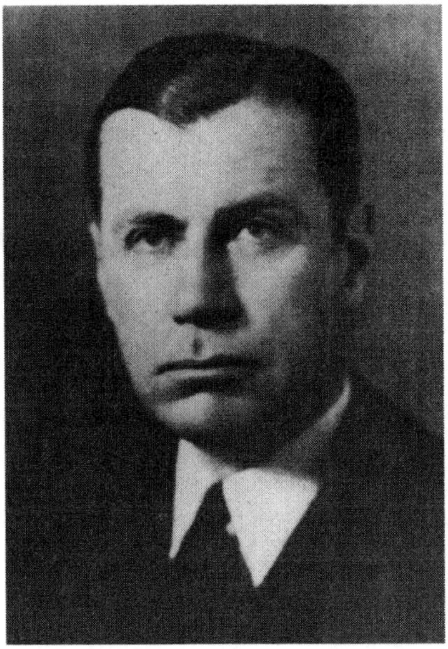

Figure 1-16. William Rienhoff, Jr. (1894-1981). From Meade RH, *A History of Thoracic Surgery*, 1961. Courtesy of Charles C. Thomas, Publisher, Ltd., Springfield, IL.

demonstrated that high intrathoracic anastomoses could be done routinely with success.[67,68] The safety of cervical esophagogastrostomy was confirmed shortly thereafter.[69,70] Gavriliu soon reintroduced the use of a reverse gastric tube, which became a popular means of reconstruction with some surgeons.[71,72] With time, the stomach became the standard organ for use in esophageal reconstruction, particularly for patients who underwent resection for cancer.[73]

Jejunum

The utility of small bowel for use in esophageal reconstruction was well recognized before the 1940s, but prior successes had been achieved only through the use of extrapleural routes. Reinhoff performed the first successful intrathoracic esophagojejunostomy in 1942 and reported the case fully in 1946 (Figure 1-16).[74] His one-stage operation accomplished what Longmire and Ravitch had struggled to achieve for years both in the laboratory and in clinical work.[75] Based on the work of Roux, Herzen, Yudin, and Reinhoff, Harrison described the first reconstruction of the entire esophagus with jejunum using a transpleural route in 1949.[76] Robertson and Serjeant made a major contribution to esophageal surgery in their 1950 description of the substernal route for use in reconstruction, which remains a favorite technique of many surgeons today.[77]

Until the 1950s, esophageal replacement was performed for anatomic deficiencies that were most often secondary to atresia, caustic injury, or resection or obstruction related to cancer. Indications expanded to include use of jejunal interposition as a substitute for the lower esophageal sphincter following the report of Merendino and Dillard in 1955,[78] who suggested that a short, isoperistaltic length of jejunum could protect the esophagus from acid-peptic injury. A striking technical innovation was also described at about this time. Androsov and a group of engineers in Moscow developed techniques for small vessel anastomoses using metal clips, and used this method to supply blood from the internal mammary vessels to an interposed segment of intestine in 11 patients.[79] An alternative technique for providing blood supply was described by Kasai, who used a short segment of jejunum on a long vascular pedicle to perform an isolated reconstruction of the cervical esophagus.[80] Follow-up by Allison, Wooler, and Gunning of patients undergoing jejunal interposition at least 3 years previously demonstrated normal nutritional intake and work capacity in most patients, confirming the utility of small bowel as an esophageal substitute for benign disease.[81]

Colon

The colon was the last organ to be successfully used as an intrathoracic esophageal replacement. The reasons for this are likely related to concerns about the reliability of its blood supply, its contents, and the size mismatch between the colon and the esophagus. Few attempts at esophagocologastrostomy were reported prior to the 1950s. A variety of segments had been used, including right, transverse, and left colon. Rudler's collective review, published in 1951, describes 28 cases in which there were 8 operative deaths, while anastomotic leakage occurred in 13 of the 20 survivors.[82]

Orsoni and Lemaire were among the first to describe the routine use of the transverse and descending colon for reconstruction, including its placement through both posterior mediastinal and substernal routes.[83] Goligher and Robin reviewed the attributes of various reconstructive organs in 1954 and concluded that the left colon was best suited for reconstruction of the pharynx and esophagus after pharyngectomy.[84] Subsequent large experiences were published in which either the right[85] or left[86] colon was championed as the segment of choice for interposition. Over time, esophageal replacement using the left colon as described by Belsey held sway by virtue of its smaller diameter and more reliable blood supply.

References

1. Meade RH. **A History of Thoracic Surgery**. Springfield, IL, Charles C. Thomas, 1961.

2. Mikulicz J. Ein Fall von Resection des Carcinomatosen Oesophagus mit Plastischen Ersatz des excirdirten Stuckes. *Prager Med Wschr* 1886;11:93-94.
3. Czerny. Neue Operationen. Zbl Chir 1877;4:433-434.
4. Torek F. The first successful case of resection of the thoracic portion of the oesophagus for carcinoma. *Surg Gynecol Obstet* 1913;16:614-617.
5. Zaaijer. Erfolgreiche transpleurale Resektion eines Cardiacarcinoms. *Beitr Klin Chir* 1913;83:419-430.
6. Jackson C. Peptic ulcer of the esophagus. *JAMA* 1910;55:1857-1858.
7. Gross SW. Gastrostomy, oesophagostomy, internal oesophagotomy, combined oesophagotomy, oesophagectomy, and retrograde divulsion in the treatment of stricture of the oesophagus. *Am J Med Sci* 1884;88:58-69.
8. Biondi D. Experimental intrathoracic esophago-gastrostomy. *Policlinico* (Suppl) 1895:964.
9. Gosset. De l'oesophago-gastrostomie transdiaphragmatique. *Rev de Chir* 1903;28:694-707.
10. Beck C, Carrell A. Demonstration of specimens illustrating a method of formation of a prethoracic esophagus. *Ill Med J* 1905;7:463-464.
11. Hirsch M. Plastischer Ersatz des Oesophagus aus dem Magen. *Zbl Chir* 1911;38:1561-1564.
12. Kirschner. Ein neues Verfahren der Oesophagoplastik. *Arch Klin Chir* 1920;114:606-663.
13. Wullstein L. Ueber antethorakale Oesophago-Jejunostomie und Operationen nach gleichem Prinzip. *Dtsch Med Wschr* 1904;30:734-736.
14. Bircher E. Ein Beitrag zur plastischen Bildung eines neuen Oesophagus. *Zbl Chir* 1907;34:1479-1482.
15. Lexer. Oesophagoplastik. *Dtsch Med Wschr* 1908;34:574.
16. Garre C. Ueber Oesophagus-Resection und Oesophagoplastik. *Langenbeck's Arch Klin Chir* 1898;57:719-722.
17. Denk W. Zur Radikaloperation des Oesophaguskarzinoms. *Zbl Chir* 1913; 40:1965-1968.
18. Payr. Antethorakaler Oesophagusplastik. *Munchen Med Wschr* 1917;64:783.
19. Jianu A. Ueber Oesophagoplastik. *Deutsch Ztschr Chir* 1914;131:397-403.
20. Halpern JO. Zur Frage von der Speiserohrenplastik. *Zbl Chir* 1913;40:1834.
21. Meyer W. Ein Vorschlag bezuglich der Gastrostomie und Gastrostomie und Oesophagoplastik nach Jianu-Roepke. *Zbl Chir* 1913;40:267-268.
22. Lotheissen G. Zur Behandlung der Speiserohrenstrikturen. *Zbl Chir* 1913;40:1969-1971.
23. Lotheissen G. Ueber plastischen Ersatz der Speiserohre, insbesondere aus dem Magen. *Beitr Klin Chir* 1922;126:490-531.
24. Fink F. Ueber plastischen Ersatz der Speiserohre. *Zbl Chir* 1913;40:545-547.
25. Roux. L'oesophago-jejuno-gastrostomose, nouvelle operation pour retrecissement infranchissable de l'oesophage. *Semaine Med* 1907;27:37-40.
26. Herzen P. Eine Modifkation der Roux'schen Oesophago-jejuno-gastrostomie. *Zbl Chir* 1908;35:219-222.
27. Kelling G. Oesophagoplastik mit Hilfe des Querkolon. *Zbl Chir* 1911; 36:1209-1212.
28. Vulliet H. De l'oesophagoplastie et des ses diverses modifications. *Samaine Med* 1911;31:529-530.

29. Roith O. Die Einseitige antethorakale Oesophagoplastik aus dem Dickdarm. *Deutsch Ztschr Chir* 1923-1924;183:419-423.
30. Ochsner A, Owens N. Anterothoracic oesophagoplasty for impermeable stricture of the oesophagus. *Ann Surg* 1934;100:1055-1091.
31. Meyer W. Oesophagogastrostomy after intrathoracic resection of the oesophagus. *Ann Surg* 1909;50:175-189.
32. Macewen W. Clinical observations on the introduction of tracheal tubes by the mouth instead of performing tracheotomy or laryngotomy. *Br Med J* 1880;II:122-124, 163-165.
33. O'Dwyer J. Intubation of the larynx. *New York Med J* 1885;42:145-147.
34. O'Dwyer J. Two cases of croup treated by tubage of the glottis. *New York Med J* 1885;42:605-607.
35. Matas R. Intralaryngeal insufflation. *JAMA* 1900;34:1371-1375, 1468-1473.
36. Tuffier, Hallion. Etude experimentale sur la chirurgie du poumon. Sur les effets circulatoires de la respiration artificielle par insufflation et de l'insufflation maintenue du poumon. *Compt Rend Soc Biol* 1896;48:1047-1050.
37. Jackson C. The recent progress of endoscopic methods as applied to the larynx, trachea, bronchi, esophagus and stomach. *Laryngoscope* 1913;23:721-760.
38. Meltzer SJ, Auer J. Continuous respiration without respiratory movements. *J Exp Med* 1909;11:622-625.
39. Elsberg CA. The value of continuous intratracheal insufflation of air in thoracic surgery: with description of an apparatus. *Med Record* 1910;77:493-495.
40. Rowbotham ES, Magill I. Anaesthetics in the plastic surgery of the face and jaws. *Proc R Soc Med* 1920-1921;14:21-27.
41. Gale JW, Waters RM. Closed endobronchial anesthesia in thoracic surgery: preliminary report. *J Thorac Surg* 1932;1:432-437.
42. Magill IW. Endotracheal anaesthesia. *Proc R Soc Med* 1928;22:83-88.
43. Griffith HR, Johnson E. The use of curare in general anesthesia. *Anesthesiology* 1942;3:418-421.
44. Cullen SC. The use of curare for the improvement of abdominal muscle relaxation during inhalation anesthesia. *Surg Gynecol Obstet* 1943;14:261-266.
45. Harroun P, Hathaway HR. The use of curare in anesthesia for thoracic surgery. Preliminary report. *Surg Gynecol Obstet* 1946;82:229-231.
46. Stephens HB, Harroun P, Beckert FE. The use of curare in anesthesia for thoracic surgery. *J Thorac Surg* 1947;16:50-61.
47. Lilienthal H. Carcinoma of the thoracic oesophagus. Successful resection. *Ann Surg* 1921;74:116-120.
48. Hedblom CA. Combined transpleural and transperitoneal resection of the thoracic oesophagus and the cardia for carcinoma. *Surg Gynecol Obstet* 1922;35:284-287.
49. Eggers C. Resection of the thoracic portion of the esophagus for carcinoma. Report of a successful case. *Arch Surg* 1925;10:361-373.
50. Eggers C. Carcinoma of the thoracic portion of the oesophagus. *Surg Gynecol Obstet* 1930;50:630-634.
51. Turner GG. Excision of the thoracic oesophagus for carcinoma, with construction of an extrathoracic gullet. *Lancet* 1933;2:1315-1316.
52. Ohsawa T. Surgery of the oesophagus. *Arch Jap Chir* 1933;10:605-695.

53. Marshall SF. Carcinoma of the esophagus: successful resection of the lower end of the esophagus with reestablishment of esophageal gastric continuity. *Surg Clin N Am* 1938;18:643-648.
54. Adams WE, Phemister DB. Carcinoma of the lower thoracic esophagus. Report of a successful resection and esophagogastrostomy. *J Thorac Surg* 1937-8;7:621-632.
55. Yudin SS. The surgical construction of 80 cases of artificial esophagus. *Surg Gynecol Obstet* 1944;78:561-583.
56. King ESJ. Oesophagectomy for carcinoma of the thoracic oesophagus. *Br J Surg* 1935;23:521-529.
57. Eggers C. Experiences with carcinoma of the esophagus. *J Thorac Surg* 1933; 2:229-246.
58. Edwards AT, Lee ES. Extirpation of the oesophagus for carcinoma. *J Laryngol Otol* 1936;51:281-292.
59. Brunn H, Stephens HB. Carcinoma of the thoracic esophagus. A report of the successful removal in one case. *J Thorac Surg* 1937-8;7:38-42.
60. Wookey H. The surgical treatment of cancer of the pharynx and upper esophagus. *Surg Gynecol Obstet* 1942;75:499-506.
61. Wookey H. The surgical treatment of cancer of the hypopharynx and the oesophagus. *Br J Surg* 1948;35:249-266.
62. Ladd WE. The surgical treatment of esophageal atresia and tracheoesophageal fistulas. *N Engl J Med* 1944;230:625-637.
63. Watson WL, Converse JM. Reconstruction of cervical esophagus. *Plast Reconstr Surg* 1953;11:183-196.
64. Bricker EM, Burford TH. Experiences with tubed pedicle grafts in esophageal reconstruction following resection for cancer. *Ann Surg* 1957;145:979-992.
65. Churchill ED, Sweet RH. Transthoracic resection of tumors of the stomach and esophagus. *Ann Surg* 1942;115:897-920.
66. Sweet RH. Surgical management of carcinoma of midthoracic esophagus. Preliminary report. *N Engl J Med* 1945;233:1-7.
67. Lewis I. The surgical treatment of carcinoma of the oesophagus, with special reference to a new operation for growths of the middle third. *Br J Surg* 1946-7;34:18-31.
68. Sweet RH. Carcinoma of the superior mediastinal segment of the esophagus. *Surgery* 1948;24:929-938.
69. Garlock JH. Resection of thoracic esophagus for carcinoma located above arch of aorta: cervical esophagogastrostomy. *Surgery* 1948;24:1-8.
70. Rapant V, Hromada J. Surgical treatment of corrosive stenoses of the thoracic part of the esophagus by a single-stage palliative anastomosis. *J Thorac Surg* 1950;20:454-473.
71. Gavriliu D, Georgescu L. Esofagoplastie directa cu material gastric (procedeu personal). *Rev St Med* 1951;3:33-36.
72. Gavriliu D, Georgescu L. Esophagoplastie viscerala directa. *Chirurgia* 1955; 4:104-138.
73. le Roux BT. An analysis of 700 cases of carcinoma of the hypopharynx, the oesophagus, and the proximal stomach. *Thorax* 1961;16:226-255.
74. Reinhoff WF Jr. Intrathoracic esophagojejunostomy for lesions of the upper third of the esophagus. *South Med J* 1946;39:928-940.

75. Longmire WP Jr, Ravitch MM. A new method for constructing an artificial esophagus. *Ann Surg* 1946;123:819-834.
76. Harrison AW. Transthoracic small bowel substitution in high stricture of the esophagus. *J Thorac Surg* 1949;18:316-326.
77. Robertson R, Sarjeant TR. Reconstruction of esophagus. *J Thorac Surg* 1950;20:689-705.
78. Merendino KA, Dillard DH. The concept of sphincter substitution by an interposed jejunal segment for anatomic and physiologic abnormalities at the esophagogastric junction. *Ann Surg* 1955;142:486-509.
79. Androsov PI. Blood supply of mobilized intestine used for an artificial esophagus. *Arch Surg* 1956;73:917-926.
80. Kasai M, Abo S, Makino K, et al. Reconstruction of the cervical esophagus with a pedicled jejunal graft. *Surg Gynecol Obstet* 1965;121:102-106.
81. Allison PR, Wooler GH, Gunning AJ. Esophagojejunogastrostomy. *J Thorac Surg* 1957;33:738-748.
82. Rudler JC. Sur 28 oesophagoplastics prethoracique avec le colon, partiques pour cancer de l'oesophage. *Rev Chir* 1951;70:193.
83. Orsoni P, Lemaire M. Technique des oesophagoplasties par le colon transverse et descenant. *J Chirurgie* 1951;67:491-505.
84. Goligher JC, Robin IG. Use of left colon for reconstruction of pharynx and oesophagus after pharyngectomy. *Br J Surg* 1954-5;42:283-290.
85. Brain RHF, Reading PV. Colon transplantation into the pharynx and cervical oesophagus. *Br J Surg* 1966;53:933-942.
86. Belsey R. Reconstruction of the esophagus with left colon. *J Thorac Cardiovasc Surg* 1965;49:3-55.

Chapter 2

Reparative Surgery of the Esophagus

One of the most difficult decisions to make when treating patients with benign esophageal problems is whether to resect the esophagus or preserve and repair it. Factors that influence the decision include the patient's age and general performance status, the functional status of the esophagus, the anatomic extent of pathologic changes in the esophagus, and the availability of appropriate tissues for repair or replacement. It is best never to throw something away unless it can be replaced. No organ or tissue can ever completely duplicate the function of the normal esophagus, making its preservation an important consideration in esophageal surgery. This chapter provides an overview of indications for surgical approaches to patients in whom the esophagus is to be preserved and repaired.

Rationale for Esophageal Preservation

Esophageal preservation should be considered for patients who have benign disease, predominantly normal esophageal anatomy, and preserved esophageal function. The potential advantages of leaving the esophagus *in situ* include preservation of peristalsis, maintenance of gastric function, absence of redundancy of the intrathoracic alimentary tract conduit, and lack of disturbance of the swallowing mechanism (Table 2-1). Typical clinical situations in which esophageal preserving surgery is often appropriate include the presence of a benign, localized stricture, esophageal shortening due to peptic esophagitis or of congenital origins, esophageal perforation in the absence of malignant disease, and failure of surgical control of pathologic gastroesophageal acid reflux (Table 2-2).

Table 2-1.
Selection of Patients for Esophageal Reconstruction.

Potential Advantages
Preserved peristaltic function
Gastric reservoir capacity maintained
Negligible redundancy of intrathoracic conduit
Swallowing mechanism undisturbed
Potential Disadvantages
Susceptibility of mucosa to irritation by digestive juices
Potential for malignant degeneration

Table 2-2.
Criteria for Esophageal Preserving Operations.

Esophageal preservation - possible
Peptic stricture
Esophageal shortening
Failed surgery for reflux
Esophageal preservation - inappropriate
Squamous cell carcinoma
Achalasia
Scleroderma
Partial esophageal - salvage
Adenocarcinoma
Barrett's dysplasia

Some of the general concepts addressed here are covered in greater detail in Chapter 8.

Preservation of Peristaltic Function

Maintenance of peristaltic function is one of the most important indications for esophageal preservation. Resection necessitates replacement with stomach, small bowel, or colon under most circumstances. As will be seen, none of these esophageal replacement organs possesses peristaltic activity remotely comparable to that of the esophagus. The stomach is a good example. Gastric motility is separated into fundic, antral, and pyloric phases.[1,2] Activity in the fundus (the primary region of gastric reservoir function) is characterized by initial relaxation to accommodate ingested food, followed by a slow increase in tone that propels food toward the antrum. The gastric antrum functions to both grind and pump food by means of phasic and intermittent peristaltic contractile activity. The pylorus regulates food movement into the duodenum, and closes completely during the antral stroke.[2-4] These nonperistaltic activities are partially under vagal control, which is disrupted during esophagectomy.

The colon similarly lacks cohesive peristaltic activity. Major functions of the colon include absorption, slow aboral movement of luminal contents, retention of fecal material until defecation, and rapid movement of fecal material during defecation.[5,6] Contractions of the colon that permit these functions are classified as individual phasic contractions, organized groups of contractions, and special propulsive contractions. Individual phasic contractions (both long- and short-duration types) are poorly coordinated and generally do not propagate. They are under myogenic, neural (central nervous system, autonomic nervous system, and enteric nervous system), paracrine, and other pharmacologic control. Organized groups of contractions are collections of individual phasic contractions that appear as alternating periods of quiescence and contractile activity at any single site in the colon.[7] This activity does not propagate or propel fecal material to the front of the complex. The enteric nervous system is likely a major mechanism of grouping of this activity. Special propulsive contractions occur in the human only once or twice per day, are likely stimulated by mechano- and chemo-receptors in the colon wall, and are linked to defecation. It is apparent that the normal function of the colon does not include regular peristaltic activity.

Of the possible esophageal substitutes in common use, peristalsis-like activity is a possible characteristic of only the jejunum. As in the colon, smooth muscle activity in the jejunum is characterized by different types of contractions, one being individual phasic contractions. The jejunum possesses only a single type of individual phasic contraction, which is under myogenic, neural, and chemical control. Such contractions are often phase-locked due to the existence of strong cell-to-cell coupling of electrical activity and to similarity of intrinsic frequencies in adjacent segments. Organized groups of contractions, which normally occur in the fasting state and are characterized by orderly aboral migration, appear to support a cleaning function and the movement of bile to the ileum for enterohepatic circulation. Organized groups of contractions that extend over relatively long distances are known as phase II activity or migrating motor complexes (MMCs). These usually originate in the duodenum and can propagate to the terminal ileum.[8,9] Contractions propagating over long distances (MMCs) are suppressed in the postprandial period.[10] The jejunum also exhibits two other types of migrating contractions, giant and individual migrating contractions, that extend over intermediate distances. The former are similar to those that occur in the rest of the gastrointestinal tract. Individual migrating contractions occur in the fed and the postprandial state, and about 50% propagate over shorter distances (10 to 20 cm).[9,11,12] This peristalsis-like activity is substantially diminished when the jejunum is used as an esophageal substitute,[13] and jejunal contractile activity is not neurally linked to primary peristaltic activity of the esophagus or to the swallowing cascade under such conditions.

Because the peristaltic function of the esophagus cannot be duplicated by any of the traditional reconstructive organs following esophagectomy, food transit through the new alimentary tract is necessarily dependent on gravity. This requires patients to eat in an upright position and to maintain such a position for some time after completing a meal. In addition, elevation of the head of the bed is often necessary to prevent nocturnal regurgitation and aspiration. Such requirements are burdensome and adversely affect the patient's quality of life. These considerations underscore the importance of esophageal preservation under selected circumstances.

Maintenance of Gastric Function

The stomach is a complex organ with many discrete functions. These include expanding to receive food after a meal, grinding and mixing the food, production of digestive juices, discrimination between solids and liquids, and delivery of foods into the duodenum at rates that are related to their fat content and are appropriate to pancreatic digestion and intestinal absorption. The rates of gastric emptying for solids and liquids differ substantially.[14] Liquids initially distend the proximal stomach leading to contractions that raise intraluminal pressure and move them into the duodenum.[15,16] Solids are managed primarily by the distal stomach, which grinds them into small particles in an acid-peptic medium and releases the resulting chyme through the pylorus.[1,17] These processes are influenced by the volume, temperature, acidity, osmolarity, and chemical nature of the gastric contents.[18-20] In addition, proximal gastric motility is controlled by the vagal system, while distal motility is influenced by both vagal and sympathetic fibers. Hormonal influences, particularly those due to cholecystokinin, gastrin, and steroid hormones, are also important in controlling gastric reservoir and emptying activities.[21-23] When the stomach is used as a reconstructive organ, these complex functions are substantially diminished or are lost entirely. This necessitates much slower ingestion of food and smaller meals at a sitting, and often results in some weight loss.

Avoidance of Intrathoracic Alimentary Tract Redundancy

In patients who have undergone esophageal replacement, there is a tendency for redundancy of the reconstructive organ to develop, particularly in the intrathoracic portion. Redundancy can lead to stasis of food movement within the replacement segment. Food accumulation within the esophagus causes early satiety, resulting in weight loss over a period of time. Bacterial overgrowth may also occur in areas of food stasis. In addition, intrasegmental shuttling often develops, and reflux of food from the segment into the esophagus is common. This can ultimately lead to regurgitation and aspiration, with their attendant serious potential consequences, including pneumonia, lung abscess, and pulmonary fibrosis.

Preservation of Swallowing Function

Operations that require a cervical anastomosis necessitate dissection in the region of nerves that coordinate swallowing function and initiate esophageal peristalsis, including the inferior and superior laryngeal, trigeminal, facial, hypoglossus, ansa hypoglossus, and glossopharyngeal nerves, and the pharyngeal plexus. Injury to these nerves leads to cervical and, in some instances, oropharyngeal dysphagia, particularly during the early postoperative period. Such abnormalities adversely affect swallowing and result in pulmonary aspiration, pooling of food in the vestibules, pharyngooral or pharyngonasal regurgitation, and a globus-type sensation. In contrast, esophageal preservation operations do not normally require a cervical approach, minimizing these potentially disastrous complications.

Potential Disadvantages to Esophageal Preservation

Several potential disadvantages to esophageal preservation also must be kept in mind. The esophageal mucosa is susceptible to injury by digestive juices. The absence of a lower esophageal sphincter, or its severe dysfunction, may allow pathologic gastroesophageal reflux to occur. Similar problems can develop if there is delayed gastric emptying, with increasing intragastric pressure overcoming the resistance of a normal or near-normal lower esophageal sphincter. These problems can result in the development of a peptic stricture, and underscore the importance of reflux control when a decision regarding reconstruction versus replacement is under consideration.

There is a strong tendency for malignant degeneration in certain esophageal conditions that should be considered when selecting between preservation and resection. The likelihood of developing a squamous cell cancer in a patient with achalasia is increased perhaps by as much as 10 to 30 times that in the normal population.[24-28] The risk of squamous cell cancer in patients with prior caustic esophageal injury is also greatly increased, perhaps by as much as a factor of 1000.[29,30] Similarly, the risk of adenocarcinoma developing in Barrett's mucosa is increased by a factor of 25 to 40.[31] Consideration of these risks is important when deciding on definitive surgical therapy for a benign esophageal problem, as they may influence an otherwise difficult choice.

Contraindications to Esophagus-Preserving Operations

Primary esophageal cancers should be managed without regard to potential benefits of preserving esophageal function. Once the most appropriate surgical therapy is provided, subsequent replacement is performed based on the extent of esophageal resection and the available replacement organs. For patients with squamous cell carcinoma of the esophagus, a potentially curative operation includes a near-total esophagectomy because of the high incidence of field changes within the mucosa and of second primary cancers associated with such changes. In contrast, adenocarcinomas of the esophagus or esophagogastric junction do not necessarily require a subtotal esophagectomy in order to be potentially curative, and a similar argument can be made when operating for high grade dysplasia in Barrett's mucosa.

A patient whose caustic esophageal injury is not extensive but who requires operative correction of a nondilatable stricture probably would benefit from esophageal resection rather than attempts at preservation. Such patients are often young and have an incidence of carcinomatous degeneration in the esophagus that is much higher than that in the normal population. Resection theoretically eliminates this risk if performed before invasive carcinoma develops. In addition, resection, rather than bypass, is indicated in most patients because of the risk of esophageal shortening leading to hiatal herniation, peptic esophagitis, and hemorrhage or anemia that cannot be controlled with bypass surgery.

Severe esophageal dysmotility, which is present in patients with achalasia, progressive systemic sclerosis, mixed connective tissue disease, amyloidosis and Chagas' disease, is a strong contraindication to esophageal preservation operations. Problems of stasis, intrathoracic shuttling, regurgitation, and aspiration are common when a severely dysfunctional esophagus is left *in situ*. Preoperative assessment of esophageal motility is very important as an aid in determining the fate of an abnormally functioning esophagus.

Specific Indications

Esophageal Stricture

Benign localized esophageal strictures develop most commonly as a result of peptic injury. The primary means of treating most such strictures is dilation and medical therapy. Intensive acid suppression therapy combined with dilation results in successful management of peptic strictures in nearly 80% of patients. Complications develop in only 2% of patients, only some of whom have perforations (see below).[32] Less than half of the remaining 20% of patients require operative intervention, and the majority of these individuals undergo standard fundoplication with successful control of reflux. The occasional patient will have a nondilatable peptic stricture and preserved esophageal function, making that individual a candidate for esophageal preservation by means of an esophagoplasty (see Chapter 4). Esophagoplasty should also be considered for patients who suffer perforation at the time of dilation of a peptic stricture, particularly if the patient satisfies the criteria of early diagnosis, minimal contamination, and substantially preserved esophageal function.

Nondilatable strictures may also develop as a result of radiation fibrosis, moniliasis or other infections, drug-induced injuries, or other causes.[33] These strictures often measure more than several centimeters in length, and thus are not usually amenable to esophagoplasty. However, under unusual circumstances, patients with localized strictures of other than peptic origin are candidates for esophagoplasty if the above criteria are met.

Shortened Esophagus

Esophageal shortening usually develops due to severe peptic or caustic injury. The transmural fibrosis and subsequent contracture result in a decrease in overall esophageal length and, in most patients, produce a Type I (sliding) hiatal hernia. Patients with esophageal shortening due to caustic stricture typically have a long region of esophageal narrowing that is not suitable to preservation operations. Patients with shortening due to peptic esophageal strictures, on the other hand, are often candidates for preservation operations and present challenging surgical problems.

The amount of esophageal shortening due to peptic stricture is quite variable, as is the degree of fibrosis. If the stricture is not dilatable, a "lengthening" procedure combined with a patch esophagoplasty would be required for esophageal preservation. Unfortunately, such a procedure is unlikely to be of long-term benefit because of the technical difficulties in establishing an adequate antireflux barrier in such patients. In the absence of an antrectomy and bile diversion operation, the resultant high degree of persistent reflux would create new inflammation and fibrosis, culminating in worsening of the shortening and stricture.

In patients with dilatable strictures and esophageal shortening, extensive esophageal mobilization is often sufficient to permit a standard intra-abdominal fundoplication without undo tension on the esophagus or the fundoplication wrap. If such cannot be accomplished, a lengthening esophagoplasty may be performed as originally described by Collis and subsequently modified by others (see Chapter 3).[34-36] This operation creates a "neoesophagus" from the lesser curvature of the stomach, leaving the gastric fundus intact to enable the construction of any of a variety of fundoplication wraps.

Failed Antireflux Operations

Patients with failed antireflux operations present formidable challenges to the esophageal surgeon. Causes for recurrent symptoms following fundoplication surgery include esophageal dysmotility, disruption of the wrap resulting in an inadequate lower esophageal high pressure zone, a combination of these two, and mechanical problems in the presence of an intact wrap such as a slipped wrap or too tight a wrap.[37-42] Caution must always be exercised in approaching these problems, because recurrent symptoms, even though they are strongly suggestive of gastroesophageal reflux, may be unrelated to the prior fundoplication operation. It is important to make an accurate diagnosis under these circumstances, which requires a complete evaluation, including endoscopy, contrast radiography, esophageal motility and pH monitoring, and, in some patients, scintigraphic assessment of gastric emptying.

Most patients with recurrent gastroesophageal reflux after fundoplication surgery require only medical therapy, including dietary management, weight loss counseling, prokinetic agents, and acid suppression therapy. In some patients reoperation is necessary, for which the primary option is a repeat fundoplication, possibly combined with a lengthening procedure. In other patients the function of the esophagus is largely destroyed due to severe fibrosis resulting from peptic esophagitis, and repeat fundoplication in these individuals often provides unsatisfactory results. In such patients other surgical options include resection and reconstruction or esophageal preservation with acid suppression and duodenal diversion. The latter operation is also indicated in selected patients who have had multiple prior operations in the region of the hiatus, and in whom it is anticipated that further dissection would be extremely difficult. Acid suppression is achieved by vagotomy and antrectomy with reconstruction accomplished using a Billroth II gastrojejunostomy, and a Roux-en-Y limb provides diversion of duodenal contents. Although the moderate amount of experience with this operation that has been reported is favorable, caution must be used in selecting candidates.[43-46] The operation, while sparing the esophagus, carries the risk of postoperative complications such as dumping, diarrhea, and regurgitation, and is as formidable a procedure as esophagectomy. It does not directly correct the pathophysiology of gastroesophageal reflux disease, and sacrifices one of the primary organs used for esophageal reconstruction. Because acid suppression and duodenal diversion are not directly applicable to surgery of the esophagus, no detailed description of the operation is provided in this book. However, this procedure should be kept in mind as an alternative therapy for complicated reflux problems in patients in whom esophagectomy is inappropriate.

Esophageal Perforation

Esophageal perforation results most commonly from iatrogenic injury during diagnostic endoscopy or intraluminal interventional procedures such as dilation, laser therapy, sclerosis, extraction of foreign bodies, and placement of stenting prostheses. Perforation may also develop under a variety of other circumstances, such as barogenic trauma (including Boerhaave's syndrome), penetrating trauma, caustic injury, foreign body ingestion, and intraoperative injury. Early diagnosis and intervention is the mainstay of therapy for esophageal perforation. Selection of appropriate intervention depends upon the etiology of the perforation, the presence of any preexisting esophageal pathology, the time interval between perforation and diagnosis, the patient's overall condition, and the findings at the time of operation.

In many instances of esophageal perforation it is appropriate to preserve the esophagus. This is usually possible in the presence of benign disease when the function of the esophagus is largely preserved, when the patient's general condition is favorable, and when there is minimal contamination of the pleura and mediastinum. Under such circumstances the treatment is straightforward, requiring primary repair reinforced with a flap (pleura, pericardial fat, or intercostal muscle) or by fundoplication. If circumstances do not permit primary repair but esophageal preservation is still an option, an exclusion procedure or simple drainage may be indicated. In many situations it is not appropriate to attempt to preserve the esophagus. Examples include the presence of a cancer of the esophagus or esophagogastric junction, the finding of a large, irreparable perforation, or the development of substantial mediastinal contamination. Under such circumstances, esophagectomy with eventual reconstruction is the appropriate therapy.

In selected cases of perforation, usually when such has occurred during dilation of a benign stricture, simple repair of the esophagus is insufficient. Primary closure under such circumstances would result in a continuing problem with the stricture, requiring repeated dilations in the postoperative period to restore luminal diameter and function. In such instances it is possible to perform a patch esophagoplasty (see Chapter 4). This can be accomplished with a diaphragmatic or gastric patch, but should be considered only when the perforation is diagnosed early, when there is minimal intraoperative contamination, and when the lengths of the stricture and perforation are not prohibitive.

References

1. Read NW, Houghton LA. Physiology of gastric emptying and pathophysiology of gastroparesis. *Gastroenterol Clin N Am* 1989;18:359-373.
2. Cullen JJ, Kelly KA. Gastric motor physiology and pathophysiology. *Surg Clin N Am* 1993;73:1145-1160.
3. Keinke O, Ehrlein H-J. Effect of oleic acid on canine gastroduodenal motility, pyloric diameter and gastric emptying. *Q J Exp Physiol* 1983;68:675-686.
4. Raybould HE, Holzer P, Thiefin G, et al. Vagal afferent innervation and regulation of gastric function. In: **Sensory Nerves and Neuropeptides in Gastroenterology**. Costa M, et al. (eds). New York, Plenum Press, 1991, pp 109-127.
5. Sarna SK. Physiology and pathophysiology of colonic motor activity. *Dig Dis Sci* 1991;36:827-862.
6. O'Brien MD, Phillips SF. Colonic motility in health and disease. *Gastroenterol Clin N Am* 1996;25:147-162.
7. Sarna SK. Colonic motor activity. *Surg Clin N Am* 1993;73:1201-1223.
8. Sarna SK. Cyclic motor activity; migrating motor complex: 1985. *Gastroenterology* 1985;89:894-913.
9. Husebye E. The patterns of small bowel motility: physiology and implications in organic disease and functional disorders. *Neurogastroenterol Mot* 1999;11:141-161.
10. Quigley EMM. Gastric and small intestinal motility in health and disease. *Gastroenterol Clin N Am* 1996;25:113-145.
11. Sarna SK, Soergel KH, Harig JM, et al. Spatial and temporal patterns of human jejunal contractions. *Am J Physiol* 1989;257:G423-G432.
12. Kunze WAA, Furness JB. The enteric nervous system and regulation of intestinal motility. *Ann Rev Physiol* 1999;61:117-142.
13. Johnson CP, Sarna SK, Cowles VE, et al. Motor activity and transit in the autonomically denervated jejunum. *Am J Surg* 1994;167:80-88.
14. Siegel JA, Urbain J-L, Adler LP, et al. Biphasic nature of gastric emptying. *Gut* 1988;29:85-89.
15. Wilbur BG, Kelly KA. Effect of proximal gastric, complete gastric, and truncal vagotomy on canine gastric electric activity, motility and emptying. *Ann Surg* 1973;178:295-303.
16. Strunz UT, Grossman MI. Effect of intragastric pressure on gastric emptying and secretion. *Am J Physiol* 1978;235:E552-E555.
17. Meyer JH, Thompson JB, Cohen MB, et al. Sieving of solid food by the canine stomach and sieving after gastric surgery. *Gastroenterology* 1979;76:804-813.
18. Minami H, McCallum RW. The physiology and pathophysiology of gastric emptying in humans. *Gastroenterology* 1984;86:1592-1610.
19. Paraskevopoulos JA, Houghton LA, Eyre-Brooke I, Johnson AG, Read NW. Effect of composition of gastric contents on resistance to emptying of liquids from stomach in humans. *Dig Dis Sci* 1988;33:914-918.

20. Sun WM, Houghton LA, Read NW, Grundy DG, Johnson AG. Effect of meal temperature on gastric emptying of liquids in man. *Gut* 1988;29:302-305.
21. Debas HT, Farooq O, Grossman MI. Inhibition of gastric emptying is a physiological action of cholecystokinin. *Gastroenterology* 1975;68:1211-1217.
22. Strunz UT, Code CF, Grossman MI. Effect of gastrin on electrical activity of antrum and duodenum of dogs. *Proc Soc Exp Biol Med* 1979;161:25-27.
23. Hutson WR, Roehrkasse RL, Wald A. Influence of gender and menopause on gastric emptying and motility. *Gastroenterology* 1989;96:11-17.
24. Peracchia A, Segalin A, Bardini R, et al. Esophageal carcinoma and achalasia: Prevalence, incidence and results of treatment. *Hepato-Gastroenterol* 1991;38:514-516.
25. Aggestrup S, Holm JC, Sorensen HR. Does achalasia predispose to cancer of the esophagus? *Chest* 1992;102:1013-1016.
26. Meijssen MAC, Tilanus HW, van Blankenstein M, et al. Achalasia complicated by oesophageal squamous cell carcinoma: A prospective study in 195 patients. *Gut* 1992;33:155-158.
27. Sandler RS, Nyren O, Ekborn A, et al. The risk of esophageal cancer in patients with achalasia. *JAMA* 1995;274:1359-1362.
28. Streitz JM Jr, Ellis FH Jr, Gibb SP, et al. Achalasia and squamous cell carcinoma of the esophagus: analysis of 241 patients. *Ann Thorac Surg* 1995;59:1604-1609.
29. Csikos M, Horvath O, Petri A, et al. Late malignant transformation of chronic corrosive oesophageal strictures. *Langenbecks Arch Chir* 1985;365:231-238.
30. Isolauri J, Markkula H. Lye ingestion and carcinoma of the esophagus. *Acta Chir Scand* 1989;155:269-271.
31. Tytgat GN. Incidence of cancer in esophageal columnar metaplasia (Barrett's esophagus). *Dis Esoph* 1992;1:29-35.
32. Ferguson MK. Medical and surgical management of peptic esophageal strictures. *Chest Surg Clin N Am* 1994;4:673-695.
33. Bonavina L, DeMeester TR, McChesney L, et al. Drug-induced esophageal strictures. *Ann Surg* 1987;206:173-183.
34. Collis JL. An operation for hiatus hernia with short esophagus. *J Thorac Cardiovasc Surg* 1957;34:768-773.
35. Pearson FG, Cooper JD, Patterson GA, et al. Gastroplasty and fundoplication for complex reflux problems. *Ann Surg* 1987;206:473-481.
36. Adler RH. Collis gastroplasty: Origin and evolution. *Ann Thorac Surg* 1990;50:839-842.
37. Collard JM, Romagnoli R, Kestens PJ. Reoperation for unsatisfactory outcome after laparoscopic antireflux surgery. *Dis Esoph* 1996;9:56-62.
38. Ellis FH Jr, Gibb SP, Heatley GJ. Reoperation after failed antireflux surgery. Review of 101 cases. *Eur J Cardiothorac Surg* 1996;10:225-231.
39. Stein HJ, Feussner H, Siewert JR. Failure of antireflux surgery: Causes and management strategies. *Am J Surg* 1996;171:36-40.
40. Deschamps C, Trastek VF, Allen MS, et al. Long-term results after reoperation for failed antireflux procedures. *J Thorac Cardiovasc Surg* 1997;113:545-551.
41. Ferguson MK. Pitfalls and complications of antireflux surgery. *Chest Surg Clin N Am* 1997;7:489-511.

42. Horgan S, Pohl D, Bogetti D, et al. Failed antireflux surgery. *Arch Surg* 1999;134:809-817.
43. Salo JA, Ala-Kulju KV, Heikkinen LO, et al. Treatment of severe peptic esophageal stricture with Roux-en-Y partial gastrectomy, vagotomy, and endoscopic dilation. *J Thorac Cardiovasc Surg* 1991;101:649-653.
44. Fekete F, Pateron D. What is the place of antrectomy with Roux-en-Y in the treatment of reflux disease? Experience with 83 total duodenal diversions. *World J Surg* 1992;16:349-353.
45. Bonavina L, Fontebasso V, Bardini R, et al. Surgical treatment of reflux stricture of the oesophagus. *Br J Surg* 1993;80:317-320.
46. Ellis FH Jr, Gibb SP. Vagotomy, antrectomy, and Roux-en-Y diversion for complex reoperative gastroesophageal reflux disease. *Ann Surg* 1994;220:536-543.

Chapter 3

Collis Gastroplasty and Other Lengthening Procedures

Esophageal lengthening procedures are sometimes used in the management of esophageal shortening which results from a variety of causes. Cicatricial contracture of a peptic stricture will sometimes result in the development of a Type I (so-called "sliding") hiatal hernia. In such cases the Type I hernia is fixed and, as a result, the term "sliding" is obviously a misnomer. Other causes of esophageal shortening include caustic esophageal injury, fibrosis due to irradiation, focal injury secondary to medications, and congenital hypoplasia. Initial therapy consists of esophageal dilation and treatment of underlying causes of esophageal inflammation. Management of strictures that cannot be satisfactorily dilated includes esophagoplasty or resection, both of which are among the topics of the remaining chapters of this book. The object of the present chapter is to illustrate methods of "lengthening" the esophagus by means of a plastic operation, permitting its preservation.

Dilatable strictures accompanied by esophageal shortening form a watershed where the art and science of esophageal surgery diverge. Decisions regarding appropriate management of such problems are daunting, and few experimental data are available that help to clarify the clinical issues. At one end of the spectrum lies conservative management, which includes intermittent esophageal dilation and ongoing medical therapy. Unfortunately, such treatment is often doomed to failure, with worsening of the esophageal shortening and development of an end-stage condition ultimately requiring esophageal resection. Surgical options include either resection with reconstruction, lying at the far end of the spectrum, or a lengthening gastroplasty, which represents a more conservative surgical option. The latter technique preserves the entire esophagus and leaves

From Ferguson MK: *Reconstructive Surgery of the Esophagus* Armonk, NY: Futura Publishing Company, Inc., © 2002.

the stomach largely intact, which is an advantage since, if the operation is unsuccessful, it does not "queer the pitch" for a further attack on the lesion, permitting resection and reconstruction when necessary.[1]

Extension of the esophageal tube by gastroplasty is not universally accepted as an appropriate option for management of esophageal shortening. However, it appears to have gained favor during the 1980s, more than 20 years following its introduction. Gastroplasty is one of the primary ways by which esophageal preservation is possible even in the face of severe fibrosis and shortening, and, as such, it merits a thorough and objective review.

Historical Background

Efforts Preceding Introduction of the Gastroplasty

Gastroesophageal acid reflux was not recognized as a cause for heartburn and benign strictures of the distal esophagus until publication of the experimental work of Wangensteen in 1949 and the landmark clinical paper of Allison in 1951.[2,3] During the subsequent decade most surgical efforts focused on correction of the anatomic defect of hiatus hernia rather than on prevention of gastroesophageal reflux. It was known that only a small percentage of patients with a hiatus hernia had symptoms of any sort. The majority of those with symptoms were affected by gastroesophageal reflux, and therapy of reflux problems was not standardized.

Reflux patients without strictures typically were managed by reduction of the hernia and crural repair of the type originally described by Allison,[3] and subsequently modified using approaches typical of those summarized by Tanner and Humphreys.[4,5] Other options for management of reflux included anterior gastropexy,[6] pyloroplasty or other measures such as gastric drainage procedures to improve gastric emptying,[7-9] transposition of the esophageal hiatus to the dome of the diaphragm,[10-12] reconstitution of the cardioesophageal angle,[13-16] and construction of cardioesophageal valves using local tissues or rotation of a pedicled flap of the ileocecal valve to the region of the esophagogastric junction.[17-19]

Patients who had reflux complicated by stricture presented even greater technical challenges. Options for surgical therapy included resection with low or high intrathoracic esophagogastrostomy[20-22] and short segment resection accompanied by either interposition of a short segment of jejunum or colon,[23-25] low intrathoracic esophagogastrostomy and antrectomy,[26] or Roux-en-Y esophagojejunostomy.[27] Needless to say, such operations were attended by a high rate of mortality, although long-term control of reflux symptoms was believed to be satisfactory.

This brief overview of surgical efforts during the late 1940s and 1950s, aimed at correcting anatomic defects in patients with hiatal hernia and relieving reflux symptoms, underscores the lack of understanding during this period of the pathophysiologic mechanisms that underlie gastroesophageal reflux. Most physicians of that time believed that reflux was due to a mechanical defect of the crura or of the phrenoesophageal membrane.[13,15] Support for these beliefs came from initial success observed following crural repair for symptomatic hiatal hernia, and from the lack of recognized reflux that developed following modified Heller myotomy for achalasia when the phrenoesophageal membrane was not disrupted. In addition, a number of individuals suggested that another factor in controlling reflux was the acuity of the angle at which the esophagus inserts into the stomach (the angle of His).[13,15,16]

Reflux problems accompanied by complications such as stricture and esophageal shortening engendered interesting debate among surgeons of the time. Vigorous discussion typically ensued when the problem of acquired esophageal shortening arose at surgical meetings. The discussion following the presentation of Burford and Lischer on treatment of short esophagus at the American Surgical Association in 1956 is such an example, during which several prominent surgeons all but denied the existence of such an entity.[7]

The Collis Gastroplasty

It was into this fray that J. Leigh Collis of Birmingham, England, entered when he proposed his operation for esophageal lengthening. He expressed the concern that the more radical operations in use at that time, namely esophagectomy and gastric pullup or bowel interposition, were poorly tolerated by many patients, and that continued conservative management of symptoms through pharmacologic therapy and dilation was destined to failure. The rationale for development of this technique, therefore, was to fill the need for an operation that did "not disorganize the patient's digestive apparatus too much and which [was] easily tolerated by even a frail and aged person."[28] Collis was aware that standard operations for reflux and hiatal hernia up to that time had a high rate of recurrence, and felt that the one factor that could control reflux by itself was the acute angle of implantation of the esophagus into the stomach. He achieved this in his standard operation by suturing the crura anterior to the esophagogastric junction, increasing the acuity of this angle.[15] In patients with peptic esophageal shortening and a fixed hiatal hernia, such a procedure was technically difficult and less effective, leading to the development of the gastroplasty as a means to reduce the bulk of the intrathoracic pouch, permitting the standard crural repair to be performed subsequently.

The initial Collis gastroplasties were performed with the patient in a right lateral decubitus position, rolled slightly posteriorly. A thoracoabdominal incision was made from the umbilicus to the edge of the trapezius muscle, and the seventh or eighth rib was resected. After opening the diaphragm laterally, the esophagus and stomach were mobilized. The gastroplasty was performed by dividing and oversewing the stomach between two bowel clamps, creating a narrow tube of stomach parallel to the lesser gastric curvature (Figure 3-1). Results of the operation in 11 patients were reported, among whom there was one postoperative death and one subphrenic abscess.[28] A sufficient period of follow-up was available in eight patients, of whom seven had good results. Interestingly, Collis reported that symptoms of Parkinsonism and narcolepsy were also improved in two patients following this operation. The discussion that followed the presentation of this paper at the 1957 meeting of the American Association for Thoracic Surgery was favorable, and contained a certain note of envy, as more than one discussant voiced the wish that they had the imagination to invent such an operation.

Unfortunately, simple lengthening of the esophageal tube combined with a crural repair did not promote satisfactory long-term control of gastroesophageal reflux. In his summary of the first 30 cases of gastroplasty, Collis himself was somewhat unenthusiastic about the overall results, in that reflux symptoms were only partially controlled in the majority of patients, and 30% of patients had what most surgeons would consider an unsatisfactory outcome.[29]

Modifications to the Collis Gastroplasty

It was at about this time that improved manometric techniques disclosed the existence of an intrinsic lower esophageal high pressure zone,[30,31] and experimental work demonstrated that wrapping the esophagus created an antireflux barrier.[32] Interestingly, clinical efforts were proceeding in parallel with this experimental work, shortly culminating in the landmark publications of Nissen and Belsey on fundoplication in the management of gastroesophageal reflux.[33,34]

Credit for combining a standard fundoplication operation with the Collis lengthening procedure goes to Pearson and his group at the University of Toronto.[35] The rationale for this operation was to employ the lengthening gastroplasty described by Collis, and combine it with a more effective technique for maintaining the appropriate intra-abdominal length of esophagus and acuity of the angle of His, namely the Belsey fundoplication. Results in the first 24 patients operated upon beginning

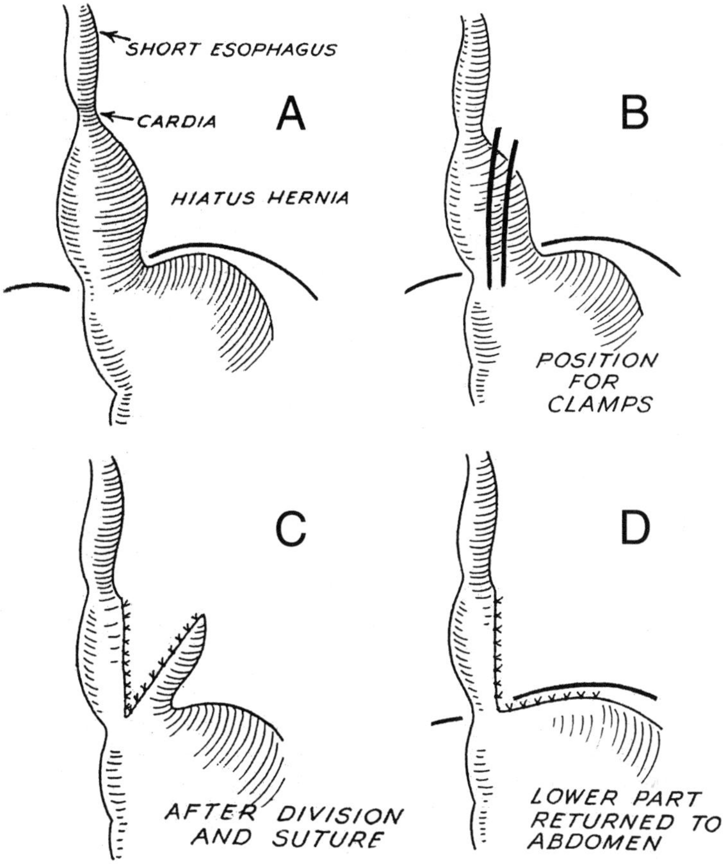

Figure 3-1. Collis' original gastroplasty, illustrating esophageal shortening (A); an additional portion of the stomach has been drawn up into the chest, and bowel clamps have been applied to outline a narrow stomach tube (B); the stomach has been divided and oversewn along the length of the clamps, creating a connecting tube between the esophagus and the stomach proper (C); the enlarged gastric fundus has been returned to the abdomen, creating an acute angle between the connecting tube and the stomach proper. A standard crural repair was performed at this point in the operation. [Reproduced from Collis JL. An operation for hiatus hernia with short esophagus. *Thorax* 1957;12:181–188, with permission from the publisher.]

in 1964 were initially reported in 1970, and demonstrated abolition of symptomatic reflux in 22 patients and restoration of normal swallowing function in 17 patients. The initial reaction to this operation was favorable, and it was adopted at a number of surgical centers. Orringer and Sloan reported a technical modification in 1974, employing a stapling device to close the edges of the gastroplasty incision, which was widely adopted thereafter.[36]

In subsequent reports from Toronto, the indications for use of the Collis-Belsey fundoplication had expanded to include not only peptic shortening of the esophagus but recurrent hiatus hernia, panmural esophagitis without stricture, and reflux problems associated with primary motor disorders.[37] Of 33 patients with peptic strictures operated upon more than 5 years prior to review, results were good or excellent in 25 of 26 patients, while 5 had died of unrelated causes and 2 were lost to follow-up. Other centers reported similar initial results,[38,39] but longer follow-up suggested that use of the Collis-Belsey approach was not so favorable. In 1977, Orringer and Sloan reported the results of surgery on 83 patients, in whom 19% had symptomatic reflux and 30% had reflux on esophageal pH testing postoperatively, and cautioned that further assessment of long-term results was warranted before the procedure was enthusiastically adopted.[40] In contrast, the Toronto group reported continuing favorable results with the Collis-Belsey operation, which they attributed to technical differences in performance of the operation.[41]

The response of Orringer and Sloan to their poor results following the Collis-Belsey operation was to create a higher amplitude, lower esophageal high-pressure zone around the gastroplasty tube using a total fundoplication: the so-called Collis-Nissen operation.[42] Evaluation of results in the first 28 patients demonstrated satisfactory increases in lower esophageal high pressure zone amplitudes and length, and the operation was subsequently adopted by many surgeons in preference to the Collis-Belsey procedure.

Additional technical modifications to the gastroplasty included its performance using a linear stapling device to fashion the gastric tube without cutting between the staple lines, the formation of a V-Y as opposed to a linear gastroplasty, and the creation of a funnel-like tube by performing a cardioplasty. The so-called uncut gastroplasty was originally introduced by Demos in the early 1970s and was independently reported by others shortly thereafter.[43-45] The technique has been combined most often with a total fundoplication wrap, while in selected instances a partial fundoplication wrap has also been employed.[46] This method has been adopted by some surgeons because of the theoretical benefits of a technically simpler operation and a reduced possibility of fistula formation.[47] The V-Y gastroplasty was developed in Bristol in an effort to increase the amount of fundic tissue available for wrapping the neoesophagus, but was in all other elements similar to the Collis-Belsey operation as originally described by Pearson.[48] The cardioplasty operation as described by Vankemmel is similar to the uncut gastroplasty except that the staple line is not placed parallel to the lesser curvature of the stomach. Instead, it is angled from the fundus towards the lesser curve to narrow the outlet at the bottom of the swallowing passage, and a subsequent fundoplication is performed.[49]

Table 3-1.
Current Indications for Gastroplasty and Fundoplication.

- Accepted
  - Peptic stricture with esophageal shortening
  - Type III hiatal hernia with esophageal shortening
  - Reoperation for gastroesophageal reflux
  - Advanced Type I hiatal hernia
- Controversial
  - Peptic stricture without apparent esophageal shortening
  - Barrett's esophagus requiring fundoplication
  - Gastroesophageal reflux requiring fundoplication

Four methods are now frequently used approaches to gastroplasty in the management of peptic esophageal stricture with esophageal shortening: Collis-Belsey, Collis-Nissen, uncut gastroplasty and total fundoplication, and, rarely, uncut gastroplasty and partial fundoplication.

Indications

The gastroplasty operation was originally devised to treat esophageal shortening due to peptic stricture, and it is discussed here in that context. However, current usage of cut and uncut gastroplasties includes indications that are much broader (Table 3-1). Peptic stricture with esophageal shortening remains the single strongest indication for gastroplasty and fundoplication, despite the fact that it is no longer the most common reason for performing this operation. Esophageal shortening also develops occasionally in association with a Type III hiatal hernia (paraesophageal hernia with the esophagogastric junction displaced into the mediastinum), although mobilization of the esophagus during repair of such hernias demonstrates that adequate esophageal length remains in most such cases.

In addition to esophageal shortening, other manifestations of gastroesophageal reflux comprise the majority of indications for gastroplasty and fundoplication. These include mild esophageal stricture without obvious radiographic esophageal shortening, but in which subtle shortening nevertheless may be present. The history of a prior antireflux operation suggests that additional surgery will be more difficult and the results of surgery will not be as good as in previously unoperated patients. Esophageal fibrosis is common in such patients as a result of both peptic injury and prior operation, and gastroplasty is used to maximize the likelihood of operative success. Advanced forms of Type I (sliding) hiatal hernia is another indication for gastroplasty that is sometimes mentioned, suggesting that esophageal mobilization will be inadequate to restore a proper intra-abdominal length of esophagus. Less established indications for gastroplasty include the presence of Barrett's esophagus in patients with gastroesophageal reflux requiring operation, uncomplicated gastroesophageal reflux requiring operation, and obesity in patients requiring surgery for reflux problems.

It is evident from this latter group of indications that the gastroplasty operation is being used by some surgeons as a component of the operation of choice for almost all reflux patients. Whether this is an effective means to surgically manage reflux routinely and whether results of such operations in patients without severe complications of reflux are similar to results of simple fundoplication remain to be seen. The fact that a large number of patients are operated upon using gastroplasty techniques for other than "traditional" indications likely skews the results of such operations. This fact must be kept in mind in reviewing the outcome of gastroplasty surgery.

The Gastroplasty Operation

Patient Preparation

Careful preoperative evaluation is necessary for patients who are candidates for possible gastroplasty. This includes the performance and/or review of tests necessary to confirm the clinical diagnosis and to assess the relevant anatomy and function of the stomach and esophagus. Such tests may include barium swallow, assessment of gastric emptying using endoscopy, contrast upper gastrointestinal radiographic examination or scintigraphic measurement of gastric emptying time, esophageal pH study, and an assessment of esophageal motility to evaluate the function of the body and sphincters and to rule out the existence of primary motility disorders.

Patients with a stricture should have dilations performed preoperatively. This determines whether the stricture is dilatable, permits assessment of the likelihood of the stricture being dilated to a sufficient size intraoperatively, and limits the amount of dilation that is necessary intraoperatively. There is also speculation that repetitive preoperative dilation of strictures in patients with esophageal shortening may result in esophageal lengthening preoperatively, thus obviating the need for gastroplasty in some patients.

Because gastroplasty operations are most commonly performed in patients with complex problems, the decision to proceed with gastroplasty is often not made until intraoperative exploration and esophageal mobilization are complete. In addition, other surgical options, including the need for resection and reconstruction, are frequently left open until the time of the operation. For these reasons, careful counseling of the patient with regards to a variety of possible surgical interventions is appropriate. Bowel preparation is performed preoperatively in patients who have even a small chance of needing esophagectomy and reconstruction.

Standard (Open) Surgical Technique

The usual operative approach is through a left thoracotomy. The patient is positioned under general anesthesia in a right lateral decubitus position. A double-lumen endotracheal tube or bronchial blocker is used to permit collapse of the ipsilateral lung. Alternatively, the lung can be retracted without being collapsed to provide sufficient exposure of the operative field. A lateral thoracotomy is performed, dividing the latissimus dorsi muscle but sparing the serratus anterior muscle, and the chest is opened in the seventh intercostal space. In a patient with a very low-lying diaphragm, an eighth-interspace incision may provide better exposure. A 1-cm section of the inferior rib may be taken from near the transverse process (beneath the paraspinous muscles) to permit greater distraction of the ribs without causing a fracture.

The pulmonary ligament is divided and the lung is retracted cephalad. The distal esophagus is dissected from the mediastinum and is encircled with a rubber drain, taking care to leave the vagus nerves in contact with the esophagus. While using the drain to elevate the esophagus from the posterior mediastinum, the dissection is carried caudal to the level of the esophagogastric junction. Distal to this, a hernia sac is usually found that is incised anteriorly, permitting entry into the peritoneal cavity. Anterior medial and lateral attachments of the phrenoesophageal membrane are divided with scissors or electrocautery. Posteromedially and posteriorly there are attachments to gastrohepatic omentum and retroperitoneal tissues that are divided between clamps and ligated. In particular, an artery communicating between the left gastric artery and the inferior diaphragmatic artery (Belsey's artery) must be clamped and divided. Similar division of attachments to the splenic hilum posterolateral is often necessary. Care is taken to identify and preserve the vagus nerves, which are prone to injury during this phase of the dissection.

The esophagus is mobilized cephalad to the level of the inferior pulmonary vein. If necessary, additional length is gained by mobilizing it as far as the aortic arch. If an esophageal stricture is present, it is dilated using mercury-filled rubber (Maloney) bougies passed orally. Dilation to a minimum size of 50 Fr is necessary to ensure adequate relief of dysphagia postoperatively.

At this point, the surgeon must decide how the operation will proceed. If the esophagus can be dilated satisfactorily, and if there is adequate peristaltic function based on preoperative assessment of esophageal motility, a fundoplication operation is appropriate. If there is sufficient length of esophagus as a result of intraoperative mobilization to permit a fundoplication wrap to rest in an intra-abdominal location without tension, a standard fundoplication wrap is performed. If the length of the esophagus is not sufficient, then a gastroplasty is performed, followed by fundoplication. If the preoperative and intraoperative assessments combined suggest that fibrosis has progressed to such an extent that useful function of the esophagus cannot be restored, then a resection is performed, followed by reconstruction.

When a fundoplication operation is to be performed, crural sutures are placed posteriorly but are left untied until the fundoplication has been completed. This permits reapproximation of the crura and calibration of the hiatal orifice without having to displace the esophagus. In preparation for gastroplasty, the stomach is mobilized into the chest using gentle traction and several proximal short gastric vessels are divided. In patients who have had prior surgery in this region, mobilization of the stomach through the hiatus alone may not be technically possible. In such instances the diaphragm is opened peripherally, leaving a 1- to 2-cm rim of diaphragm on the chest wall to facilitate its closure at the conclusion of the operation. This maneuver gives sufficient exposure to the upper abdomen to permit completion of the operation in all except the most difficult of cases.

The esophagogastric fat pad is excised. A large bougie (50–60 Fr) is passed orally into the stomach, and the fundus and greater curvature are retracted laterally. To perform the Collis-type gastroplasty, a linear cutting stapler (5–6 cm) is fired on the greater curvature side of and adjacent to the bougie, parallel to the lesser curvature. The staple line is reinforced with a running suture (Figure 3-2). An uncut gastroplasty is performed using a linear cutting stapler with the blade removed, or with a linear stapling device without an aligning pin, positioning the stapler in a similar fashion (Figure 3-3).

Following completion of the gastroplasty, a total or partial fundoplication is performed (Figures 3-4, 3-5) and the wrap is reduced into the abdomen. The crural sutures are then tied, making certain that the hiatus is closed only tight enough to permit passage of a finger-tip alongside the esophagus. The stomach is drained initially with a nasogastric tube, and an intercostal tube is placed to drain the pleural space.

Minimally Invasive Techniques

Minimally invasive techniques for performing a Collis-type gastroplasty have recently been described.[50-53] The most common method is

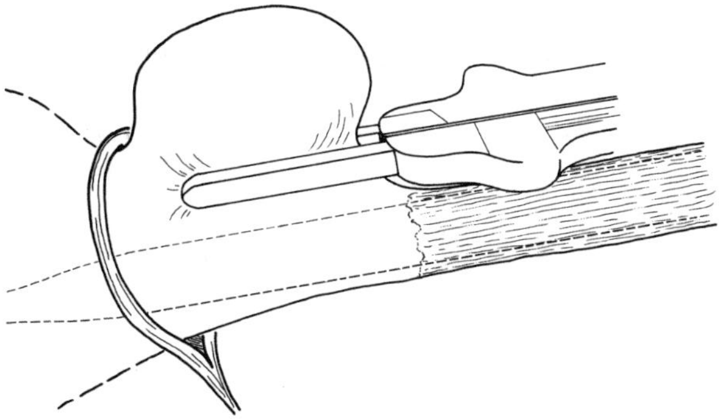

A

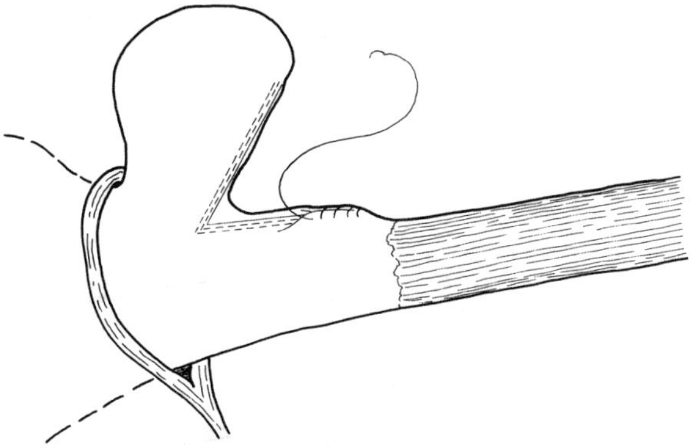

B

Figure 3-2. Standard gastroplasty performed using a left transthoracic approach with a linear cutting stapler positioned adjacent to a bougie within the esophagus and stomach (**A**); the staple line is reinforced with a running suture (**B**).

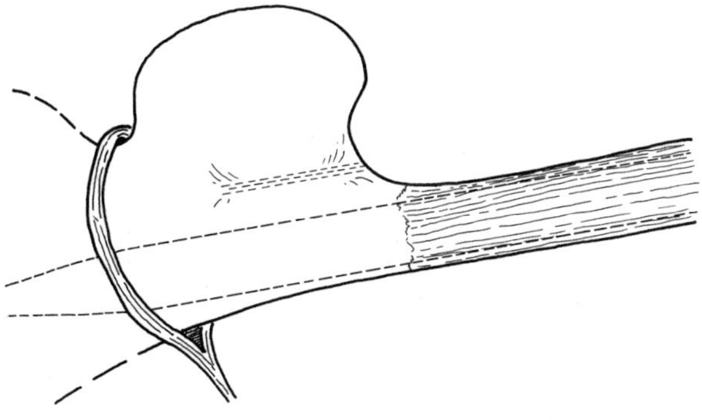

Figure 3-3. An uncut gastroplasty is performed with a standard linear stapler or with a linear cutting stapler from which the blade has been removed.

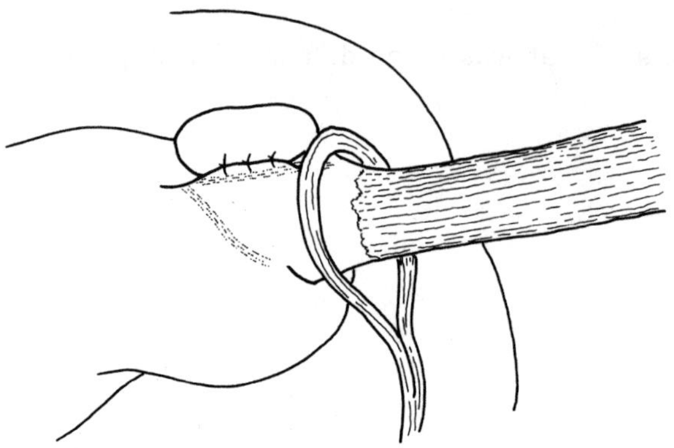

Figure 3-4. A total fundoplication performed after a Collis gastroplasty.

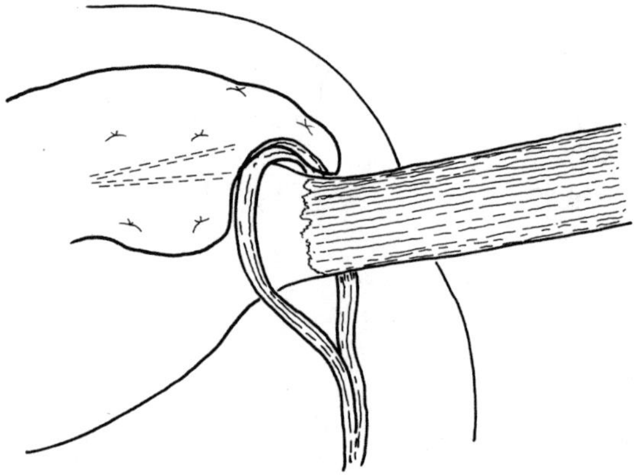

Figure 3-5. A partial fundoplication performed after a Collis gastroplasty.

laparoscopic gastroplasty. A standard laparoscopic approach is begun in the same fashion as for any fundoplication operation, placing a telescope port, a liver retractor port, and two or three operating ports in the upper abdomen. Once the proximal stomach and distal esophagus have been mobilized completely, and the surgeon's judgment is that there is true esophageal shortening, the gastroplasty procedure is begun. A large bougie is passed down the esophagus and is positioned immediately adjacent to the lesser gastric curvature. A spot on the stomach is marked with electrocautery 3 cm from the esophagogastric junction and 1 cm from the bougie. A 2-cm incision is made in the abdominal wall. A heavy monofilament suture with a straight needle is passed through the anvil of a 21-mm circular stapler and the anvil and suture are brought into the abdomen through the accessory incision. The needle is passed through the posterior wall of the stomach and is brought out through the anterior wall at the site that was marked. The anvil is pulled through after it. The stapler is passed through a large port and is connected to the anvil, after which it is fired, creating a circular, sealed hole in the stomach (Figure 3-6). A 30-mm linear cutting stapler is then inserted through this hole, oriented cephalad, and is fired adjacent to the dilator. The staple line may be oversewn for added security. A standard fundoplication is then performed.

Alternatively, the gastroplasty portion of the operation may be performed with thoracoscopic assistance. The patient is positioned semilateral with the left side rolled up. The standard laparoscopic portion of the operation is performed to complete the mobilization of the stomach and esophagus. When it is determined that a lengthening procedure is necessary, the patient is rotated to the right, the left lung is deflated, and thoracic ports are placed for the telescope and for two instruments. The mediastinal pleura is divided over the esophagus, exposing the esophagogastric junction. A large bougie is passed down the esophagus and is positioned adjacent to the lesser curvature of the stomach. A linear cutting stapler is positioned at the esophagogastric junction immediately adjacent to the dilator. The stapler is fired, and the staple line may be oversewn for added security. A standard laparoscopic fundoplication is then performed.

Postoperative Care

Drainage tubes are typically removed within a few days of the operation. If satisfactory clinical progress is evident, a liquid diet is begun, and the diet is advanced as tolerated over the subsequent few days. Dysphagia is a common sequela of complex operations for esophageal disease, but it typically resolves within weeks of surgery. Patients are counseled to expect some swallowing difficulties in the early postoperative period. Some surgeons routinely perform a contrast esophagram to evaluate for a possible leak prior to beginning the patient on an oral diet.

Operative Complications

The risk of leakage from the gastroplasty is the primary factor that distinguishes the gastroplasty and fundoplication operation from fundoplication alone. In some patients a small fistula tract is evident at the time a contrast radiograph is performed which is appropriately managed by keeping the patient free of oral intake and on intravenous alimentation until the leak has sealed. Larger leaks, especially those that are accompa-

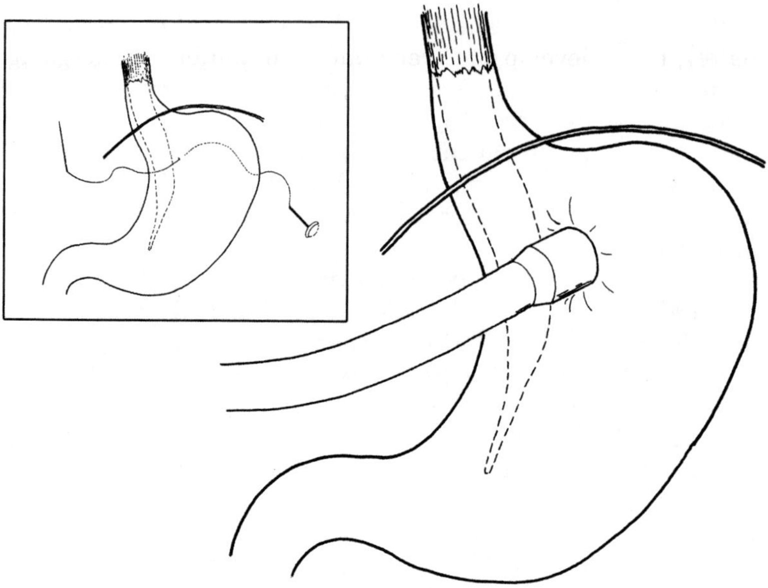

A

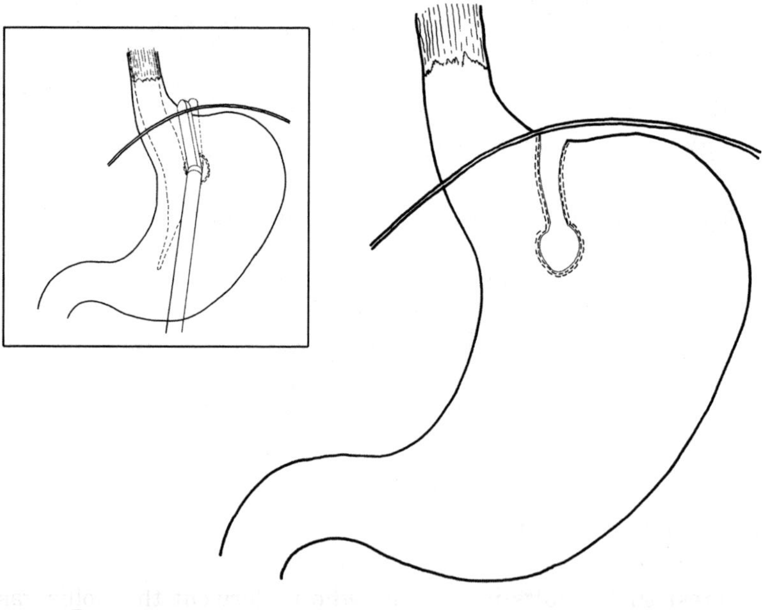

B

Figure 3-6. A minimally invasive approach for Collis gastroplasty uses standard laparoscopic port sites. A circular stapler is positioned adjacent to a large bougie in the esophagus and stomach (A), creating a sealed hole through the stomach; a linear cutting stapler is passed through this hole and is fired to complete the gastroplasty (B).

nied by clinical signs of infection, require more aggressive intervention. Fortunately, leaks develop in fewer than 2% of patients undergoing cut or uncut gastroplasty and fundoplication,[54-63] a rate that is similar to that reported for fundoplication alone.[64]

Other common complications of gastroplasty and fundoplication are wound infection and atelectasis and/or pneumonia, each of which has an overall incidence of less than 2%.[54-63] Less frequent problems include pulmonary embolus, bowel obstruction or prolonged ileus, intra-abdominal abscess, myocardial infarction, incidental splenectomy, postoperative bleeding, and acute recurrence of the hiatal hernia, each of which has an overall incidence of less than 1%. The mortality rate for gastroplasty and fundoplication is less than 1%.[54-63,65]

Results of Gastroplasty and Fundoplication

Moderate and long-term results are available for a large number of patients who have undergone gastroplasty and fundoplication. Unfortunately, the broad range of indications used for these operations precludes any formal analysis of results specific to a single indication such as peptic stricture with esophageal shortening. The variety of techniques used to assess postoperative outcome also makes the comparison of results among various centers quite difficult. In reports in which objective studies are used to assess outcome, these data are used in preference to those representing qualitative analysis of outcome. In some reports there are no quantitative data available. With these caveats in mind, the results of gastroplasty and fundoplication are summarized in Tables 3-2 and 3-3. A good outcome is classified as one in which the patient was asymptomatic or had minor residual symptoms. Patients with fair results include those with persistent dysphagia requiring dilation more than a few months postoperatively, symptomatic heartburn requiring therapy, or other notable residual or new symptoms, but who remain improved following operation. Patients with poor results are those with major residual symptoms following operation or who suffered an operative death.

Results of the Collis gastroplasty and its "cut" modifications have been reported by a large number of authors and demonstrate an overall good outcome in about 85% of patients, while fair results were observed in nearly 10% and poor results were identified in 7% (Table 3-2).[56-63,65,66] It is of interest that results in patients who underwent the Collis gastroplasty and fundoplication for esophageal shortening due to peptic stricture and in whom no prior operation had been performed experienced outcomes similar to all other operated patients. There does not seem to be any difference in results comparing patients who had partial fundoplication to those who had total fundoplication.

Table 3-2.
Results of Collis Gastroplasty and Fundoplication.

Reference	Year	Patients Operated	Patients Followed	Period of Follow-up (years)	Type of Fundoplication	Deaths	Results (%) Good	Fair	Poor
Henderson, et al.[56]	1985	351	335	5–8.5	Total	0	312 (93)	13 (4)	10 (3)
Tomas-Ridocci, et al.[a 65]	1985	46	46	1–3	Total	0	36 (78)	10 (22)	0
Pearson, et al.[a 57]	1987	215	215	1–20	Partial	0	199 (93)	10 (4)	6 (3)
Thayer, et al.[b 58]	1988	70	68	1–13	Partial or total	0	40 (59)	11 (16)	17 (25)
Stirling, et al.[59]	1989	353	261	1–12	Total	1	195 (75)	34 (13)	32 (12)
Beauchamp, et al.[60]	1989	58	55	1–5	Total	1	47 (85)	2 (4)	6 (11)
Sancho-Fornos, et al.[61]	1989	46	46	>3	Total	0	39 (85)	5 (11)	2 (4)
Testart, et al.[c 62]	1991	49	32	4–10	Partial	3	24 (75)	3 (9)	5 (16)
Jeyasingham, et al.[d 63]	1993	58	48	0.6–10.5	Partial	3	33 (69)	12 (25)	3 (6)
Rieger, et al.[66]	1994	11	11	0.5–15	Total	0	8 (73)	0	3 (27)
		1257	1117			8	933 (84)	100 (9)	84 (7)

[a]Previously unoperated patients with acquired esophageal shortening due to peptic stricture
[b]Ten patients had an uncut Collis-Nissen operation
[c]Barrett's esophagus without esophageal shortening
[d]V-Y gastroplasty

Table 3-3.
Results of Uncut Gastroplasty and Fundoplication.

Reference	Year	Patients Operated	Patients Followed	Period of Follow-up (years)	Type of Fundoplication	Deaths	Results (%) Good	Fair	Poor
Evangelist, et al.[45]	1978	48	48	0.3–4.4	Total	0	47 (98)	0	1 (2)
Keenan, et al.[54]	1984	20	20	5 (mean)	Total	0	11 (55)	5 (25)	4 (20)
Demos[47]	1984	82	80	2–12	Total	0	71 (89)	6 (8)	3 (3)
Piehler, et al.[55]	1984	136	131	0.8–3.5	Total	0	110 (84)	11 (8)	10 (8)
Vankemmel, et al[a].[67]	1989	10	10	2–9	Partial	0	8 (80)	1 (10)	1 (10)
		296	289			0	247 (85)	23 (8)	19 (7)

[a]Cardioplasty

Results of uncut gastroplasties combined with fundoplication are very similar to those of the more traditional Collis-type gastroplasty and fundoplication. Over 85% of patients had a good outcome, 8% had a fair outcome, and 7% had a poor outcome (Table 3-3).[45,47,54,55,67] Almost all procedures were performed using a total fundoplication, making a comparison between types of fundoplication impossible.

Other Concerns

Dysphagia Resulting from Creation of an Inert Tube

Following the initial descriptions of the gastroplasty-fundoplication operations, some individuals expressed concern that the interposition of an inert gastric tube between the stomach and esophagus would be a frequent cause of postoperative dysphagia, particularly in patients in whom distal esophageal peristaltic function was poor.[68] In fact, manometric studies performed postoperatively usually demonstrate not only a relatively normal high pressure zone at rest in the region of the gastroplasty tube, but adequate relaxation to deglutition as well.[47,56,57,59,61,65] Indeed, early studies demonstrated that the responses of the gastric fundus to stimulation were similar to those of the esophagus.[68] This information recently has been corroborated by the careful anatomic evaluations of Liebermann-Meffert and others, who demonstrated that the anatomic correlates of the lower esophageal high pressure zone were located to a great extent along the lesser curvature of the stomach.[69]

Stability of the Uncut Gastroplasty

There is considerable experience with stapling of the stomach during operations for morbid obesity and of the esophagogastric junction in the management of esophageal perforation by "esophageal exclusion."[71] In many patients in whom through-and-through staple lines are placed without division of the mucosa, the staple lines separate over time. In esophageal surgery, this staple line separation takes a matter of weeks and is likely promoted to some extent by the peristaltic activity of the esophagus. Gastric staple lines separate over a longer period of time, possibly due to the more constrained underlying motility patterns of the stomach. Separation of the staple lines and recanalization of the previously stapled area is possible because placing a staple line without dividing the mucosa does not promote healing of the apposing tissues to each other.

Delayed separation of the staple line is not of concern in patients in whom a "cut" gastroplasty has been performed because the divided mucosal edges heal together, making the separation between the "neoesophagus" and gastric fundus permanent. Theoretically, there is cause for concern that the staple line of an uncut gastroplasty may separate over time because the mucosal edges have not been cut. This type of complication has not been reported, and the vanishingly small likelihood of such a problem may be due to the fact that nearly all uncut gastroplasties are accompanied by a total fundoplication, which may serve to reinforce the staple line and prevent its separation.

Risk of Carcinoma

The growing recognition of the relationship between Barrett's esophagus and adenocarcinoma of the esophagus has caused concern on the part of some surgeons that gastroplasty may predispose patients to the development of adenocarcinoma. Indeed, in the discussion of Pearson's 1970 presentation of the Collis-Belsey operation there is concern expressed over the types of cells contained in the gastroplasty tube.[1] In discussion of a subsequent presentation by Pearson and his colleagues, the gastroplasty tube was referred to as an iatrogenic Barrett's esophagus, and the concern over the increased risk of cancer in these patients was again expressed.[72]

The extent of risk imposed by creating a gastroplasty tube in all likelihood is very small. In fact, the tube is not an "iatrogenic Barrett's esophagus," because, at least at the time of its formation, it contains normal gastric fundic epithelium, whereas none of the three types of metaplastic epithelium that comprise Barrett's mucosa are found within it. A total of seven instances of adenocarcinoma developing in patients following gastroplasty have been reported.[57,67,73] In at least half of these cases, the carcinoma was diagnosed 3 to 9 months following the gastroplasty operation, too short an interval to permit association of the gastroplasty in their development. In all but one of the remaining patients, the carcinomas were thought to arise in true Barrett's epithelium, cephalad to the gastroplasty tube. Longer follow-up in a large number of patients will be necessary to settle this controversy, but evidence that supports the increased risk of cancer in these patients is currently lacking.

References

1. Belsey R. Discussion of reference 35
2. Wangensteen OH, Leven NL. Gastric resection for esophagitis and stricture of acid-peptic origin. *Surg Gynecol Obstet* 1949;88:560-570.
3. Allison PR. Reflux esophagitis, sliding hiatal hernia, and the anatomy of repair. *Surg Gynecol Obstet* 1951;92:419-431.

4. Tanner NC. Treatment of oesophageal hiatus hernia. *Lancet* 1955;19:1050-1055.
5. Humphreys GH II, Ferrer JM Jr, Wiedel PD. Esophageal hiatus hernia of the diaphragm. *J Thorac Surg* 1957;34:749-767.
6. Boerema VI, Germs R. Gastropexia anterior geniculata wegen Hiatusbruch des Zwerchfells. *Zentralblatt Chir* 1955;39:1585-1590.
7. Burford TH, Lischer CE. Treatment of short esophageal hernia with esophagitis by Finney pyloroplasty. *Ann Surg* 1956;144:647-652.
8. MacLean LD, Wangensteen OH. The surgical treatment of esophageal stricture. *Surg Gynecol Obstet* 1956;103:5-14.
9. Fisher HC, Johnson ME. Esophageal hiatal hernia a manifestation of peptic esophagitis. *AMA Arch Surg* 1957;75:660-673.
10. Merendino KA, Varco RL, Wangensteen OH. Displacement of the esophagus into a new diaphragmatic orifice in the repair of para-esophageal and esophageal hiatus hernia. *Ann Surg* 1949;129:185-197.
11. Effler DB, Collins EN. Complications and surgical treatment of hiatus hernia and short esophagus with thoracic stomach. *JAMA* 1951;147:305-308.
12. Effler DB, Ballinger CS. Complications and surgical treatment of hiatus hernia and short esophagus. *J Thorac Surg* 1951;22:235-247.
13. Barrett NR. Hiatus hernia. *Br J Surg* 1954;42:231-244.
14. Sealy WC, Carver G. Sliding hiatal hernia--symptoms, pathogenesis, and results of treatment. *JAMA* 1957;164:655-658.
15. Collis JL, Kelly TD, Wiley AM. Anatomy of the crura of the diaphragm and the surgery of hiatus hernia. *Thorax* 1954;9:175-189.
16. Wooler G. Reconstruction of the cardia and fundus of the stomach. *Thorax* 1956;11:275-280.
17. Dillard DH, Griffith CA, Merendino KA. The surgical construction of an esophageal valve to replace the "cardiac sphincter." An experimental study. *Surg Forum* 1954;5:306-314.
18. Watkins DH, Prevedel A, Harper FR. A method of preventing peptic esophagitis following esophagogastrostomy. *J Thorac Surg* 1954;28:367-382.
19. Najarian JS, Murray DH Jr, Buster CD, Grimes OF. Utilization of the ileocecal valve as a substitute for the "cardio-esophageal sphincter." *Surg Forum* 1956;7:344-348.
20. Sweet RH. A consideration of certain benign lesions of the esophagus. *Surgery* 1956;40:447-458.
21. Valdoni P. Traitement radical des stenoses oesophagiennes. *Presse Med* 1951;59:1216-1218.
22. Sweet, RH, Robbins LL, Gephart T, et al. The surgical treatment of peptic ulceration and stricture of the lower esophagus. *Ann Surg* 1954;139:258-268.
23. Allison PR, Wooler GH, Gunning AJ. Esophagojejunogastrostomy. *J Thorac Surg* 1957;33:738-748.
24. Girvin GW, Merendino KA. Cardiac sphincter substitution by interpositioned jejunum. *AMA Arch Surg* 1956;72:241-246.
25. Merendino KA, Dillard DH. The concept of sphincter substitution by an interposed jejunal segment for anatomic and physiologic abnormalities at the esophagogastric junction. *Ann Surg* 1955;142:486-509.

26. Ellis FH Jr, Andersen HA, Clagett OT. Treatment of short esophagus with stricture by esophagogastrectomy and antral excision. *Ann Surg* 1958;148:526-536.
27. Barnes WA, McElwee RS. Surgical treatment of non-neoplastic lesions at the esophago-gastric junction. *Ann Surg* 1953;137:523-529.
28. Collis JL. An operation for hiatus hernia with short esophagus. *J Thorac Surg* 1957;34:768-778.
29. Collis JL. Gastroplasty. *Thorax* 1961;16:197-206.
30. Fyke FE Jr, Code CF, Schlegel JF. The gastroesophageal sphincter in healthy human beings. *Gastroenterologia* 1956;86:135-150.
31. Fleshler B, Hendrix TR, Kramer P, Ingelfinger FJ. Resistance and reflex function of the lower esophageal sphincter. *J Appl Physiol* 1958;12:339-342.
32. Adler RH, Firme CN, Lanigan JM. A valve mechanism to prevent gastroesophageal reflux and esophagitis. *Surgery* 1958;44:63-76.
33. Nissen R. Gastropexy and "fundoplication" in surgical treatment of hiatal hernia. *Am J Dig Dis* 1961;6:954-961.
34. Skinner DB, Belsey RHR. Surgical management of esophageal reflux and hiatus hernia. *J Thorac Cardiovasc Surg* 1967;53:33-54.
35. Pearson FG, Langer B, Henderson RD. Gastroplasty and Belsey hiatus hernia repair. *J Thorac Cardiovasc Surg* 1971;61:50-63.
36. Orringer MB, Sloan H. An improved technique for the combined Collis-Belsey approach to dilatable esophageal strictures. *J Thorac Cardiovasc Surg* 1974;68:298-302.
37. Pearson FG, Henderson RD. Long-term follow-up of peptic strictures managed by dilatation, modified Collis gastroplasty, and Belsey hiatus hernia repair. *Surgery* 1976;80:396-404.
38. Orringer MB, Sloan H. Collis-Belsey reconstruction of the esophagogastric junction. *J Thorac Cardiovasc Surg* 1976;71:295-303.
39. Urschel HC, Razzuk MA, Wood RE, et al. An improved surgical technique for the complicated hiatal hernia with gastroesophageal reflux. *Ann Thorac Surg* 1973;15:443-451.
40. Orringer MB, Sloan H. Complications and failings of the combined Collis-Belsey operation. *J Thorac Cardiovasc Surg* 1977;74:726-735.
41. Pearson FG, Cooper JD, Nelems JM. Gastroplasty and fundoplication in the management of complex reflux problems. *J Thorac Cardiovasc Surg* 1978;76:665-672.
42. Orringer MB, Sloan H. Combined Collis-Nissen reconstruction of the esophagogastric junction. *Ann Thorac Surg* 1978;25:16-21.
43. Demos NJ, Smith N, Williams D. New gastroplasty for strictured short esophagus. *New York State J Med* 1975;75:57-59.
44. Bingham JAW. Hiatus hernia repair combined with the construction of an anti-reflux valve in the stomach. *Br J Surg* 1977;64:460-465.
45. Evangelist FA, Taylor FH, Alford JD. The modified Collis-Nissen operation for control of gastroesophageal reflux. *Ann Thorac Surg* 1978;26:107-111.
46. Payne WS. Surgical management of reflux-induced oesophageal stenoses: Results in 101 patients. *Br J Surg* 1984;71:971-973.
47. Demos NJ. Stapled, uncut gastroplasty for hiatal hernia: 12-year follow-up. *Ann Thorac Surg* 1984;38:393-399.

48. Reilly KM, Jeyasingham K. A modified Pearson gastroplasty. *Thorax* 1984;39:67-69.

49. Vankemmel M. Etude comparee schematique de quatre procedes de correction du reflux gastro-oesophagien par voie abdominale. *J Chir (Paris)* 1982;119:295-301.

50. Swanstrom LL, Marcus DR, Galloway GQ. Laparoscopic Collis gastroplasty is the treatment of choice for the shortened esophagus. *Am J Surg* 1996;171:477-481.

51. Jobe BA, Horvath KD, Swanstrom LL. Postoperative function following laparoscopic Collis gastroplasty for shortened esophagus. *Arch Surg* 1998;133:867-874.

52. Johnson AB, Oddsdottir M, Hunter JG. Laparoscopic Collis gastroplasty and Nissen fundoplication. A new technique for the management of esophageal foreshortening. *Surg Endosc* 1998;12:1055-1060.

53. Luketich JD, Raja S, Fernando HC, et al. Laparoscopic repair of giant paraesophageal hernia: 100 consecutive cases. *Ann Surg* 2000;232:608-618.

54. Keenan DJM, Hamilton JRL, Gibbons J, et al. Surgery for benign esophageal stricture. *J Thorac Cardiovasc Surg* 1984;88:182-188.

55. Piehler JM, Payne WS, Cameron AJ, et al. The uncut Collis-Nissen procedure for esophageal hiatal hernia and its complications. *Probl Gen Surg* 1984;1:1-14.

56. Henderson RD, Marryatt GV. Total fundoplication gastroplasty (Nissen gastroplasty): Five-year review. *Ann Thorac Surg* 1985;39:74-79.

57. Pearson FG, Cooper JD, Patterson GA, et al. Gastroplasty and fundoplication for complex reflux problems. *Ann Surg* 1987;206:473-481.

58. Thayer JO Jr, Gibb SP, Ellis FH Jr. Gastroplasty and fundoplication for severe gastroesophageal reflux with esophageal shortening. *Dis Esoph* 1988;1:153-158.

59. Stirling MC, Orringer MB. Continued assessment of the combined Collis-Nissen operation. *Ann Thorac Surg* 1989;47:224-230.

60. Beauchamp G. The Collis-Nissen procedure. In **Benign Lesions of the Esophagus and Cancer**. Giuli R, McCallum RW (eds): Springer-Verlag, Paris, 1989, pp 463-466.

61. Sancho-Fornos S, Magallon CR, Carrillo AP, et al. The advantage of Collis-Nissen procedure via an abdominal or thoracic approach. In **Benign Lesions of the Esophagus and Cancer**. Giuli R, McCallum RW (eds): Springer-Verlag, Paris, 1989, pp 466-471.

62. Testart J, Kartheuser A, Peillon C, et al. L'operation de Collis pour brachyoesophage. *Gastroenterol Clin Biol* 1991;15:512-518.

63. Jeyasingham K, Bhatnagar NK, Peppas G, et al. A continuous 10-year assessment of the results of surgery for shortened esophagus. In **Recent Advances in Diseases of the Esophagus**. Nabeya K, Hanaoka T, and Nogami H (eds): Springer-Verlag, Tokyo, 1993, pp 84-90.

64. Urschel JD. Gastroesophageal leaks after antireflux operations. *Ann Thorac Surg* 1994;57:1229-1232.

65. Tomas-Ridocci M, Paris F, Carbonell-Antoli C, et al. Total fundoplication with or without gastroplasty for gastroesophageal reflux: Comparative study. *Ann Thorac Surg* 1985;39:508-511.

66. Rieger NA, Jamieson GG, Britten-Jones R, Tew S. Reoperation after failed antireflux surgery. *Br J Surg* 1994;81:1159-1161.
67. Vankemmel M, Goachet C, Brandt MF. Are there still indications for cardioplasty? In: **Benign Lesions of the Esophagus and Cancer**. Giuli R, McCallum RW (eds), Springer-Verlag, Paris, 1989, pp 488-493.
68. DeMeester TR. Discussion of reference 53.
69. Lind JF, Duthie HL, Schlegel JF, Code CF. Motility of the gastric fundus. *Am J Physiol* 1961;210:197-202.
70. Liebermann-Meffert D, Allgower M, Schmidt P, Blum AL. Muscular equivalent of the lower esophageal sphincter. *Gastroenterology* 1979;76:31-38.
71. Bardini R, Bonavina L, Pavanello M, et al. Temporary double exclusion of the perforated esophagus using absorbable staples. *Ann Thorac Surg* 1992;54:1165-1167.
72. Skinner DB. Discussion of reference 53.
73. Groome JW, Peppas G, Jeyasingham K. Carcinoma developing in the neooesophagus following gastroplasty. *Eur J Cardio-thorac Surg* 1992;6:220-222.

Chapter 4

Patch Esophagoplasty

Patch esophagoplasty is a procedure in which autologous tissue is used to reconstruct a full-thickness, partially-circumferential defect in the esophagus. Such defects may be due to trauma, excision of a benign tumor that involves only a portion of the esophageal circumference, and longitudinal esophagotomy as therapy for a benign annular stricture. The most common of the problems for which patch esophagoplasty is useful is peptic stricture, for which reconstruction has been accomplished with a variety of gastric patches. Repair of defects due to other causes has been reported infrequently. A wide variety of surgical techniques also has been described, with the result that no single technique for one particular indication has achieved widespread acceptance. This chapter summarizes these two broad categories of repair, focusing on the gastric patch esophagoplasties employed in the management of peptic stricture.

During the first half of the twentieth century, available methods for managing focal esophageal abnormalities included esophageal bypass, limited or subtotal esophageal resection, and esophagoplasty.[1-7] Simple esophagoplasty, the only original means by which the full extent of the esophagus could be preserved, first was described as a treatment for peptic stricture. The operation was performed by opening the stricture longitudinally and closing the incision transversely. This technique of simple esophagoplasty often resulted in a persistent peptic stricture due to the continued presence of gastroesophageal reflux that produced the stricture in the first place. Following the introduction of patch esophagoplasty using the stomach, the original technique of limited esophagoplasty was largely abandoned, and patch esophagoplasty became an accepted method for establishing an adequate lumen in a strictured esophagus.

The main advantage of patch esophagoplasty, as originally developed, was preservation of the remaining esophagus and its peristaltic activity, particularly in patients with focal esophageal abnormalities. In addition,

---

From Ferguson MK: *Reconstructive Surgery of the Esophagus* Armonk, NY: Futura Publishing Company, Inc., © 2002.

this technique was minimally disruptive to other intrathoracic and intra-abdominal organs, minimizing iatrogenic problems and maintaining other surgical options if patch esophagoplasty failed. However, as use of this technique became more frequent, numerous problems associated with it were recognized, which have resulted in its limited application in current practice. Most aspects of this technique are of historical interest only. Nevertheless, its use is still appropriate for the rare patient for whom other reconstructive methods are not feasible.

Historical Background

Efforts Preceding Introduction of the Patch Esophagoplasty

Most early methods of managing obstructive esophageal disease, including peptic stricture, caustic injury, congenital disorders, and esophageal cancer, required at least one esophageal anastomosis. This often was a high-risk aspect of the operation due to the lack of a serosal esophageal layer and to the perceived poor blood supply of the esophagus, both of which were thought to contribute to a high rate of anastomotic leak and subsequent mortality.[8-10] Clinical and laboratory initiatives were brought to bear on identifying techniques to improve anastomotic healing or avoiding anastomoses altogether. Efforts during the 1940s and 1950s focused on identifying means to reinforce esophageal anastomoses with autologous tissues. Such tissues included pedicled or free grafts of lung, pleura and pericardium, as well as free grafts of omentum and peritoneum.[11-22] Under most circumstances, it appeared that pedicled or free grafts would adhere to the esophagus, but that the addition of such grafts to an adequately performed anastomosis did not improve its strength or the risk of leakage.

Autologous tissues, with or without supportive prosthetic material, were also used to close partially circumferential full thickness esophageal defects and to bridge complete gaps in the esophagus. Tissues typically used included fascia, skin, dermal grafts, pedicled intercostal muscle, pericardium, diaphragm, and omentum, and repairs were performed both experimentally and clinically.[23-27] These operations occasionally produced gratifying results, but most often culminated in death of the patient due to breakdown of the repair and subsequent sepsis.

Simple esophagoplasty using the technique of Heineke-Mikulicz for pyloroplasty was originally introduced by Wendel as a method of managing achalasia.[28] It was subsequently used sporadically in the treatment of short annular esophageal strictures that were presumably of peptic origin. Limited reports prior to 1960 include at least 11 patients, of whom

4 experienced short-term relief of dysphagia, 1 died, 3 required repeated dilations, and 3 needed reoperation for resection of the stricture.[3,7,29] The failure of simple esophagoplasty in these patients was likely related to the preexisting advanced degree of underlying inflammation in the esophagus, the total destruction of the antireflux mechanism by the longitudinal esophagotomy, and the transposition of the esophagogastric junction into the thoracic cavity that necessarily accompanied esophagoplasty on many occasions.

Development of the Fundic (Thal) Patch Esophagoplasty

One of Alan Thal's prominent clinical and research interests was peptic esophagitis and its complications. He was dissatisfied with the results after incision of the esophagogastric junction and simple esophagoplasty, which promoted free reflux into an already injured esophagus. Believing that resection and interposition, particularly as championed by Merendino and others,[6,30,31] was unnecessarily complex, he sought a more simple solution to these problems. Early efforts resulted in the development of a canine model of distal esophageal stricture with which the authors demonstrated the feasibility of using a fundic patch for esophagogastroplasty (Figure 4-1).[32] This technique had distinct advantages over simple esophagoplasty in that the partial gastric wrap served to recreate the normal barrier to reflux, limiting acid exposure of the distal esophagus.[33]

The operation as originally described included exposure of the esophagus and cardia through an abdominal incision. A longitudinal incision was made across the esophagogastric junction measuring 4 cm in length on the esophagus and 3 cm in length on the stomach. While the margins of the incision were separated by stay sutures, the anterior wall of the stomach was pulled cephalad and sewn to the edges of the defect in two layers, lining the defect with gastric serosa.[33] A subsequent modification of the technique included a split-thickness skin graft over the gastric serosa for use in lining the esophagus (Fig 4-2).[32,34] This technique was used clinically to repair spontaneous ruptures of the esophagus and to reconstruct the esophagogastric junction in patients with peptic esophageal stricture, achalasia, and hiatal hernia.[34-36] Results of Thal's early efforts demonstrated a good outcome in 18 of 22 (82%) patients suffering from peptic esophageal stricture with one operative death.[34]

Development of Other Patch Esophagoplasties

Since Thal's initial reports, other techniques of gastric patch esophagoplasties have been described for management of distal esophageal stric-

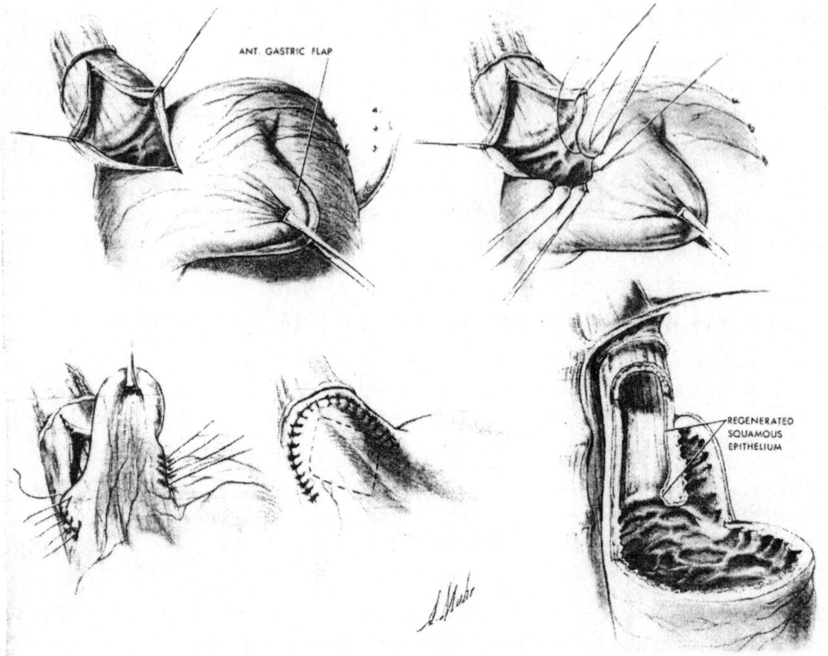

Figure 4-1. The original technique for Thal patch application for management of esophageal stricture [Reprinted with permission from the American College of Surgeons (*Surg Gynecol Obstet* 1965;120:1225–1231.)]

ture. These include use of a segment of gastric antrum or the greater curve of the stomach as a pedicled gastric patch.[37,38] Both techniques base the vascularized patch on the left or right gastroepiploic vessels, respectively, and position the patch with the mucosa lining the esophagus. A fundoplication is added below the level of the patch to reduce acid reflux. Using these techniques, results in a very small number of patients have been satisfactory.

Use of other tissues to repair esophageal defects other than those created surgically in the management of peptic stricture has been reported sporadically, echoing the early efforts at use of autologous material to repair or reinforce the esophagus.[39-42] These techniques include use of pedicled flaps of intercostal muscle, pericardium, and diaphragm for management of congenital fistula, congenital stenosis, and perforation of the esophagus.

Indications for Patch Esophagoplasty

Common indications for patch esophagoplasty are listed in Table 4-1. In each instance there is either a strong rationale to preserve the

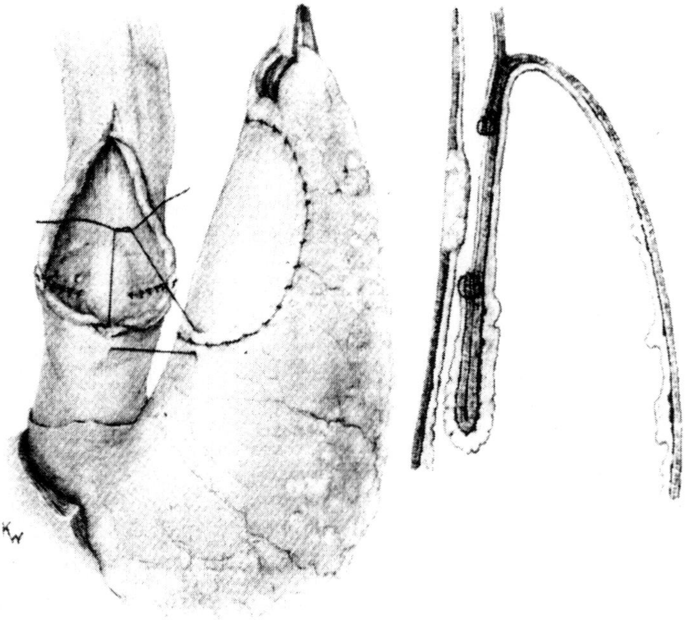

Figure 4-2. The modified technique for Thal patch application, including a split thickness skin graft to line the esophageal lumen (from ref 34, reproduced with permission from the publisher).

Table 4-1.
Indications for Patch Esophagoplasty.

Strictures	
	Peptic
	Inflammatory, nonpeptic
	Congenital
	Healed esophageal perforation
Perforations	
	Secondary to dilation
	Barogenic
Esophageal fistula	
	Congenital
	Acquired, benign

esophagus or a contraindication to esophageal resection. The most common situation in which patch esophagoplasty is performed is for a distal peptic esophageal stricture that fails to respond adequately to maximum conservative therapy, including aggressive dilation and intensive acid suppression therapy. These strictures must be dense enough to otherwise require esophagectomy and reconstruction. In such situations, patch esophagoplasty is used when the patient is considered a poor candidate for more aggressive surgical therapy for either anatomic or physiologic reasons.

Other problems that are amenable to patch esophagoplasty include those secondary to a local inflammatory process caused by ingested pills, isolated congenital strictures, and stenoses due to healing of esophageal perforation. Patch esophagoplasty is of use in the acute management of esophageal perforation, particularly when the perforation is located near the esophagogastric junction, as in the case of barogenic rupture and perforation resulting from dilation of a peptic stenosis or, rarely, after pneumatic dilation for achalasia.

The Patch Esophagoplasty Operation

Patient Preparation

Patients who are to undergo elective patch esophagoplasty for management of a peptic stricture are treated for an extended period preoperatively with acid suppression medication such as H_2 receptor blockers or proton pump inhibitors to reduce as much as possible the degree of intramural esophageal inflammation. Careful preparation of the bowels with cathartics and antibiotics is also indicated to permit jejunal or colon interposition, should it be determined intraoperatively that patch esophagoplasty is not appropriate. Operations for congenital or acquired fistulae are preceded by a period of pulmonary toilet to decrease the likelihood of a postoperative pneumonia developing. Because patch esophagoplasty is a clean contaminated procedure, all patients are given perioperative antibiotics.

Surgical Techniques

Gastric (fundic) patch esophagoplasty for peptic stricture

The operation is performed through a left thoracotomy, entering the chest in the seventh interspace. After dividing the pulmonary ligament and retracting the lung superiorly, the distal esophagus is mobilized from its bed. The phrenoesophageal membrane is divided circumferentially at the hiatus, and the proximal stomach is mobilized by dividing attachments to the diaphragm and several short gastric vessels. The retroperitoneal space is entered and the descending branch of the inferior phrenic artery (Belsey's artery) is divided.

A full-thickness longitudinal incision is made through the stricture, extending past the lower esophageal sphincter to the gastric fundus, if necessary. A large bougie is passed through the mouth and into the stomach to maintain an appropriate esophageal diameter. A split-thickness skin graft is sutured to the edges of the mucosal defect with the epidermal side facing the lumen. The gastric fundus is tacked to the muscular edges of the esophageal defect. A total fundoplication is performed using the remaining gastric fundus while the bougie is still in place. Three heavy nonabsorbable sutures are placed through the anterior portion of the fundic wrap, the esophagus, and the posterior portion of the fundic wrap. The sutures are spaced 1 cm apart, producing a 2 cm wrap.

If there is sufficient esophageal length, the wrap is reduced below the diaphragm and the crura are approximated with heavy interrupted nonabsorbable sutures. In most patients, there will be insufficient esophageal length to permit reduction of the repair below the diaphragm. If this is the case, the wrap is permitted to remain in the thorax, and a sufficiently large hiatal defect is created to prevent gastric obstruction. The edges of the defect in the diaphragm are sutured to the stomach to prevent intrathoracic herniation of abdominal contents.

Other patch esophagoplasties

For localized problems affecting regions other than the gastroesophageal junction, the approach to the thoracic esophagus is through the left seventh interspace for problems in the distal esophagus or through the right fifth or sixth interspace for problems in the middle or upper esophagus. The cervical esophagus is easily approached through a collar incision, which can be extended using a partial sternotomy if additional exposure is necessary. For operations on an esophageal stricture, the defect is laid open widely; a large bougie is passed through the patient's mouth and through the defect to stent it open during its repair. Esophageal perforations or fistulae are identified, and the edges are trimmed back to healthy tissue if necessary. An autologous flap of tissue is prepared. For problems affecting the cervical esophagus, a simple flap of strap muscle or sternocleidomastoid muscle is easily prepared and will usually cover any defect without undue tension on the flap.

Middle and upper esophageal problems are best managed with an intercostal muscle flap or a flap from shoulder girdle muscles such as latissimus dorsi or serratus anterior. For intercostal muscle flaps, either one or two intercostal neurovascular bundles are included, depending on the size of the area to be covered. This typically necessitates removal of at least one rib. Development of other muscle flaps to be transposed into the chest is based on the dominant neurovascular supply to the muscle.

The latissimus dorsi muscle is based on the thoracodorsal artery and nerve, and the serratus anterior is based on the long thoracic artery and nerve. The assistance of an expert in reconstructive surgical techniques is invaluable in preparing these flaps. Once the flap is raised, it is transposed and is stitched to the edge of the esophageal defect with interrupted absorbable sutures.

Problems affecting the lower esophagus are managed with an intercostal muscle flap as described above, or with flaps of diaphragm or stomach. A full-thickness diaphragm flap is raised near the esophageal hiatus and is based medially or laterally depending on the location of the esophageal pathology. After suturing the edges of the muscle flap to the esophagus, the defect in the diaphragm is closed with heavy, interrupted, nonabsorbable sutures. Gastric patches rotated from the body or antrum also have been described. These have the advantage of an excellent blood supply based on the right gastroepiploic artery. The artery is freed from the greater curvature, preserving its branches to the region of the flap. A full-thickness patch of stomach is excised and is brought through the esophageal hiatus in a retrogastric plane. It is sutured to the esophageal defect using interrupted, absorbable stitches. The gastric defect is closed transversely.

Postoperative Care

The area of the esophagoplasty is drained, and standard pleural drains are placed for patients undergoing transpleural operations. The stomach is decompressed with a nasogastric tube for at least several days postoperatively. The duration of gastric decompression is longer for patients who undergo gastric patch esophagoplasty rather than muscle patch esophagoplasty using a chest wall muscle flap. A contrast esophagram is performed about 1 week postoperatively, and a liquid diet is begun if the radiograph shows no evidence for extravasation of contrast material.

Results of Patch Esophagoplasty

Although patch esophagoplasty has been used by a number of surgeons for several decades, only limited results have been reported. Gastric patch esophagoplasty for management of peptic stricture yields a good outcome in two-thirds of patients, and over 80% are improved after operation (Table 4-2).[34,37,38,41-45] The results are best in patients who have a concomitant fundoplication, whether or not the fundoplication is left in the thorax or is reduced into the abdomen.[44] Failure to perform a fundoplication yields poor results in the majority of patients.[43] The two variations

Table 4-2.
Results of Patch Esophagoplasty.

Indication	Technique	Reference	Year	Patients	Operative Mortality	Outcome (%) Good	Fair	Poor
Peptic stricture	Fundic patch (Thal)	Thal[34]	1968	22	1	82	0	18
	Fundic patch (Thal)	Jones et al.[43]	1971	6	--	17	0	83
	Antral patch	Hugh et al.[37]	1979	6	0	50	33	17
	Fundic patch (Thal)	Maher et al.[44]	1981	68	3	67	20	13
	Gastric patch	Schon et al.[38]	1989	3	0	100	0	0
				105	4	67	15	18
Perforation, trauma	Fundic patch (Thal)	Thal[34]	1968	6	1	83	0	17
	Diaphragm flap	Rao[41]	1974	1	0	100	0	0
	Diaphragm flap	Jara[42]	1979	1	0	100	0	0
	Diaphragm flap	Richardson et al.[45]	1994	8	0	75	25	0
				16	1	81	13	6

of the gastric pedicled patch esophagoplasty have not been performed in a sufficient number of patients to permit meaningful comparisons with the fundic patch operation, although the limited results appear similar.[37,38]

The use of a fundic patch or flap of diaphragm in the management of esophageal perforation or trauma has been reported in only a small number of patients. Over 80% of patients experienced a good result, and operative mortality was low.

Other Considerations

Two primary concerns attend the use of gastric patch esophagoplasty in the management of peptic esophageal stricture. The most important issue regards the use of the stomach in this fashion for reconstruction, particularly with regard to the use of gastric patches pedicled on the gastroepiploic arcade. Such procedures sacrifice the stomach for use as an organ for esophageal replacement by either eliminating the primary blood supply or sacrificing the fundus. In addition, the introduction of potentially acid-producing gastric mucosa into the esophagus, as in the case of the pedicled grafts, may promote peptic erosion and recurrence of the stricture.[46] The performance of an intrathoracic fundoplication, as is often necessary with the Thal-type patch, can expose the patient to the possibility of serious long-term complications such as bleeding, necrosis and perforation of the stomach,[47,48] although some surgeons argue that technical modifications substantially reduce these risks.[49-51] In recognition of these risks, the use of gastric fundic-patch techniques for managing esophageal stricture and perforation should be limited to selected patients in whom more standard approaches are precluded.

References

1. Barnes WA, Redo SF. Evaluation of esophago-jejunostomy in the treatment of lesions at the esophago-gastric junction. *Ann Surg* 1957;146:224-228.
2. Benedict EB, Nardi GL. Peptic stenosis of esophagus. *Am J Surg* 1957;93:238-241.
3. Hale HW Jr, Drapanas T. Reflux esophagitis. *Am J Surg* 1957;93:228-233.
4. Lindskog GE, Kline JL. The problem of hiatus hernia complicated by peptic esophagitis. *N Engl J Med* 1957;257:110-113.
5. Mustard RA. Reflux oesophagitis. *Can Med Assoc J* 1957;76:811-821.
6. Merendino KA, Thomas GI. The jejunal interposition operation for substitution of the esophagogastric sphincter. *Surgery* 1958;44:1112-1115.
7. Hayward J. The treatment of fibrous stricture of the oesophagus associated with hiatal hernia. *Thorax* 1961;16:45-55.

8. Macmanus JE, Dameron JT, Paine JR. The extent to which one may interfere with the blood supply of the esophagus and obtain healing on anastomosis. *Surgery* 1950;28:11-23.
9. Shek JL, Prietto CA, Tuttle WM, et al. An experimental study of the blood supply of the esophagus and its relation to esophageal resection and anastomoses. *J Thorac Surg* 1950;19:523-533.
10. Swenson O, Merrill K Jr, Peirce EC II, et al. Blood and nerve supply to the esophagus. *J Thorac Surg* 1950;19:462-476.
11. Holman CW, McSwain B. Transthoracic esophagogastrostomy. *Surgery* 1942;11:882-885.
12. Thompson SA, Pollock B. The use of free omental grafts in the thorax. *Am J Surg* 1945;70:227-231.
13. Nissen R. Bridging of esophageal defect by pedicled flap of lung tissue. *Ann Surg* 1949;129:142-147.
14. Deaton WR Jr, Bradshaw HH. Lung-pleura graft for esophagoesophageal anastomosis. *J Thorac Surg* 1950;20:166-168.
15. Kleinsasser LJ, Cramer I, Warshaw H. Anastomosis of the cervical esophagus: Experimental evaluation of peritoneal grafts. *Surgery* 1950;28:438-442.
16. Warshaw H, Kleinsasser LJ. Anastomosis of the thoracic esophagus: III. Experimental evaluation of peritoneal grafts, one-layer anastomosis. *Surg Forum* 1950;53-56.
17. Cramer I, Kleinsasser LJ. Anastomosis of the cervical esophagus: Experimental evaluation of peritoneal grafts. *Arch Surg* 1951;63:243-246.
18. McSwain B, Byrd B Jr, Langa AM, Haber A. The use of the parietal pleural graft in experimental esophageal anastomosis. *Surg Gynecol Obstet* 1955;100:205-206.
19. Adler RH. The use of pericardial grafts with a thrombin-fibrinogen coagulum in esophageal surgery. *Surgery* 1956;39:906-916.
20. Roth M. Use of a lobe of the lung to secure sutures of the esophagus. *J Thorac Cardiovasc Surg* 1961;41:342-347.
21. Hopper CL, Berk PD, Howes EL. Strength of esophageal anastomoses repaired with autogenous pericardial grafts. *Surg Gynecol Obstet* 1963;117:83-86.
22. Bryant LR. Experimental evaluation of intercostal pedicle grafts in esophageal repair. *J Thorac Cardiovasc Surg* 1965;50:626-633.
23. Rob CG, Bateman GH. Reconstruction of the trachea and cervical oesophagus. *Br J Surg* 1949;37:202-205.
24. Edgerton MT. One-stage reconstruction of the cervical esophagus or trachea. *Surgery* 1952;31:239-250.
25. Ross RR. Repair of tracheal and esophageal defect by use of a pedicle graft. *Surgery* 1956;39:654-662.
26. Moore TC, Goldstein J. Use of intact omentum for closure of full-thickness esophageal defects. *Surgery* 1959;45:899-904.
27. Petrovsky BV. The use of diaphragm grafts for plastic operations in thoracic surgery. *J Thorac Cardiovasc Surg* 1961;41:348-355.
28. Wendel W. Zur chururgie des Oesophagus. *Arch Klin Chir* 1910;93:311-329.
29. Sauerbruch F, O'Shaughnessy L. **Thoracic Surgery**. A Revised and Abridged Edition of Sauerbruch's Die Chirurgie der Brustorgane. London, Edward Arnold, 1937, p 322.

30. Skinner HH, Merendino KA. An experimental evaluation of an interposed jejunal segment between the esophagus and the stomach combined with upper gastrectomy in the prevention of esophagitis and jejunitis. *Ann Surg* 1955;141:201-207.
31. Holt CJ, Large AM. Surgical management of reflux esophagitis. *Ann Surg* 1961;153:555-562.
32. Tsukamoto M, Thal AP. Correction of experimental esophageal stricture with the use of the skin-lined fundic patch. *J Thorac Cardiovasc Surg* 1966;52:682-689.
33. Thal AP, Hatafuku T, Kurtzman R. A new method for reconstruction of the esophagogastric junction. *Surg Gynecol Obstet* 1965;120:1225-1231.
34. Thal AP. A unified approach to surgical problems of the esophagogastric junction. *Ann Surg* 1968;168:542-550.
35. Thal AP, Hatafuku T. Improved operation for esophageal rupture. *JAMA* 1964;188:826-828.
36. Thal AP, Hatafuku T, Kurtzman R. New operation for distal esophageal stricture. *Arch Surg* 1965;90:464-472.
37. Hugh TB, Lusby RJ, Coleman MJ. Antral patch esophagoplasty. *Am J Surg* 1979;137:221-225.
38. Schon GR, Nieves ASS, Marcucci JC. Gastric vascular pedicle patch esophagoplasty for stricture. *Ann Thorac Surg* 1989;48:356-358.
39. Dooling JA, Zick HR. Closure of an esophagopleural fistula using onlay intercostal pedicle graft. *Ann Thorac Surg* 1967;3:553-557.
40. Vidne B, Levy MJ. Use of pericardium for esophagoplasty in congenital esophageal stenosis. *Surgery* 1970;68:389-392.
41. Rao KVS, Mir M, Cogbill CL. Management of perforations of the thoracic esophagus. *Am J Surg* 1974;127:609-612.
42. Jara FM. Diaphragmatic pedicle flap for treatment of Boerhaave's syndrome. *J Thorac Cardiovasc Surg* 1979;78:931-933.
43. Jones EL, Booth DJ, Cameron JL, et al. Functional evaluation of esophageal reconstructions. *Ann Thorac Surg* 1971;12:331-346.
44. Maher JW, Hocking MP, Woodward ER. Long-term follow-up of the combined fundic patch fundoplication for treatment of longitudinal peptic strictures of the esophagus. *Ann Surg* 1981;194:64-69.
45. Richardson JD, Tobin GR. Closure of esophageal defects with muscle flaps. *Arch Surg* 1994;129:541-548.
46. Hugh TB, Lusby RJ, Coleman MJ. Gastric patch esophagoplasty: An experimental study. *Am J Surg* 1979;137:226-227.
47. Richardson JD, Larson GM, Polk HC Jr. Intrathoracic fundoplication for shortened esophagus. *Am J Surg* 1982;143:29-35.
48. Mansour KA, Burton HG, Miller JI Jr, et al. Complications of intrathoracic Nissen fundoplication. *Ann Thorac Surg* 1981;32:173-178.
49. Pennell TC. Supradiaphragmatic correction of esophageal reflux strictures. *Ann Surg* 1981;193:655-665.
50. Maher JW, Hocking MP, Woodward ER. Supradiaphragmatic fundoplication. *Am J Surg* 1984;147:181-186.
51. Collard JM, De Koninck XJ, Otte JB, et al. Intrathoracic Nissen fundoplication: Long-term clinical and pH-monitoring evaluation. *Ann Thorac Surg* 1991;51:34-38.

Chapter 5

Preliminary Considerations

Most patients who require esophageal reconstruction initially undergo an elective or semi-elective esophageal resection by the surgeon who is to perform the reconstruction. The most common indications for resection are carcinoma, trauma, and end-stage benign esophageal disease. Esophageal reconstruction for such patients usually is performed under the same anesthetic without undue additional operating time or morbidity. The functional results of a one-stage approach to resection and reconstruction are very good. Under some circumstances, however, delayed esophageal reconstruction is necessary. Examples of such situations include severe mediastinal soilage following delayed recognition of an esophageal perforation, hemodynamic compromise accompanying coagulative esophageal necrosis after caustic ingestion, and cardiovascular instability in the elderly patient undergoing esophagectomy for cancer. The staged approach to reconstruction often necessitates placement of additional drains, feeding tubes, and other appliances that may have an unanticipated and detrimental effect on subsequent attempts at reconstruction.

Regardless of whether the reconstruction is to be accomplished under the same anesthetic or in a staged fashion, contemplation of the necessity for esophageal replacement provides the surgeon with an invaluable opportunity to carefully plan procedures performed prior to reconstruction. This allows the surgeon to conduct the preliminary procedures in a manner that interferes as little as possible with the principles guiding subsequent reconstruction, while, at the same time, permits expeditious completion of the necessary initial operative steps, including resection. The considerations that affect eventual reconstruction include the choice of access incisions used for performing the resection, the length of esophagus that is removed, the amount of stomach that is resected, the placement of drainage tubes within organs and/or cavities, and the insertion of enteral feeding tubes. In addition, there is a host of other seemingly minor techni-

From Ferguson MK: *Reconstructive Surgery of the Esophagus* Armonk, NY: Futura Publishing Company, Inc., © 2002.

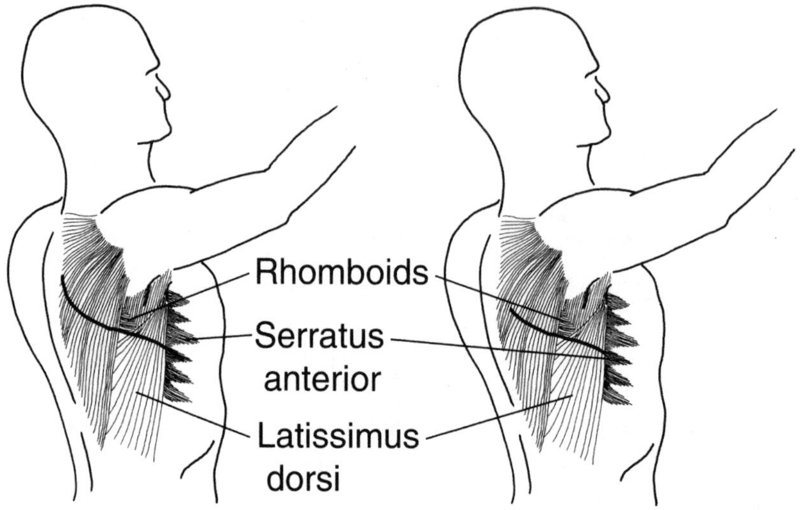

Figure 5-1. A standard lateral thoracotomy incision (right) provides exposure similar to that gained through a posterolateral thoracotomy (left) while preserving the serratus anterior and rhomboid muscles.

cal factors that can potentially have an unexpected and, in some situations, a profound impact on the success of subsequent reconstruction.

Incisions

Transthoracic operations on the esophagus are most commonly performed for resection of esophageal cancer, and typically require exposure of most of the intrathoracic esophagus. Many of these resections are performed through a standard lateral or posterolateral thoracotomy. This incision requires division of muscles of the chest wall and shoulder girdle that have potential use in reconstructive esophageal operations, including latissimus dorsi, serratus anterior, and, occasionally, rhomboid major and trapezius. Little exposure is gained by dividing the latter three muscles. A similar degree of operative exposure is provided by a standard lateral thoracotomy, which requires division of the latissimus dorsi muscle only (Figure 5-1). This incision preserves the other muscles, which are sometimes useful in the management of postoperative pleural space problems, chest wall defects, and anastomotic leaks or disruptions.[1-5] New approaches to esophagectomy under direct vision using thoracoscopic techniques also provide the advantage of sparing chest wall and shoulder girdle muscles.[6-9]

The thoracotomy incision is best performed through an intercostal space rather than through the bed of a resected rib, as sometimes is depicted in older surgical atlases. This technique has the advantage of being more likely to preserve the associated neurovascular bundle and sacrifices little of the intercostal muscle. The use of intercostal muscle flaps based on the intercostal neurovascular bundle has been described in the salvage of esophageal reconstructions complicated by leak, necrosis, or infection.[10,11] Preservation of this tissue reserves it for possible future use should complications develop in the early postoperative period.

Routine intra-abdominal exposure is best provided by an upper midline laparotomy, although there is increasing experience with the use of laparoscopic techniques for the abdominal portion of esophagectomy.[12,13] This incision, in contrast to paramedian, subcostal, or chevron incisions, does not necessitate division of either rectus abdominis muscle or the superior epigastric arteries on which they are based. Preservation of these muscles and their blood supply may be invaluable in subsequent reconstruction of low anterior chest wall or abdominal wall complications resulting from wound infection or dehiscence. Because these complications are fortunately rare, the decision to use a midline incision should be tempered by the pulmonary condition of the individual patient. Upper midline abdominal incisions cause greater impairment of ventilation than do subcostal incisions, and should be avoided in patients with severe respiratory insufficiency.

Cervical exposure of the esophagus is best achieved through a modified collar incision or through an incision made parallel to the anterior border of the sternocleidomastoid muscle. Once the platysma is divided, it is usually not necessary to divide either the sternocleidomastoid muscle or the strap muscles (with the possible exception of the omohyoid muscle) to gain adequate exposure of the cervical esophagus. The strap muscles are preserved to facilitate possible future esophageal reconstruction. The muscles most importantly preserved are the sternohyoid and sternothyroid. These long, thin muscle groups are particularly useful in wrapping anastomoses and for reinforcing primary closure of wounds of the esophagus. They are also often used as an interposition of well-vascularized tissue between the trachea and esophagus to avoid fistula formation, or between the carotid artery and esophagus to avoid potentially fatal bleeding problems.

Preservation of the Omentum

The omentum is not usually regarded with the amount of respect it is due, despite the fact that the omentum has been used for years as tissue for reconstruction in a wide variety of situations. Patching of perforated duodenal ulcers, reinforcement of intra-abdominal anastomoses, and buttressing of splenic repairs with omentum have been performed for decades.[14] More recently the omentum has been used to provide well-vascularized autologous tissue for intrathoracic problems.[15,16] The first successful lung transplants were accomplished, in part, through reinforcement of bronchial and tracheal suture lines with omentum.[17] The risks of complications after tracheotracheal anastomoses following tracheal resection, and bronchial stump closures in the face of radiation damage, infection, or relative ischemia have also been reduced by wrapping with omentum.[18,19] Local ischemic problems are aided by angiogenic factors produced by the omentum, which appear to stimulate vessel ingrowth and promote healing.[20,21] The omentum also provides bulk that facilitates the management of intrathoracic space problems such as those that exist after lung resection or that accompany empyema.[22]

Despite these facts, the omentum is often approached with disregard, and is sometimes removed, transected, or inadvertently injured during the course of intra-abdominal operations. In addition to this thoughtless handling of the omentum, it is sometimes intentionally removed as part of an en bloc esophagectomy for management of carcinomas of the esophagus or esophagogastric junction on the premise that doing so will make the lymphatic dissection more complete. However, there is no evidence that this extension of the cancer operation reduces the likelihood of local recurrence or contributes to long-term survival. Because the omentum is a valuable tissue that can serve a variety of functions in the surgical patient, its preservation should be considered during any intra-abdominal operation.

Omental flaps for reconstructive purposes are based on the main blood supply to the omentum, the right gastroepiploic artery. Unfortunately, this vessel also serves as the main blood supply to the stomach when this organ is mobilized as an esophageal replacement. Therefore, it is not possible to create both a large independent omental flap and a standard gastric tube for esophageal reconstruction. It is possible, however, to retain a moderate-sized omental flap on the stomach during its preparation as a replacement organ (Figure 5-2). This provides soft tissue with which to wrap the anastomosis between the esophagus and stomach, helping to ensure its healing without a leak.[23-25] Unnecessary sacrifice of any of the omentum, therefore, should be avoided.

Extent of Gastric Resection

Resection of part of the stomach is an integral portion of most esophagectomy operations. A small amount of gastric cardia is removed during operations for benign disease, even when the whole stomach is to be used for reconstruction, to eliminate the possibility of any retained squamous epithelium in the stump, which would predispose the patient to ulceration

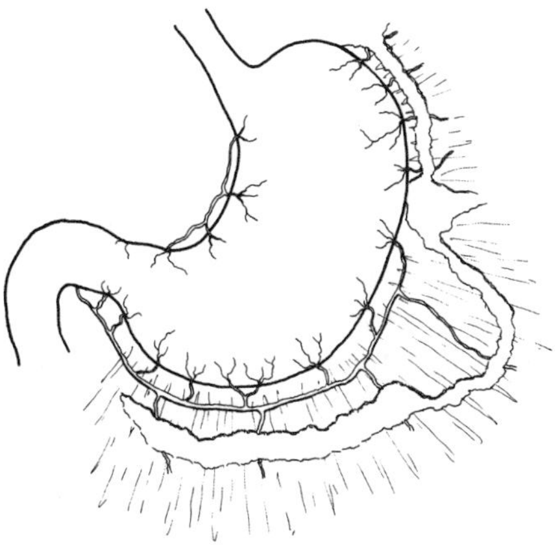

Figure 5-2. Preservation of a small flap of omentum on the greater curvature of the stomach, vascularized by the right gastroepiploic artery. This can be used to reinforce a subsequent esophagogastric anastomosis.

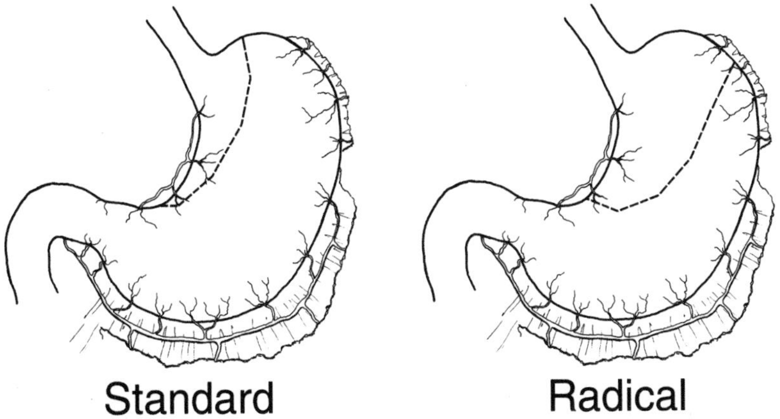

Figure 5-3. The extent of gastric resection necessary when treating benign esophageal disease, while performing a standard esophagectomy (5-cm margin from gross tumor), and during radical en bloc esophagectomy (10-cm margin from gross tumor).

at that site. In fact, many surgeons advocate the creation of a gastric tube for use in reconstruction, which is formed by resecting the cardia and lesser curve, eliminating concerns regarding retained gastric mucosa. More extensive resections are performed routinely for cancers of the distal esophagus and cardia. For standard esophagectomy operations, a 5-cm margin of normal tissue distal to the gross extent of tumor is recommended, along with resection of the lesser curve, the left gastric artery, and all associated lymph nodes (Figure 5-3).[26]

Any of these standard resections permit the stomach to be used as a replacement organ for the entire esophagus. The maximum length of the stomach after it is prepared for pull-up is determined by the length from the pylorus to the gastric fundus (the position of the cardia being relatively unimportant in determining this length) and by the degree of mobilization of the first three portions of the duodenum that can be achieved. Therefore, during any of these standard operations on the esophagus and esophagogastric junction, it is important that nothing be done to disturb the gastric fundus or its remaining blood supply.

For radical en bloc esophagectomy, the extent of gastric resection that is recommended is quite different. The margin of normal tissue which serves as the distal margin of resection is 10 cm, which often requires removal of a more substantial amount of stomach than does standard esophagectomy, often including the gastric fundus.[27,28] Some surgeons advocate performance of a total gastrectomy for tumors that arise in the cardia and for so-called gastroesophageal junctional cancers.[29,30] If these techniques are used, use of the stomach for reconstruction is precluded, necessitating the construction of a colonic or jejunal interposition.

Extent of Esophageal Resection

The extent of esophageal resection is usually dictated by the underlying esophageal disease, by routes available for reconstruction, and by the personal preferences of the surgeon. The latter among these should be the least important consideration, because surgeons should be capable of utilizing a variety of techniques to maximize the functional outcome after esophagectomy. The length of the native esophagus remaining after resection is a major determinant of long-term successful function. For patients with benign diseases such as peptic stricture or distal esophageal perforation, in whom the function of the majority of the esophageal body is likely to be relatively normal, every attempt is made to preserve the esophagus. When esophageal reconstruction is to be accomplished under the same anesthetic as that used for esophagectomy, this enables the performance of an intrathoracic anastomosis using a stomach pull-up or bowel interposition. Even when the esophagus is badly damaged due to perforation and liquifactive necrosis accompanying contamination of the mediastinum, it is not necessary to dispose of the entire intrathoracic esophagus even if a staged, extramediastinal reconstruction is planned. Instead, the intrathoracic portion of the esophagus is mobilized into the neck and then is tunneled subcutaneously onto the chest wall, preserving most of the length of the esophagus for use in future reconstruction.[31]

Placement of Enteral Feeding Tubes

The placement of enteral feeding tubes at the time of esophageal operations greatly facilitates the provision of enteral nutrition during the early postoperative period, even in patients who experience a satisfactory postoperative course and return to a regular diet without complication.[32] More importantly, such routes of caloric administration are invaluable in the management of patients who experience perioperative complications, such as respiratory insufficiency and anastomotic leak, that prevent adequate oral intake of calories. Enteral feeding under these circumstances obviates the need for intravenous alimentation, provides more complete nutrition, and helps to prevent septic complications related to transmural migration of bacteria.

Enteral feeding tubes should be inserted in a manner that does not interfere with esophageal reconstruction. The advantages of gastrostomy tubes are ease of insertion, ease of replacement once the tract has become well formed, and the ability to give bolus feedings. Unfortunately, there are several theoretical disadvantages to placing a gastrostomy tube for enteral feedings. Performance of a double pursestring around the gastrostomy site narrows the body of the stomach somewhat. Using a Witzel technique[33] further narrows the body of the stomach, making subsequent reconstruction using the stomach considerably more difficult. Because the stomach, when used for esophageal reconstruction, relies on intramural collaterals for its blood supply from the right gastroepiploic artery, interruption of even a small part of this collateral supply can endanger the viability of the proximal stomach and may threaten the integrity of the anastomosis.

Jejunal feeding tubes have the disadvantages of being technically more difficult to place, often require fluoroscopy to assure appropriate positioning when replacement is necessary, and require pumps to provide a continuous flow of feedings. Their advantages are that they are well tolerated, the tubes can be placed at any site in the proximal jejunum without concern over the patient's ability to tolerate feedings, and reconstruction is generally not interfered with using this approach. The last point is particularly important, because a feeding tube insertion site can be selected that is distal to the region from which a jejunal autograft is to be taken, placing the site distal also to the ultimate jejunojejunostomy that is used to reestablish alimentary tract continuity.

Gastric Drainage

It is often necessary to decompress the stomach after the initial portion of a staged operation on the esophagus, such as after an urgent

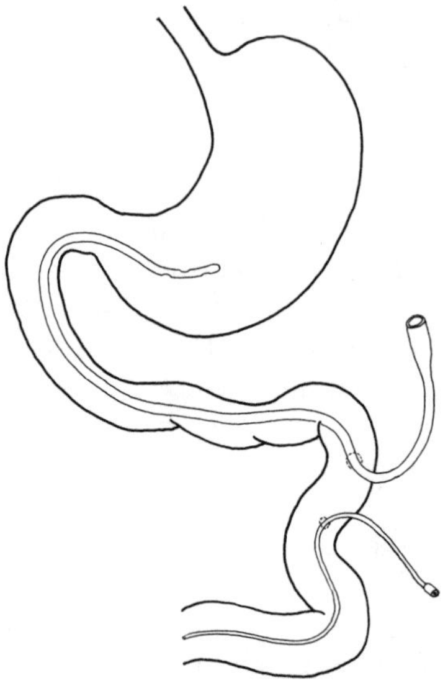

Figure 5-4. Drainage of the stomach retrograde using a jejunal insertion site avoids the use of a gastrostomy tube, which can interfere with the use of the stomach for esophageal reconstruction.

esophagectomy for esophageal perforation. Gastric decompression reduces the likelihood that the closure of the stomach at the cardia will break down in the presence of contamination from the perforation. The same caveats described earlier with reference to gastrostomy feeding tubes also apply to gastric drainage tubes. Therefore, it is sometimes wise to forego placement of a gastrostomy drainage tube and, instead, use retrograde drainage through a jejunostomy (Figure 5-4). This provides adequate gastric decompression without interfering with the size or vascularity of the stomach, and does not compromise eventual use of the jejunum for reconstruction if such is necessary. If use of the latter technique is not feasible and a gastrostomy is necessary, it should be performed as a Stamm gastrostomy through a double purse-string only, which is then sutured to the peritoneum.[34]

References

1. Miller JI, Mansour KA, Nahai F, et al. Single-stage complete muscle flap closure of the post-pneumonectomy empyema space: A new method and possible solution to a disturbing complication. *Ann Thorac Surg* 1984;38:227-231.
2. Arnold PG, Pairolero PC. Intrathoracic muscle flaps: An account of their use in the management of 100 consecutive patients. *Ann Surg* 1990;211:656-660.
3. Ali I, Unruh H. Management of empyema thoracis. *Ann Thorac Surg* 1990;50:355-359.
4. Tobin GR, Mavroudis C, Howe WR, et al. Reconstruction of complex thoracic defects with myocutaneous and muscle flaps. *J Thorac Cardiovasc Surg* 1983;85:219-228.

5. Arnold PG, Pairolero PC. Chest wall reconstruction. Experience with 100 consecutive patients. *Ann Surg* 1984;199:725-732.
6. Akaishi T, Kaneda I, Higuchi N, et al. Thoracosopic en bloc total esophagectomy with radical mediastinal lymphadenectomy. *J Thorac Cardiovasc Surg* 1996;112:1533-1541.
7. Law S, Fok M, Chu KM, Wong J. Thoracoscopic esophagectomy for esophageal cancer. *Surgery* 1997;122:8-14.
8. Peracchia A, Rosati R, Fumagalli U, Bona S, Chella B. Thoracoscopic dissection of the esophagus for cancer. *Int Surg* 1997;82:1-4.
9. Watson DI, Jamieson GG, Devitt PG. Endoscopic cervico-thoraco-abdominal esophagectomy. *J Am Coll Surg* 2000;190:372-378.
10. Bryant LR. Experimental evaluation of intercostal pedicle grafts in esophageal repair. *J Thorac Cardiovasc Surg* 1965;50:626-633.
11. Richardson JD, Martin LF, Borzotta AP, et al. Unifying concepts in the treatment of esophageal leaks. *Am J Surg* 1985;149:157-162.
12. Luketich JD, Nguyen NT, Weigel T, et al. Minimally invasive approach to esophagectomy. *JSLS* 1998;2:243-247.
13. Watson DI, Davies N, Jamieson GG. Totally endoscopic Ivor Lewis esophagectomy. *Surg Endosc* 1999;13:293-297.
14. Marschall MA, Cohen M. The use of greater omentum in reconstructive surgery. *Surg Ann* 1994;26:251-268.
15. Mathisen DJ, Grillo HC, Vlahakes GJ, et al. The omentum in the management of complicated cardiothoracic problems. *J Thorac Cardiovasc Surg* 1988;95:677-684.
16. Liebermann-Meffert DMI, Siewert JR. The role of the greater omentum in intrathoracic transposition. *Neth J Surg* 1991;43:154-160.
17. Cooper JD. The evolution of techniques and indications for lung transplantation. *Ann Surg* 1990;212:249-256.
18. Balderman SC, Weinblatt G. Tracheal autograft revascularization. *J Thorac Cardiovasc Surg* 1987;94:434-441.
19. Nakanishi R, Shirakusa T, Takachi T. Omentopexy for tracheal autografts. *Ann Thorac Surg* 1994;57:841-845.
20. Goldsmith HS, Griffith AL, Kupferman A, et al. Lipid angiogenic factor from omentum. *JAMA* 1984;252:2034-2036.
21. Beelen RHJ. The greater omentum: Physiology amd immunological concepts. *Neth J Surg* 1991;43:145-149.
22. Shirakusa T, Ueda H, Takata S, et al. Use of omental flap in treatment of empyema. *Ann Thorac Surg* 1990;50:420-424.
23. Goldsmith HS, Kiely AA, Randall HT. Protection of intrathoracic esophageal anatomoses by omentum. *Surgery* 1968;63:464-466.
24. Fekete F, Breil P, Ronsse H, et al. EEA stapler and omental graft in esophagogastrectomy. *Ann Surg* 1981;191:825-830.
25. Kai Z, Yihua Y. Use of pedicled omentum in oesophagogastric anastomosis: Analysis of 100 cases. *Ann R Coll Surg Engl* 1987;69:209-211.
26. Akiyama H, Tsurumaru M, Kawamura T, et al. Principles of surgical treatment for carcinoma of the esophagus. *Ann Surg* 1981;194:438-446.
27. Skinner DB. En bloc resection for neoplasms of the esophagus and cardia. *J Thorac Cardiovasc Surg* 1983;85:59-71.

28. Skinner DB, Little AG, Ferguson MK, et al. Selection of operation for esophageal cancer based on staging. *Ann Surg* 1986;204:391-401.
29. Holscher AH, Schuler M, Siewert JR. Surgical treatment of adenocarcinomas of the gastroesophageal junction. *Dis Esoph* 1988;1:35-49.
30. DeMeester TR, Zaninotto G, Johansson K-E. Selective therapeutic approach to cancer of the lower esophagus and cardia. *J Thorac Cardiovasc Surg* 1988;95:42-54.
31. Orringer MB, Stirling MC. Esophagectomy for esophageal disruption. *Ann Thorac Surg* 1990;49:35-43.
32. Gerndt SJ, Orringer MB. Tube jejunostomy as an adjunct to esophagectomy. *Surgery* 1994;115:164-169.
33. Witzel. *Zentrabl Chir* 1891;18:601.
34. Stamm. *Med News* 1894;65:324.

Chapter 6

Planning Esophageal Replacement

The short- and long-term implications of the timing and techniques used in reconstruction of the esophagus are more important for patients than are the timing and techniques of esophageal resection. Although this claim initially may appear to be overstated, a brief analysis of the relevant facts demonstrates that it is true. Examination of the most common indication for esophagectomy, carcinoma of the esophagus and cardia, demonstrates that long-term survival is independent of the technique of resection. Despite the fact that several types of potentially curative resections are performed frequently, there are currently no data from randomized, prospective trials that demonstrate the superiority of the transhiatal, exclusive left transthoracic, or combined thoracic and abdominal approaches with regard to operative morbidity, surgical mortality, or survival. Similarly, the superiority of a radical en bloc esophagectomy versus a standard esophagectomy has not been established for the treatment of esophageal carcinoma. The extent of nodal dissection, including such examples as routine lymphadenectomy, two-field extended nodal dissection, and three-field extended dissection, has not been shown conclusively to be a determinant of long-term survival from esophageal cancer. The timing of resection has not had a substantial influence on long-term outcome either. Whether the resection is performed before or after radiation therapy, chemotherapy, or combined chemoradiotherapy, has not affected survival or disease-free survival in most reports.

In contrast to this, the timing and techniques of esophageal reconstruction determine to a great extent both short-term morbidity and long-term outcomes for these patients, as will be seen in Chapter 7. As a result, planning of esophageal replacement is of utmost importance. The issues of primary importance are whether reconstruction should be performed initially or be delayed, the appropriate timing of intervention should

From Ferguson MK: *Reconstructive Surgery of the Esophagus* Armonk, NY: Futura Publishing Company, Inc., © 2002.

delayed replacement be selected, interval management of the patient prior to staged reconstruction, and preparation of the patient prior to reconstruction.

Concurrent versus Staged Replacement

Concurrent replacement of the esophagus refers to its replacement under the same anesthetic as for the operation in which the esophagus is removed. Typically this occurs during esophagectomy and reconstruction for carcinoma, and is also performed for treatment of benign problems such as complicated gastroesophageal reflux or an end-stage esophageal motility disorder such as achalasia (Table 6-1). Under these circumstances the surgeon and patient recognize preoperatively that an esophagectomy is planned. Accordingly, appropriate preparations are made prior to the operation so that reconstruction can be performed with maximum safety and reliability. Concurrent replacement may also be appropriate even though preoperative preparation has not been possible. Examples are esophageal perforation during dilation for end-stage peptic esophagitis, or barogenic esophageal rupture (diagnosed early) that results in an irreparable esophagus. If there is minimal soilage of the mediastinum, if the stomach is available for use as a reconstructive organ, and if the patient's physiologic condition permits, esophageal replacement may be performed under the same anesthetic as for the esophagectomy without undue risk to the patient.

There are many advantages to performing a concurrent reconstruction compared to a staged resection and reconstruction. When only a single hospitalization is necessary, overall hospital length of stay is decreased. Similarly, because no recuperative period is necessary between operations, as would be the case if a staged reconstruction were performed, the period of functional disability is shortened, permitting earlier return to baseline performance status and normal activities. In the case of operations performed for cancer, there is no substantial "down time" during which adjuvant postoperative therapy must be avoided, allowing earlier initiation of postoperative chemotherapy or radiotherapy when indicated. The psychological benefits to the patient of this approach are obvious. Moreover, there are important economic reasons to perform reconstruction expeditiously when medically warranted.

In contrast, staged reconstruction of the esophagus is often necessary to minimize operative morbidity and mortality, even though it may lengthen a patient's overall duration of hospitalization and increase the interval to full recovery. A typical example is the patient in whom the recognition of an esophageal perforation is delayed and whose esophagus is so damaged that its preservation is impossible. When the diagnosis of

Table 6-1.
Indications and Contraindications for Esophageal Resection Followed by Immediate Replacement.

Indications	
	Planned esophagectomy for carcinoma, peptic esophagitis, or end-stage motility disorder
	Perforation with minimal soilage when esophagectomy is necessary, posterior mediastinum used for reconstruction
	Perforation with moderate soilage when esophagectomy is necessary, nonanatomic route used for reconstruction
Contraindications	
	Perforation or necrosis with severe mediastinitis
	Cardiovascular instability during esophagectomy
	Prolonged operation with substantial intercompartmental fluid shifts
	Failed initial attempt at reconstruction, remaining organs not prepared
	Bleeding diathesis, including emergency operation for bleeding varices
	Aspiration pneumonia or other acute pulmonary dysfunction

esophageal perforation is delayed sufficiently, severe mediastinitis usually precludes esophageal reconstruction at the time of initial operation. If reconstruction were to be attempted, the additional time and dissection necessary to prepare the reconstructive organ would expose the patient to increased risk of ongoing infectious problems and additional cardiopulmonary morbidity. In addition, the inflammation in the mediastinum would increase the risk of suture line breakdown and anastomotic leakage or disruption.

Other situations in which delayed reconstruction may be appropriate include the patient who develops cardiovascular instability during esophagectomy; pulmonary compromise from aspiration accompanying high-grade esophageal obstruction; inability to perform gastric reconstruction in the face of an unprepared alternative reconstructive organ such as the colon; and a prolonged operation leading to compartmental fluid shifts that result in severe edema of the reconstructive organ. Evidence for inadequate blood flow to the organ to be used for reconstruction should prompt the surgeon to stage the repair, which will often lead to an improvement in blood flow.[1] In addition, staging the reconstruction may limit overall operative morbidity by decreasing pulmonary complications and by reducing the incidence of anastomotic leak.[2-3] However, an interval delay of several weeks is usually necessary to achieve these benefits, as delaying the performance of an anastomosis for 2 or 3 days appears to have no particular advantage.[4] In balance, delayed reconstruction will result in an increase in the overall duration of hospitalization, cost of medical care, and time until return to full activity. However, when viewed in the context of the potential risk to a patient's life, and the likely increase in operative morbidity and duration of hospitalization that would result if primary reconstruction was attempted, delayed replacement sometimes has a clear advantage over concurrent reconstruction.

Timing of Delayed Esophageal Replacement

The appropriate interval to wait before performing a staged esophageal reconstruction is quite variable. A number of factors enter into the analysis, and the surgeon's judgment is most important in the decision regarding the final timing of the operation (Table 6-2). Considerations include the presence of ongoing infection or inflammation; the time interval between the initial operation and the planned reconstructive operation and how this would affect the extent and vascularity of adhesions; the status of the reconstructive organ; the patient's nutritional, cardiovascular, and overall performance status; and the patient's mental preparedness for the rigors of an additional major operation.

Local Inflammation and Infection

No reconstructive procedure should be undertaken until all ongoing inflammation has subsided and there is no active infection. Infection in patients requiring staged esophageal reconstruction is most commonly due to esophageal perforation with concomitant mediastinitis and empyema. The next most common cause for infection in these patients is failed primary reconstruction, which may be due to ischemia, necrosis of the reconstructive organ, or anastomotic breakdown. Components of the initial intervention for the acute process consist of early operative intervention (including drainage) and broad spectrum antibiotic coverage. Reconstruction is not scheduled until the chest radiograph shows no evidence for effusion, pulmonary infiltrate, or mediastinitis. A computed tomogram of the chest and upper abdomen is often useful in assessing whether there is significant pleural thickening, residual pleural fluid, pericardial effusion, or mediastinitis, some of which may be difficult to detect on a plain chest radiograph. The patient's white blood cell count is monitored periodically until it is normal and the differential shows no left shift. There is little evidence that monitoring acute phase reactants, such as sedimentation rate, C-reactive protein, and complement, is of value in determining the appropriate timing of an operation.[5,6] All wounds should be clean and granulating, without signs of ongoing infection or inflammation. Ideally, all wounds should be completely epithelialized prior to reoperation to avoid cross contamination of wounds and to limit metabolic demands for wound healing.

Table 6-2.
Factors that Affect the Timing of Staged Esophageal Reconstruction.

Ongoing inflammation
Concurrent infection
Status of postoperative adhesions
Performance status
Psychological status
Function of reconstructive organ
Nutritional status
Immune status
Cardiopulmonary status

Adhesions

The greatest concern about adhesions with respect to staged reconstructive surgery of the esophagus is avoidance, when feasible, of the fibroproliferative and vascular phases of adhesion development. When synchronous reconstruction is not performed or fails, pleural and intra-abdominal adhesions begin to form as a result of trauma to mesothelial surfaces. The initial inflammatory phase is characterized by an influx of inflammatory cells into the area of injury, with migration of polymorphonuclear leukocytes and monocytes in response to the release of local and circulating cytokines. Histamine release causes increased vascular permeability and leads to fibrin deposition. The monocytes transform into macrophages that ingest debris, release additional humoral factors, and stimulate local fibroblasts. The second, or proliferative, phase is established 4 or 5 days postoperatively and is characterized by fibroblast proliferation and neovascularization through cellular migration into the fibrin. Synthesis of extracellular matrix, including collagen and proteoglycans, begins. The final phase of healing begins at a variable period of weeks after the proliferative phase and is termed the maturation phase. It is characterized by a decrease in the number of fibroblasts and macrophages, and by an increase in wound strength accomplished by an increase in both wound collagen content and cross-linking. The duration of the maturation phase is poorly defined, and may be months or, in some patients, years.

The inflammatory and early proliferative phases of adhesion formation in most patients subside with absorption of the fibrinous bridges within 8 to 12 days of injury, and minimal fibrous adhesion formation occurs under these circumstances. However, if relative ischemia, foreign body deposition, or an excess supply of fibrin (as occurs when there is blood in the pleural space or peritoneal cavity) is present, the balance of these processes will favor the maturation of fibrinous adhesions into fibrous adhesions. The most acute proliferative and neovascularization effects in such cases occur during the second through fourth weeks of the healing process, making this an inopportune time to perform an elective reoperation. Attempts to reduce adhesion formation have taken many forms, including reducing the inflammatory reaction, inhibiting coagulation, promoting fibrinolysis, and maintaining a physical separation between mesothelial surfaces,[7,8] and have not proven successful. Among the simplest measures to minimize adhesion formation are to minimize tissue desiccation, mechanical trauma, and bleeding.

Function of the Reconstructive Organ

It is important to assess the function of the organ to be used for esophageal replacement prior to planning reconstructive surgery. The three organs used most commonly for reconstruction are the stomach, jejunum, and colon. The functional integrity of the stomach may be compromised by gastritis, relative ischemia, or gastroparesis related to diabetes or other causes of neural dysfunction. The functional status of small bowel and colon to be used as an interposition organ similarly may be adversely affected by ileus, inflammation, fibrosis, and other causes of altered motility. In older patients, especially those with a history of peripheral vascular occlusive disease, vascular insufficiency also may be a factor determining the functional integrity of a reconstructive organ.

Nutritional Status

Many patients who have a serious esophageal disorder experience weight loss and have nutritional deficiencies. The etiology of these problems is often complex. Mechanical or functional obstruction of the esophagus occurs in many esophageal disorders, including carcinoma, peptic stricture, and achalasia. This causes patients to modify their food intake, limiting protein and calorie ingestion in favor of fluids. Such changes in dietary habits result in depletion of energy stores and anabolic components necessary for proper wound healing. The cachexia of cancer also contributes to malnutrition through catabolic effects that are clearly paraneoplastic but otherwise remain poorly characterized. Accurate assessment of the adequacy of a patient's nutritional status is not always possible, but should consist at a minimum of measurement of serum albumin content (see below).

Immunologic Status

In patients who have recently undergone major surgery or who have suffered from chronic illness, cellular and humoral immunity are often depressed. Demonstrable abnormalities include a decrease in T-lymphocyte activation, natural killer cell function, immunoglobulin titers, interleukin-2 (IL-2) and interleukin-6 (IL-6) synthesis, and tumor-necrosis factor alpha (TNF-α), among others.[9-11] In addition, there is evidence that neutrophil bacteriocidal activity is reduced in patients with esophageal cancer, with decreased intracellular killing capacity and myeloperoxidase activity, suggesting that these patients are at increased risk for developing a surgical infection.[12] There is no evidence at present that acute measures such as administration of hyperalimentation or supplementation with exogenous factors can reverse these abnormalities.

Cardiopulmonary Status

Pulmonary status is often suboptimal in patients with severe esophageal disorders. Individuals who are to undergo esophagectomy and primary reconstruction may have pulmonary dysfunction from chronic subclinical aspiration, which is surprisingly common among patients with benign disease such as end-stage gastroesophageal reflux disorders and achalasia. It also occurs frequently in patients with esophageal obstruction secondary to cancer. Clinical and radiographic findings suggestive of acute aspiration include evidence for an infiltrate accompanied by cough and fever, whereas a history of chronic aspiration is sometimes suggested by the presence of bibasilar pulmonary fibrosis. Patients who have undergone an esophagectomy and await reconstruction often suffer from pulmonary dysfunction. Major incisions currently required for esophagectomy, such as a laparotomy or a thoracotomy, result in substantial pain, and a thoracotomy will also diminish chest wall compliance. Patients recovering from infectious problems associated with esophageal perforation or necrosis of a reconstructive organ may also have severe pleural reactions resulting in increased discomfort and fibrosis that further limit chest wall compliance. These factors lead to decreased forced vital capacity and maximum expiratory flow, and reduce a patient's ability to clear secretions.

It is possible to predict preoperatively the risk of pulmonary complications in patients who are to undergo esophagectomy and reconstruction.[13] The factors that have been demonstrated on multivariate analysis to influence the likelihood of postoperative pulmonary dysfunction include spirometry, blood arterial oxygen and carbon dioxide levels, the diffusing capacity for carbon monoxide, patient age, and tumor stage in patients undergoing esophagectomy for cancer.[14-19] Although it is unlikely that substantial improvement in any of these factors is possible preoperatively, a modicum of improvement may be gained by getting patients to stop smoking and to make sure that use of bronchodilators is instituted when appropriate. Knowledge of the impact of these factors on outcomes following esophagectomy and reconstruction will help the surgeon plan an operation intelligently and discuss specific risks with the patient.

Although cardiac dysfunction is not as common preoperatively in patients as is pulmonary dysfunction, it is nevertheless a serious problem that can have profound effects on the outcome of esophageal reconstruction. A careful history and physical examination and electrocardiogram are important in evaluating patients for cardiac dysfunction. If potential abnormalities are detected, a more thorough evaluation is warranted, such as echocardiography, a radionuclide stress test, or coronary angiography. In patients who have not had initial resection, the most likely factors that lead to cardiac dysfunction are coronary artery disease and acquired valvular heart disease. The risk of cardiac complications may be predicted by the presence of premature ventricular contractions on a preoperative electrocardiogram, patient age, and performance status. Prophylactic digitalization has not been shown to control dysrhythmias postoperatively.[20]

In patients who have had an esophagectomy and await reconstruction, dysfunction may also be due to pericardial disease, such as pericarditis or pericardial effusion, that is secondary to surgical trauma or infection. Attempting esophageal reconstruction without proper evaluation and treatment of such potential problems places patients at unnecessary risk.

Performance Status

The performance status of the patient who is a candidate for esophageal reconstruction should be optimized whenever possible. Performance status relates to a patient's ability to carry out activities of daily living and can be assessed formally using one of a number of tools such as the Karnofsky or Zubrod scales.[21-23] Although a formal assessment of performance status may be valuable in prospectively studying outcomes after esophageal resection and reconstruction, an informal evaluation may prove equally useful for clinical purposes. Patients ideally should be capable of performing most activities of daily living in a vigorous manner. The inability to do so suggests that further time and effort may be wisely expended in optimizing the patient's condition. Obviously, such guidelines apply primarily to patients with end-stage benign disease and to patients who have undergone esophagectomy and await elective reconstruction. Patients who require esophagectomy and immediate reconstruction for carcinoma, those who have high-grade esophageal obstruction putting them at risk for aspiration, and patients with severe esophageal dysfunction who are unable to maintain adequate nutrition, usually cannot afford the additional time necessary for improving their performance status prior to operation.

Psychological Status

Patients who are to have esophageal reconstruction, whether staged or concurrent with esophagectomy, need to be properly prepared from a psychological standpoint. They ideally must enter the operation with a positive view of the outcome and with an understanding of what will be required of them to help avoid postoperative complications. This mental preparation is important in enabling the patient to enthusiastically perform suggested exercises postoperatively and to resume increasing levels of activity as his or her overall postoperative condition improves. Most experienced surgeons agree that the intangible quality of a patient's cooperativeness, sensed prior to and immediately after an operation, is an important determinant of operative outcome but is difficult to define. Candid, detailed discussions of expectations on the part of the physicians, nurses, and patients alike will foster a degree of confidence and often will enable the patient to proceed through the rigors of an often difficult postoperative course with enthusiasm.

Interval Management Prior to Staged Esophageal Reconstruction

In patients in whom staged esophageal reconstruction is planned, the interval between recovery from the esophagectomy and the reconstructive operation is a valuable time to encourage rehabilitation and pursue subtle counseling in preparation for the operation ahead. Nutritional support is a necessity. This is ideally provided through enteral means, often by a jejunostomy tube placed at the time of esophagectomy. The advantages of enteral nutrition compared to parental nutrition are numerous. Enteral feedings help to maintain intestinal tissue weight and villous height and can reverse atrophy that develops as a result of reliance on parenteral nutrition. Enteral nutrition also helps to maintain the normal ability of the gut to prevent bacterial translocation, which is frequently a common denominator in septic states after major surgery and critical illnesses.[24,25] There is information that supplementation with arginine and polyunsaturated fatty acids may help to restore suppressed immune responses.[26] If enteral nutrition is not possible, then a parenteral route must be used. The goal of nutritional support is to establish positive nitrogen balance and, under optimal circumstances, produce weight gain through an increase in skeletal muscle mass. Simple tools to assess the effectiveness of these efforts include measurement of weight, weight loss, albumin, and either triceps skin fold thickness or mid-arm circumference.[27] The ability of a patient to heal wounds from a recent operation is also indicative of adequate nitrogen balance and nutritional sufficiency.

The patient's overall performance status may be improved through a supervised exercise rehabilitation program designed to increase lower extremity muscle strength and exercise capacity. This will have the added effect of improving cardiopulmonary function, quality of life, and self-reliance. Lower extremity exercise is best accomplished in an unsupervised setting by encouraging patients to do graded walking exercise, beginning at a slow pace (2-3 mile/hour) for a distance of 500-1000 yards, and increasing the distance and speed until a 2-mile walk can be accomplished in 20-30 minutes. Patients with underlying coronary artery disease, chronic obstructive pulmonary disease, or other cardiopulmonary disorder that may limit their exercise ability should undergo supervised cardiopulmonary rehabilitation in which graded exercise is performed with concomitant monitoring of blood pressure, heart rate, and oxygen saturation.

The return of a patient to activities of daily living is a strong indication that substantial psychological and physiological recovery has occurred and the patient is prepared to undergo additional major surgery. However, this recovery may take time, and often it is not possible to wait the necessary length of time for this transition to occur. Issues such as the patient's eagerness to proceed with reconstruction, difficulties attending the provision of adequate nutrition, and the ever-increasing need to consider financial implications of nutritional and cardiopulmonary exercise rehabilitation that are imposed on care givers by the health care industry must all be taken into account.

Preparation Prior to Operation

Once it is decided that the patient is in proper condition to undergo synchronous or staged reconstructive surgery, several elements of preoperative preparation are necessary. A good rule of thumb is "prepare the bowel, prepare the patient, and prepare the surgeon."

Bowel Preparation

Prior to scheduling an operation in which replacement of the esophagus is contemplated, it is useful to be certain the organ proposed for use in the reconstruction is in good functional and anatomic condition. Most patients undergo replacement with the stomach, and it is a simple matter to inquire whether there has been a history of peptic ulcer disease, upper gastrointestinal bleeding, slow gastric emptying, or other medical problems that might influence a decision to use this organ. Anatomic assessment is achieved through physical examination, barium contrast swallow and upper gastrointestinal series, and endoscopy. The ability of the surgeon to perform endoscopy to assess the stomach prior to its use in esophageal reconstruction is invaluable, as this gives a very clear impression as to the integrity of the organ and the anatomy of the pylorus.

If there is a chance that the colon will be required to achieve reconstruction, it usually should be evaluated preoperatively to rule out the existence of diverticular disease or a coexisting carcinoma. This can be accomplished with either a barium enema or colonoscopy. The latter is more expensive and often cannot be completed to the level of the cecum, but its results are more reliable than those of a radiographic study. A history and physical examination eliminates the possibility of a prior colon resection, but if one has been performed, it is always wise to obtain a copy of the operative report to discern exactly how much of the colon was removed and how reconstitution of the alimentary tract was accomplished.

There is controversy over whether angiography should be used to assess the vascular supply of the colon if its use as an esophageal replacement is contemplated. The finding of normal anatomy is reassuring and may save time during the operation in dissecting out and verifying the anatomy, but the presence of an intact marginal artery on angiography must still be accompanied by a careful intraoperative evaluation of pulses and flow in the vessels that are supplying the graft. There are small but finite risks in doing angiography, including pseudoaneurysm formation at the site of the arterial puncture, bleeding, renal complications of the contrast agent, and injury to the vessels being studied including the development of an intimal flap, which could compromise the planned operation. Angiography is best used selectively, with the candidates being those in whom a colon interposition is likely and in whom additional risk factors exist, such as advanced age, prior aortic surgery, evidence for hypertension or peripheral vascular disease, or prior partial colectomy.

Bowel preparation is necessary in most patients, even if use of the small bowel or colon is not likely. Cleansing the bowels with a mechanical preparation reduces the content of chyme and fecal matter, permitting easy retraction during a reconstructive operation employing the stomach. A traditional mechanical bowel preparation consists of feeding the patient with a low residue or clear liquid diet for several days prior to operation. Patients who are on jejunostomy tube feedings are placed on a low-residue elemental formula. Oral cathartics and saline enemas are given for 1-2 days preoperatively until the return is clear.

Mechanical cleansing can also be performed with a polyethylene glycol-electrolyte solution taken by mouth or administered by gavage at a rate of 1-2 L every hour until the rectal effluent is clear (to a maximum of 5-6 hours). This technique eliminates the need to place patients on a clear liquid diet for more than one preoperative day and does not require additional enemas to produce a clear effluent. It has been shown to be superior to more traditional techniques, producing better mechanical cleansing and leaving fewer aerobic and anaerobic bacteria in the bowel.[28,29] This preparation may also be used effectively on an outpatient basis, permitting admission of patients to the hospital on the same day as their operation.[30] Unfortunately, the latter technique cannot be used in all patients being prepared for esophageal surgery. Many patients have a relative obstruction of the esophagus that prevents their taking large amounts of fluid by mouth and prohibits the safe passage of a gavage tube. A history of severe gastroesophageal reflux, often accompanied by delayed gastric emptying, and motility disorders such as achalasia are also relative contraindications to the use of orthograde lavage. In patients who cannot drink or take such material via a feeding tube it is necessary to administer enemas until the return is clear. On occasion, even experienced surgeons find that a planned operation using the stomach for reconstruction cannot be accomplished, and in such situations it is vital that an adequate bowel preparation be performed preoperatively to permit its use in these unforseen circumstances.

In addition to a good mechanical preparation, the use of antibiotics to selectively decontaminate the bowel is standard practice. The most commonly used antibiotic regimen is erythromycin base and neomycin sulfate, but newer combinations of antibiotics or single agents such as Flagyl are gaining in popularity and have been shown to be effective in limiting the risk of postoperative infectious complications.

Most esophageal reconstructive operations are classified as clean contaminated procedures. Patients who undergo such operations have been shown to benefit from perioperative systemic antibiotics.[31,32] Use of an antibiotic dose just prior to beginning the operation, maintenance of adequate antibiotic levels throughout the operation, and possible administration of an additional dose after completion of the operation reduces wound infection rates, may lessen the incidence of other infectious complications, and reduces hospital costs.[33-36] It is important that the first dose be administered within two hours of beginning the operation to maximize efficacy and minimize the development of resistant organism caused by prolonged preoperative administration.[37,38] Single dose therapy directed at potentially contaminating organisms is the theoretical ideal for prophylactic antibiotic treatment.[39-42] The choice of antibiotic for most procedures is a second generation cephalosporin, but third generation cephalosporins (which cover gram negative organisms) should be considered for colon interpositions or if a high degree of contamination from oral flora has occurred.[31]

Patient Preparation

Preparation of the patient includes continuation of the counseling that precedes any major operation. The patient must be aware of the planned procedure, the likely problems that might occur during an operation, and the remedies for these pitfalls. The postoperative course is described in sufficient detail so that the patient will know what to expect during each phase of recovery and will understand what his or her responsibilities are during each phase. Having the patient's family or significant relations present during such preparatory discussions eliminates confusion and questions after the operation and permits them to be involved in providing support and encouragement to the patient postoperatively.

Preparation of the Surgeon

The surgeon must be prepared for a sometimes difficult and often time-consuming operation. When a case goes according to plan and no problems develop during surgery that disturb the flow of the operation, nothing is more rewarding than a successful reconstruction that ultimately restores a patient's ability to eat. However, there are many opportunities for problems during such operations and, as many surgeons know, being faced with the possibility that a reconstruction may not be accomplished can be daunting. To avoid such situations, the surgeon should be mentally prepared for all types of adversity, with contingency plans available that are designed to resolve problems with a minimum of worry and consternation. The most obvious situations are those in which the organ to be used for reconstruction is not available due to unforeseen preexisting or intraoperative problems. In other situations, the organ is available and is healthy but may not have the length needed to complete the reconstruction. In either of these situations, alternative reconstructive organs, routes, and techniques should be available to the surgeon to permit safe and successful completion of the operation. The surgeon should be mentally prepared for a potentially long operation, and it is best to reserve sufficient time to complete the operation so that no sense of hurry is present. With these caveats in mind, a good outcome is most likely.

References

1. Nabeya K, Hanaoka T, Onozawa K, et al. Two-stage esophagogastrectomy for esophageal reconstruction. In Ferguson MK, Little AG, Skinner DB (eds): **Diseases of the Esophagus, Vol I: Malignant Diseases**. Mount Kisco, NY, Futura, 1990, pp 247-252.
2. Sugimachi K, Inokuchi K, Natsuda Y, et al. Delayed anastomosis of the cervical portion of the esophagus in bypass operations for unresectable carcinoma of the esophagus. *Surg Gynecol Obstet* 1983;157:233-236.
3. Nabeya K. Esophageal reconstruction: When to perform reconstruction. *Dis Esoph* 1995;8:1-3.

4. Siewert JR, Bartels H, Lange J, et al. En bloc esophagectomy: When to reconstruct the food passage? In Ferguson MK, Little AG, Skinner DB (eds): **Diseases of the Esophagus, Vol I: Malignant Diseases**. Mount Kisco, NY, Futura, 1990, pp 253-260.
5. Christou NV, Tellado-Rodriguez J, Chartrand L, et al. Estimating mortality risk in preoperative patients using immunologic, nutritional, and acute-phase response variables. *Ann Surg* 1989;210:69-77.
6. Saito T, Kuwahara A, Shimoda K, et al. Acute phase proteins and infectious complications after surgery for esophageal cancer. *Jap J Surg* 1991;21:627-636.
7. diZerega GS. The cause and prevention of postsurgical adhesions: A contemporary update. *Prog Clin Biol Res* 1993;381:1-18.
8. Pijlman BM, Dorr PJ, Brommer EJP, et al. Prevention of adhesions. *Eur J Obstet Gynecol Reprod Biol* 1994;54:155-163.
9. Kinoshita T, Saito T, Shigemitsu Y, et al. Antibody response correlates with septic complications following esophagectomy for cancer. *J Surg Oncol* 1994;56:227-232.
10. Baxevanis CN, Papilas K, Dedoussis GV, et al. Abnormal cytokine serum levels correlate with impaired cellular immune responses after surgery. *Clin Immunol Immunopathol* 1994;71:82-88.
11. Markewitz A, Faist E, Weinhold C, et al. Alterations of cell-mediated immune response following cardiac surgery. *Eur J Cardiothorac Surg* 1993;7:193-199.
12. Saito T, Shigemitsu Y, Kinoshita T, et al. Impaired neutrophil bactericidal activity correlates with the infection occurring after surgery for esophageal cancer. *J Surg Oncol* 1992;51:159-163.
13. Ferguson MK. Preoperative assessment of pulmonary risk. *Chest* 1999;115:58S-63S.
14. Nagawa H, Kobori O, Muto T. Prediction of pulmonary complications after transthoracic oesophagectomy. *Br J Surg* 1994;81:860-862.
15. Law SY, Fok M, Wong J. Risk analysis in resection of squamous cell carcinoma of the esophagus. *World J Surg* 1994;18:339-346.
16. Tsutsui S, Moriguchi S, Morita M, et al. Multivariate analysis of postoperative complications after esophageal resection. *Ann Thorac Surg* 1992;53:1052-1056.
17. Ferguson MK, Martin TR, Reeder LB, et al. Determinants of pulmonary complications following esophagectomy. In Peracchia A, Rosati R, Bonavina L, et al. (eds): **Recent Advances in Diseases of the Esophagus**. Bologna, Monduzzi Editore, 1996, pp 527-532.
18. Chan K-H, Wong J. Mortality after esophagectomy for carcinoma of esophagus: An analysis of risk factors. *Dis Esoph* 1990;3:49-53.
19. Ferguson MK, Martin TR, Reeder LB, et al. Mortality after esophagectomy: Risk factor analysis. *World J Surg* 1997;21:599-604.
20. Ritchie AJ, Tolan M, Whiteside M, et al. Prophylactic digitalization fails to control dysrhythmia in thoracic esophageal operations. *Ann Thorac Surg* 1993;55:86-88.
21. Karnofsky DA, Burchenal JH. The clinical evaluation of chemotherapeutic agents in cancer. In MacLeod CM (ed): **Evaluation of Chemotherapeutic Agents**. New York, Columbia Press, 1949, pp 192-204.
22. Zubrod CG, Schneiderman M, Frei E III, et al. Appraisal of methods for the study of chemotherapy of cancer in man: Comparative therapeutic trial of

nitrogen mustard and triethylene thiophosphoramide. *J Chronic Dis* 1960;11:7-33.

23. Schaafsma J, Osoba D. The Karnofsky Performance Status Scale re-examined: a cross-validation with the EORTC-C30. *Qual Life Res* 1994;3:413-424.
24. Baskin WN. Advances in enteral nutrition techniques. *Am J Gastroenterol* 1992;87:1547-1553.
25. Saunders C, Nishikawa R, Wolfe B. Surgical nutrition: A review. *J R Coll Surg Edinb* 1993;38:195-204.
26. Alexander JW. Immunoenhancement via enteral nutrition. *Arch Surg* 1993;128:1242-1245.
27. McClave SA, Snider HL, Spain DA. Preoperative issues in clinical nutrition. *Chest* 1999;115:64S-70S.
28. Fleites RA, Marshall JB, Eckhauser ML, et al. The efficacy of polyethylene glycol-electrolyte lavage solution versus traditional mechanical bowel preparation for elective colonic surgery: A randomized, prospective, blinded clinical trial. *Surgery* 1985;98:708-716.
29. Fordtran JS, Santa Ana CA, Cleveland MB. A low-sodium solution for gastrointestinal lavage. Gastroenterology 1990;98:11-16.
30. Philip RS. Efficacy of preoperative bowel preparation at home. *Am Surg* 1995;61:368-370.
31. Ludwig KA, Carlson MA, Condon RE. Prophylactic antibiotics in surgery. *Annu Rev Med* 1993;44:385-393.
32. Page CP, Bohnen JM, Fletcher JR, et al. Antimicrobial prophylaxis for surgical wounds. Guidelines for clinical care. *Arch Surg* 1993;128:79-88.
33. Classen DC, Evans RS, Pestotnik SL, et al. The timing of prophylactic administration of antibiotics and the risk of surgical wound infection. *N Engl J Med* 1992;30:281-286.
34. Bricard H, Deshayes JP, Sillard B, et al. Antibiotic prophylaxis in surgery of the esophagus. *Ann Fr Anesth Reanim* 1994;13:S161-S168.
35. Waddell TK, Rotstein OD. Antimicrobial prophylaxis in surgery. Committee on Antimicrobial Agents, Canadian Infectious Disease Society. *CMAJ* 1994;151:925-931.
36. Fernandez Arjona M, Herruzo Cabrera R, Gomez-Sancha F, et al. Economical saving due to prophylaxis in the prevention of surgical wound infection. *Eur J Epidemiol* 1996;12:455-459.
37. Lizan-Garcia M, Garcia-Caballero J, Asensio-Vegas A. Risk factors for surgical wound infection in general surgery: a prospective study. *Infect Control Hosp Epidemiol* 1997;18:310-315.
38. Matuschka PR, Cheadle WG, Burke JD, et al. A new standard of care: Administration of preoperative antibiotics in the operating room. *Am Surg* 1997;63:500-503.
39. DiPiro JT. Short-term prophylaxis in clean-contaminated surgery. *J Chemother* 1999;11:551-555.
40. Esposito S. Is single-dose antibiotic prophylaxis sufficient for any surgical procedure? *J Chemother* 1999;11:556-564.
41. Novelli A. Antimicrobial prophylaxis in surgery: The role of pharmacokinetics. *J Chemother* 1999;11:565-572.
42. Polk HC, Christmas AB. Prophylactic antibiotics in surgery and surgical wound infections. *Am Surg* 2000;66:105-111.

Chapter 7

Selecting the Appropriate Esophageal Substitute

It is often said that the three "A's" of building a successful clinical practice are ability, availability, and affability. There are three "A's" that are also important in selecting an appropriate esophageal substitute: availability, anatomy, and applicability. Many organs and techniques exist for replacing the resected esophagus. The organ used most frequently is the stomach, which can be brought into the chest as a whole organ, in a tubularized form, or in a reverse tubularized form. Other organs commonly used for replacement are the colon (left, right, middle, or ileocolic segment) and the jejunum (pedicled or as a free flap). Composite replacement operations can also be performed using a combination of gastric remnant and free jejunal graft, for example. The myriad choices may initially appear daunting. However, a careful analysis of the factors that govern selection from among these choices makes the decision both rational and straightforward.

The initial factor that requires analysis is the availability of an organ, which refers to whether it is anatomically complete and is functional. Prior gastric or colon resections, for example, often preclude use of these organs as esophageal replacements. Anatomy refers to a number of technical factors that determine the suitability of an organ for use in reconstruction, and includes such things as vascular supply, length, and the relative size of the organ compared to that of the esophagus. The applicability of a particular replacement organ to an individual patient depends on a number of additional factors, including the patient's life expectancy and general condition, the technical difficulty of performing the replacement, and the short- and long-term functional characteristics of the organ to be used.

Availability

Stomach

Although the stomach is the organ most often used for esophageal replacement, there are a variety of reasons why it may not be the optimal choice in an individual patient. Prior gastric resection, ulcer disease requiring operative intervention, and loss of the right gastroepiploic artery are a few of the conditions that make use of the stomach a less-than-optimal choice (Table 7-1). Unless a well-vascularized segment of stomach of sufficient length exists and can be used to replace only the distal part of the esophagus, another organ should be selected.

Colon

The second most commonly used organ for replacement, the colon, has an even larger number of relative contraindications, foremost of which is prior resection. The mere ability to technically perform esophageal replacement surgery using a colon remnant does not mean that it should be done. For example, patients who have had a right colectomy in the past could anatomically be candidates for interposition of the left colon, because its vascular supply is based on the ascending branch of the left colic artery. However, this would necessitate a low ileosigmoid or ileorectal anastomosis, the functional results of which are only fair. Similar reconstructive options exist for patients who have had a left colectomy and undergo interposition of the right colon based on the middle colic artery. The combination of a low anastomosis with the mild dumping symptoms that frequently accompany esophagectomy can result in a very symptomatic and unhappy patient.

Diverticulosis, especially in patients with a history of diverticulitis, is another strong contraindication to use of the colon for esophageal replacement. Patients may develop symptomatic diverticulitis, the location of which may be difficult to discern early in its course. It is known that patients who develop early appendicitis initially have referred pain in the periumbilical region that migrates to the lower right quadrant before peritoneal signs develop, even when the appendix is in a retroperitoneal or intrathoracic (after colon interposition) location. Similarly, one would expect that the initial presentation of a patient with diverticulitis of the interposed colon includes nonspecific lower abdominal pain, and localization to the chest does not become apparent until transmural inflammation develops. The high frequency of mild diverticulosis in the North American adult population, however, mitigates against using its presence alone as

Table 7-1.
Relative Contraindications for Use of Organ Substitutes in Esophageal Replacement.

Stomach	
	Partial or near-total gastrectomy
	Occlusion or loss of the right gastroepiploic vessels (secondary to omentectomy or inflammation)
	Prior gastric emptying procedure: gastrojejunostomy; Finney pyloroplasty; Jaboulay duodenogastrostomy
	Prior gastrocystostomy for pancreatic pseudocyst
	Witzel-type gastrostomy
Colon	
	Partial or total colectomy
	Abdominal aortic surgery with loss of the inferior mesenteric or left colic arteries
	Atherosclerosis affecting the left, right, or middle colic arteries or the marginal artery of Drummond
	Diverticulosis
	Multiple polyps
	Portal hypertension
	Ulcerative colitis
	Familial polyposis
	Chagas' disease
	Dense fibrous adhesions
	Radiation enteritis
Jejunum	
	Crohn's disease
	Short bowel syndrome
	Radiation enteritis
	Portal hypertension
	Extensive fibrous adhesions
	Superior mesenteric artery syndrome

an absolute contraindication to the selection of the colon as an esophageal replacement, especially if other factors argue strongly for its use.

The presence of ulcerative colitis or familial polyposis, with their attendant risks of the development of adenocarcinoma of the colon, is a straightforward contraindication to the use of the colon as an esophageal replacement. More difficult is the decision to use the colon in the face of multiple small adenomatous polyps. If these can be removed endoscopically, it is appropriate to consider the colon for use as a substitute.

Factors that affect colonic motility, such as Chagas' disease or a history of colonic pseudo-obstruction, argue against the use of the colon as an esophageal substitute. There is considerable controversy over whether normal motility patterns are preserved in the stomach and colon following their use as esophageal replacements, some of which was initially discussed in Chapter 2 and is covered more completely later in this chapter.

Suffice it to say that some residual motor activity in these organs is advantageous, and the selection of an organ with a known motility disturbance is not recommended. Motility problems are also apparent in bowel that has been subjected to radiation damage. In addition to the motility disturbance, the microvascular damage that results from ionizing radiation puts these segments at higher than average risk for ischemia and necrosis.

Jejunum

The use of free or pedicled jejunal grafts as esophageal replacements is practiced routinely in a small number of medical centers. Contraindications to the use of these grafts include the presence of inflammatory bowel disease. Although Crohn's disease is known to affect the distal ileum predominantly, all portions of the alimentary tract are possible targets, and the need for multiple resections over time is well recognized. That this can result in short bowel syndrome is sufficiently cautioning to encourage surgeons to avoid the use of jejunal grafts for reconstruction when there is a history of inflammatory bowel disease. A more important concern is that the loop used for the interposition itself could develop Crohn's disease, which would be a devastating and challenging complication, to be avoided at all costs.

Portal hypertension is a relative contraindication to the use of intestinal segments for esophageal replacement. The outcomes of such operations depend in large part on the degree of hypertension that is manifest during the perioperative period. In the face of moderate to severe portal hypertension, the technical challenge of dissecting a segment to be used, while maintaining its venous drainage in a satisfactory condition, is sufficiently daunting to prohibit most surgeons from such an undertaking.

Anatomy

Factors that influence the selection of an esophageal substitute from an anatomic perspective include the vascular supply of the organ, its size and thickness relative to that of the esophagus, and the relative length of an esophageal replacement that can be constructed from the organ (Table 7-2).

Stomach

The stomach is most often prepared as a whole or a tubularized organ for pull-up. Its blood supply in this configuration is based primarily on the right gastroepiploic artery. Extensive microscopic intramural anasto-

Table 7-2.
Factors Influencing the Choice of a Reconstructive Organ.

- Anatomy
  - Vascular supply
  - Available length
  - Size (diameter) match
  - Tissue strength
- Technique
  - Technical ease of operation
  - Operative morbidity and mortality
    - Duration of operation
    - Number of anastomoses
    - Risk of vascular insufficiency
    - Recurrent nerve injury
- Motility patterns
- Other aspects of organ function
  - Acid production
  - Resistance to acid, alkali, and digestive enzymes
  - Retention of gastric reservoir capacity
- Other
  - Patient age
  - Type (and stage, if malignant) of disease

moses provide circulation to the remaining stomach after division of the short gastric arteries and the left gastric artery (whole organ) or left and right gastric arteries (tubularized organ). The right gastroepiploic artery is constant in its length and distribution and is rarely affected by atherosclerosis even when there is generalized and severe peripheral vascular disease. These factors make the blood supply reliable when the stomach is used as a whole organ or in a tubularized form, and organ necrosis is uncommon. When the stomach is prepared as a reversed tube in the manner of Gavriliu,[1] the blood supply is based primarily on intramural anastomoses from the left gastric artery through the left gastroepiploic arcade and then to the distal greater curvature, a region that is normally supplied by the right gastroepiploic vessels. In this configuration, the blood supply is not as dependable as when the blood supply is based on the right gastroepiploic arcade, a fact that leads to necrosis of the reverse gastric tube in a small percentage of patients.

The length of stomach that can be mobilized for use as a reconstructive organ is almost always sufficient regardless of the amount of esophagus that has been resected. After a thorough Kocher maneuver has been performed, which permits the pylorus to rise to almost the level of the esophageal hiatus, the fundus of the whole stomach normally reaches as high as the mandible, making it suitable for a cervical esophagogastros-

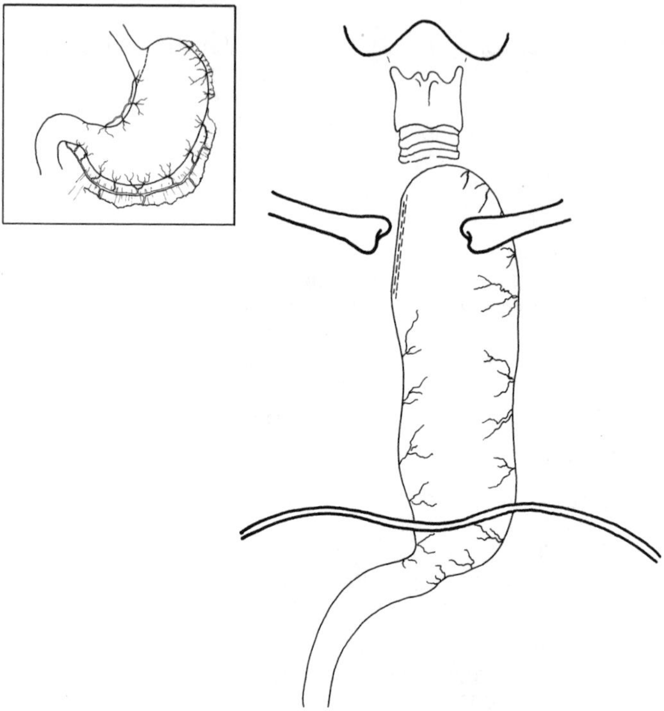

A

Figure 7-1. Relative lengths of whole (**A**) and tubularized (**B**) stomach segments used for esophageal replacement.

tomy or even a pharyngogastrostomy. The fundus is preserved when creating a standard gastric tube for esophageal replacement, no length is lost, and the length of the tube is at least as good as that of the whole stomach. Because the greater curvature of the stomach is considerably longer than is the lesser curvature, resection of the latter portion of the stomach combined with division of the right gastric artery permits even greater length to be achieved in a gastric tube as compared to the whole stomach (Figure 7-1). In contrast, the reversed gastric tube is typically shorter than either of the more standard stomach preparations (Figure 7-2). Additional length can be obtained by including the distal antrum and pylorus as part of the tube, which permits the tube to reach as high as the pharynx in most patients. However, this necessitates a much more extensive dissection and reconstruction than is required for even a standard reversed tube, and results in a higher incidence of postoperative complications.

The stomach is suited for anastomosis to the esophagus or pharynx. Whether it is used as a whole preparation or in a standard tubularized configuration, its diameter substantially exceeds that of the esophagus. This necessitates creation of a defect in the wall of the stomach that can

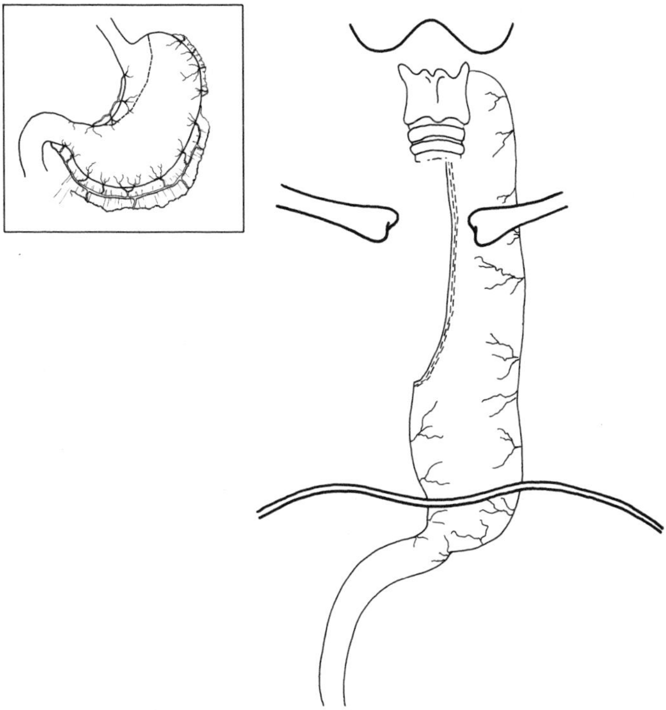

B

Figure 7-1. Continued.

be fashioned to the exact dimensions the surgeon desires, eliminating any size mismatch. In addition, since the anastomosis is typically performed along the body of the stomach rather than at the tip of the fundus, the remaining fundus serves to reinforce the posterior suture line, helping to prevent leaks and gastroesophageal reflux, as will be discussed in Chapters 9 and 15. Anastomoses performed to a reverse gastric tube are usually done in an end-to-end fashion, and the tube is created in such a way that the diameter of its proximal end (after reversal) matches that of the esophagus. The thickness of the stomach wall also lends itself to the performance of an anastomosis. Gastric tissues have good suture holding power relative to those found in the small bowel and certain parts of the colon.[2] These factors provide the reconstructive surgeon with confidence when performing esophageal replacement surgery using the stomach as a reconstructive organ.

Colon

The colon is used in a variety of configurations for esophageal replacement (Figure 7-3). In the pediatric age group the right colon is most

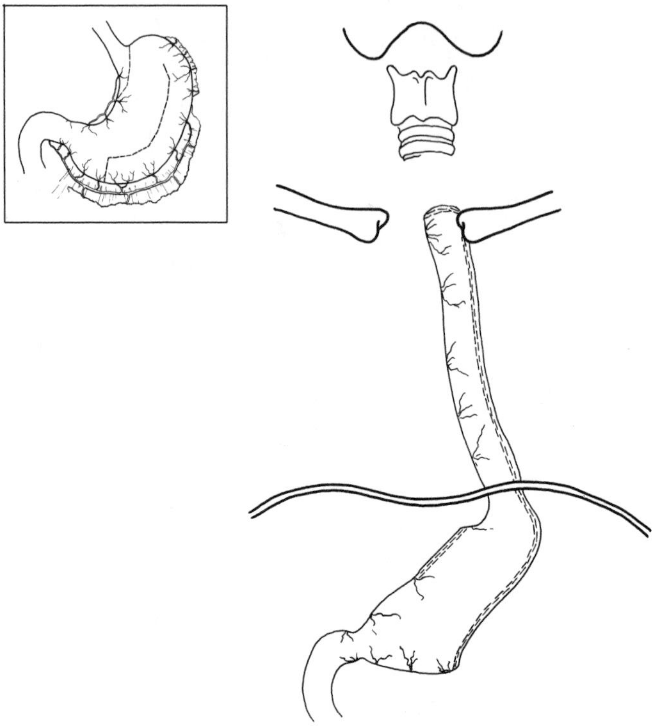

Figure 7-2. Relative length possible with construction of a reverse gastric tube used for esophageal replacement.

commonly used, and is oriented either in an antiperistaltic position based on the right colic artery, or in an isoperistaltic manner based on the middle or left colic artery.[3] Another less common option is use of an ileocolic segment placed in an isoperistaltic fashion based on the middle colic artery, preserving the ileocecal valve. It is thought by some surgeons that preservation of the ileocolic valve will help to prevent reflux from the colon into the esophagus. However, there are few data available that specifically address this issue, and the valve sometimes causes obstruction. In the adult age group, the most commonly used configurations are the left colon with or without the transverse colon based on the ascending branch of the left colic artery and placed in an isoperistaltic fashion, and the transverse colon placed in an isoperistaltic fashion and based on the middle colic artery. The arterial blood supply to all of these colon segments is reliable in young and middle-aged patients, although the supply to the left and transverse colon (from the left colic artery through the marginal artery of Drummond) is more constant than that of the right colon, which sometimes has an interrupted marginal vessel. In older patients, the colic

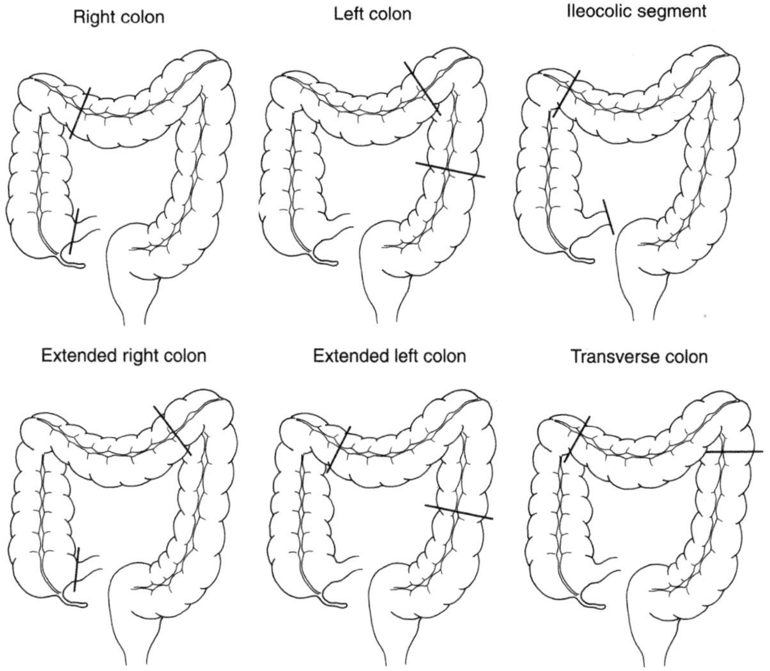

Figure 7-3. Configurations available for use of the colon as an esophageal replacement.

vessels and marginal arteries are often affected by atherosclerosis, a process that can be locally severe and preclude safe use of the colon for esophageal replacement. There is an appreciable incidence of intraoperative and early postoperative ischemia and necrosis due to arterial insufficiency, a complication that affects right colon interpositions more often than left colon interpositions.[4,5] Fortunately, this complication is almost always detected at the time of interposition. If this occurs, the colon can be discarded and an alternative method of reconstruction can be selected. Other vascular complications develop later in the early postoperative period and are more often attributed to venous congestion, a problem that is not often apparent intraoperatively.

The length of colon that can be prepared for esophageal reconstruction is related primarily to the reliability of its blood supply. Because the colon is a somewhat redundant organ, the amount needed can usually be sacrificed without undo concern about subsequent digestive function. The left and transverse colon preparations in the adult patient reliably reach to the neck for reconstruction after a near-total esophagectomy. Similarly, in the pediatric age group, right colon preparations typically reach to the neck for reconstruction of nearly the entire esophagus after resection for injury or atresia. In patients in whom a short segment of colon is necessary for use in replacing the distal esophagus, it is rare that a suitable segment cannot be found, even in the presence of atherosclerotic peripheral vascular disease.

The size of the colon relative to that of the esophagus sometimes creates problems in constructing an optimal anastomosis. The diameter mismatch is greatest for the right colon and often necessitates tailoring of the proximal end of the interposition to permit an end-to-end anastomosis. This size discrepancy is apparent when trying to place the colon through the posterior mediastinum or a substernal route, because the bulk of the right colon is much greater than that of the tubularized stomach. The discrepancy is even more evident when an ileocolic segment is constructed and the cecum is brought high into the chest prior to performing an ileoesophageal anastomosis. The size of the left and the transverse colon are much better diameter matches for the esophagus and typically permit an end-to-end anastomosis without the need for tailoring the interposition.

The thickness of the wall of the colon also lends itself to satisfactory suture placement. The left colon is thicker than the right colon in this regard, making it more suitable than the right colon in many surgeons' minds as an esophageal replacement. The suture holding power of the mucosa, the seromuscular layer, and the whole thickness of the wall of the colon are similar or slightly better than those of the stomach, and are substantially greater than for small bowel.[2]

Jejunum

The vascular supply to the jejunum is characterized by a radial, segmental arrangement that provides a challenge to the occasional esophageal reconstructive surgeon (Figure 7-4). Although the vessels are rarely affected by atherosclerotic processes to any important extent, their small diameter and inconstant arborations make the preparation of a reliably vascularized segment technically difficult. Seemingly minor technical errors may create arterial injury or venous thrombosis, resulting in ischemia that precludes use of that segment.

The length to which a jejunal graft can be extended is more limited than that of stomach or colon, largely as a result of the unique pattern of blood supply to this organ. The most common uses of jejunum for esophageal reconstruction are replacement of the distal esophagus with a pedicled graft and substitution for the cervical esophagus with a free graft. Each of these reconstructions can be performed without discarding long segments of bowel. Replacement of longer segments of the esophagus requires tailoring of the blood supply to create sufficient length of the vascular pedicle. This typically creates redundancy of the jejunum and

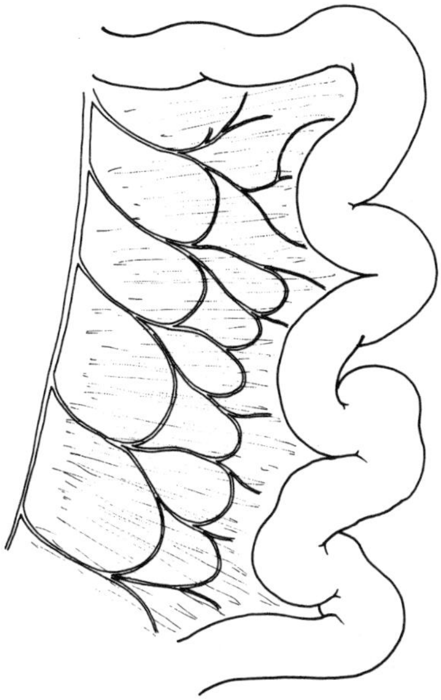

Figure 7-4. The pattern of its vascular supply limits the length of the uninterrupted jejunal segment that can be used for esophageal replacement.

requires resection of one or more segments with subsequent jejunojejunostomy to establish enteral continuity (Figure 7-5).

The jejunum provides the best diameter match for the esophagus for purposes of the anastomosis. Paradoxically, for most reconstructions of the distal esophagus the esophagojejunostomy is performed in an end-to-side fashion because of the natural tendency of the jejunum to assume a curved shape. When reconstructing the cervical esophagus, end-to-end anastomoses are preferred to avoid jejunal redundancy in the limited space available in the neck, and are usually possible because the segments of jejunum used for reconstruction are usually short and are relatively plastic. For purposes of performing an anastomosis, the thickness of the jejunum is not nearly as great as is that of the stomach or colon. The holding power of sutures through various thicknesses of the jejunum is only about half of that found in the stomach and colon.[2]

Applicability

Technical Issues

The choice of one organ over another for reconstruction depends on a number of factors (Table 7-2). The technical ease of the operation is perhaps the least important consideration. However, some surgeons do

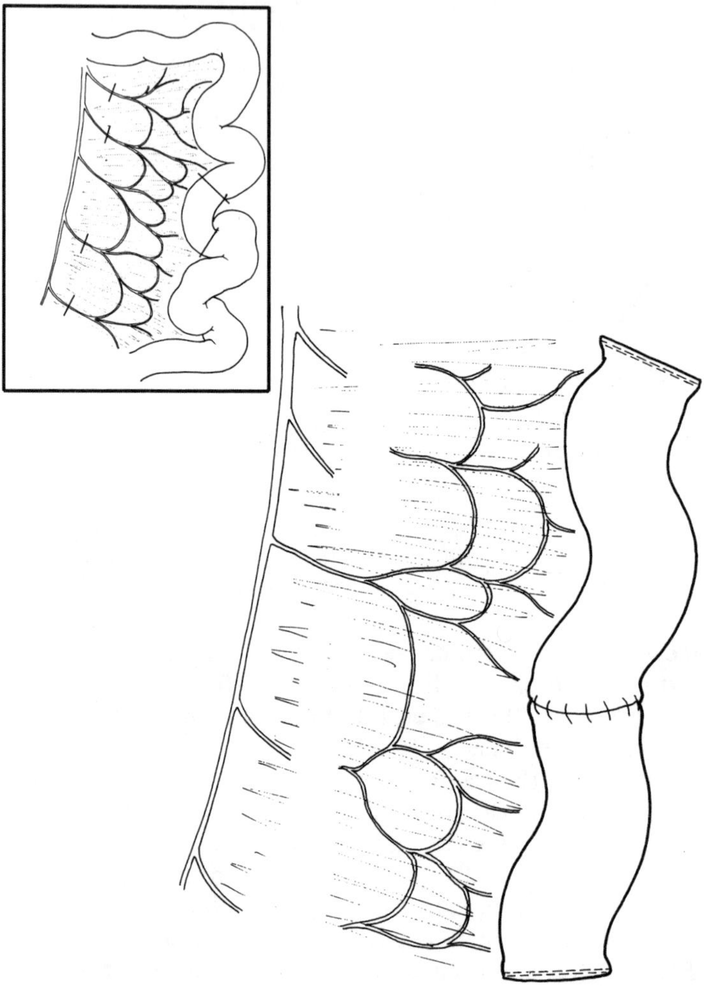

Figure 7-5. Tailoring jejunal segments on a single vascular pedicle can provide additional length.

not possess the requisite technical skills necessary to perform complex reconstructions. A specialist may be necessary to construct microvascular anastomoses for a free graft, and some medical centers do not have the personnel or equipment required for such specialized work. The technical ease of the operation is also related to whether there are preexisting problems that will affect the conduct of the operation. Prior surgery resulting in adhesions, preoperative radiation therapy or chemotherapy, portal hypertension, and similar underlying conditions can make an ordinary operation difficult and prolonged. The need to perform three anastomoses in order to accomplish a colon interposition, as compared to the necessity for only a single anastomosis required for the performance of a gastric pull-up, may add an extra hour to a procedure, increasing the duration of an operation by 20% or more. The duration of an operation in a healthy patient is not an important factor in determining operative morbidity, but most of the operations performed for esophageal replacement are not done on young, healthy patients. Therefore, time and technical factors must be considered when determining the optimal methods of esophageal replacement.

The risk of postoperative complications must also be taken into account when performing esophageal reconstructive surgery. The risk of vascular insufficiency is moderate in patients in whom colon or jejunal interpositions are performed, in contrast to the relatively low risk in patients undergoing gastric pull-up. This may be an important short-term consideration, especially in patients who have underlying cardiovascular or pulmonary disease and could not tolerate the additional stress resulting from necrosis of a reconstructive organ or an anastomotic leak. Recurrent nerve injury is a common complication of esophageal reconstruction. It occurs rarely in patients who undergo intrathoracic anastomoses and is recognized almost exclusively in patients who have a cervical anastomosis. Recurrent nerve injury is an insidious problem in the early postoperative period, interfering with effective coughing and pulmonary toilet and placing patients at risk for aspiration due to impaired intrinsic airway protection. In patients with preexisting pulmonary disease, avoidance of recurrent nerve injury may be sufficiently important that the choice of a reconstructive organ or anastomotic site will be determined by the need to avoid it.

Motility Patterns

An important issue that helps to determine the appropriate selection of an organ for reconstruction is the motility pattern of the reconstructive organ, in particular whether the replacement organ possesses peristaltic activity. This question has been investigated using a variety of techniques over a long period of time, but precious few useful data have been generated, and only brief comments can be provided that shed little light on the topic. It is useful for purposes of this discussion to briefly review the normal motility patterns of the organs used for esophageal replacement and to compare them to patterns recorded after esophageal reconstruction.

Stomach

Gastric motility is separated into fundic, antral, and pyloric phases.[6] Activity in the fundus (the primary region of gastric reservoir function) is characterized by initial relaxation to accommodate ingested food, followed by a slow increase in tone that propels food toward the antrum. The gastric antrum functions to both grind and pump food by means of phasic and intermittent peristaltic contractile activity. The pylorus regulates food movement into the duodenum, and closes completely during the antral stroke.[7] These nonperistaltic activities are partially under vagal control, which is almost always disrupted during esophagectomy.

After transposition of the whole stomach or gastric tube into the thorax, there is loss of receptive relaxation of the fundus and lack of peristaltic activity in the antrum. Emptying is dependent more on patient position and the technique used for preparing the stomach than on the composition of a meal or the presence or absence of a gastric emptying procedure. Motility studies performed postoperatively demonstrate no peristaltic activity, minimal spontaneous contractions, and few contractions associated with deglutition.[8-10]

Using scintigraphic techniques, emptying of both semisolids and liquids from the intrathoracic stomach is much slower than is tracer clearance from the normal esophagus. Interestingly, the rate of stomach emptying is substantially faster than the rate of clearance of the normal stomach in an intra-abdominal location when patients are in an upright position.[8,10-13] When patients are in a supine position, emptying of the intrathoracic stomach is very slow, and is also slow compared to that of a normal stomach in an intra-abdominal location.[13] Tracer accumulation frequently occurs above the diaphragmatic hiatus and is also sometimes seen at the level of the aortic arch. The rate of emptying of an intrathoracic stomach does not appear to be related to the presence or absence of a gastric emptying procedure, but is strongly dependent on the size of the stomach prepared as an esophageal substitute.[14] Use of a tubularized stomach results in delayed gastric emptying in fewer than 5% of patients. In contrast, use of two-thirds of the stomach is associated with an incidence of delayed emptying of 10% to 15%, whereas use of the whole stomach results in delayed gastric emptying in 35% to 40% of patients. This deficiency improves over time, however, with both tubularized and whole stomach grafts exhibiting recovery of motor activity three or more years postoperatively.[15] The route selected for passage of the intrathoracic stomach (posterior mediastinal versus substernal) does not appear to have an important influence on gastric clearance of tracer.[16]

Colon

In a manner similar to that of the stomach, the colon normally lacks cohesive peristaltic activity. Important functions of the colon include absorption, slow aboral movement of luminal contents, retention of fecal material in preparation for defecation, and rapid movement of fecal material during defecation.[17] Contractions of the colon that permit these functions are classified as individual phasic contractions, organized groups of contractions, and special propulsive contractions. Individual phasic contractions (both long- and short-duration types) are poorly coordinated and generally do not propagate. They are under myogenic, neural (central nervous system, autonomic nervous system, and enteric nervous system), and chemical control. Organized groups of contractions are collections of individual phasic contractions that appear as alternating periods of quiescence and contractile activity at any single site in the colon.[18] This activity does not propagate or propel fecal material to the front of the complex. The enteric nervous system is likely a major mechanism of grouping of this activity. Special propulsive contractions occur in the human only once or twice per day, are likely stimulated by mechano- and chemo-receptors in the colon wall, and are linked to defecation. It is apparent that the normal function of the colon does not include regular peristaltic activity.

Postoperative motility studies in patients who have had colon interposition for esophageal replacement demonstrate some simultaneous contractions and rare peristaltic contractions in the unstimulated colon.[8,19,20] Hydrochloric acid stimulation often results in coordinated contractions that progress in the aboral direction in patients with an isoperistaltic colon interposition[19,21,22] or progress in the oral direction in patients with an antiperistaltic segment interposition.[19] Similar results are found when the interposed colon is stimulated with a moderately large fluid volume.[19,23]

Scintigraphic and other functional studies in patients with a colon interposition demonstrate delayed clearance compared to that seen in the normal esophagus.[8,24-26] Clearance is somewhat slower in the interposed colon than in a gastric tube used for esophageal replacement.[25] Accumulation of tracer material occurs just above the diaphragm and sometimes at the level of the aortic arch.[8] Interestingly, there is no apparent relationship between whether the interposition is placed in an isoperistaltic or an antiperistaltic orientation and clearance time.[24]

Jejunum

Of the possible esophageal substitutes in common use, peristalsis-like activity is normally a characteristic of only the jejunum. As in the colon, smooth muscle activity in the jejunum is characterized by different types of contractions, one type being individual phasic contractions. The jejunum possesses only a single type of individual phasic contraction, which is under myogenic, neural, and chemical control. Such contractions are often phase-locked, due to the existence of strong cell-to-cell coupling of electrical activity and to similarity of intrinsic frequencies in adjacent segments. Organized groups of contractions, which normally occur in the fasting state and are characterized by orderly caudad migration, appear to support a cleaning function and the movement of bile to the ileum for enterohepatic circulation. Organized groups of contractions that extend over relatively long distances, or migrating motor complexes, usually originate in the duodenum and can propagate to the terminal ileum.[27] The jejunum also exhibits two other types of migrating contractions, giant and individual migrating contractions, that extend over intermediate distances. The former are similar to those that occur in the rest of the gastrointestinal tract, while individual migrating contractions occur in a postprandial state and propagate over shorter distances (10 to 20 cm).[28]

This peristalsis-like activity is preserved but diminished when the jejunum is used as an esophageal substitute.[29] There is controversy as to whether the contractile activity of a jejunal interposition is linked to primary peristaltic activity of the esophagus or to the swallowing cascade as assessed manometrically.[30,31] Scintigraphic examination demonstrates delayed tracer clearance compared to that of the esophagus in normal individuals.[32] Nevertheless, peristaltic activity is clinically evident in many patients with a pedicled or free jejunal graft.

Other Aspects of Organ Function

Gastric Acid Production, Acid Reflux, Alkaline Reflux

The acid production capacity of the stomach in its normal or interposed location is reduced after the requisite vagectomy that accompanies most esophagectomies. When the lesser curvature of the stomach is resected to create a gastric tube for esophageal reconstruction, the parietal cell mass in the body of the stomach is reduced, further limiting acid production by the stomach. Although acid production is by no means eliminated,[33] it is reduced in the intrathoracic stomach compared to that in the normal stomach as assessed by direct measurement of basal and stimulated gastric acid production[11,12] and by gastric pH monitoring.[10] Acid reflux from the stomach into the esophagus is not a significant clinical problem in patients who have undergone a cervical esophagogastric anastomosis, as judged by scintigraphy and esophageal pH monitoring.[8,9,12,34] In contrast, reflux of intragastric material is common in patients with a low intrathoracic esophagogastric anastomosis.[8] Interestingly, a high intrathoracic esophagogastrostomy yields fewer acid reflux problems than does a cervical anastomosis.[35] In patients with a colon or jejunal interposition, reflux from the stomach into the interposed organ is also common, and shuttling of material from the interposed organ into the esophagus occurs frequently in patients with an intrathoracic esophageal anastomosis. These interposition organs appear to be relatively resistant to injury by gastric acid and other digestive enzymes.[23,36]

Scintigraphy and pH monitoring demonstrate that alkaline reflux into the stomach is common after gastric pull-up for esophageal reconstruction.[9,10,12,33] Alkaline refluxate in this context refers to the alkaline contents of the pancreas as well as bile. Such reflux is likely related to a variety of factors, including but not limited to: 1) the reduction in gastric acid production that accompanies such operations, which would unmask previously undetected alkaline reflux; 2) the facilitation of alkaline and bile reflux by a gastric emptying procedure that is often performed in conjunction with esophageal reconstruction; and 3) the decrease in antral motility due to vagotomy. The clinical importance of this reflux is not very great. Minimal gastritis is often observed in the stomach when it is used as an esophageal substitute, whereas no such inflammation is seen in the aboral end of interposition organs such as the colon and jejunum when the distal anastomosis is performed to the stomach.

Nutrition

The nutritional consequences of esophageal reconstruction are difficult to determine with accuracy. Patient groups are often diverse, and the high incidence of esophageal cancer as an indication for esophagectomy and reconstruction complicates the long-term evaluation of outcomes in these individuals. In patients who have had a stomach pull-up for reconstruction, discoordination between gastric emptying and bile secretion is manifested by a lag between the excretion of food from the stomach and release of bile into the bowels.[11] Whether this discoordination, in addition to the well-recognized problem of accelerated gastric empyting, contributes to symptoms of dumping in some patients postoperatively is unknown at the present time. Vitamin B_{12} absorption is normal in patients with an intrathoracic stomach.[11] Absorption of other nutrients and serum levels of total protein, albumin, transferrin, and lipids are normal and are independent of whether the stomach or colon is used as a reconstructive organ.[37,38] The only significant difference between use of the stomach or colon as an esophageal replacement is the maintenance of body weight. There appears to be a greater percent loss of body weight long-term in patients reconstructed with stomach than with colon, a difference that increases over time (Fig 7-6).[37,38] Similarly, swallowing function is better long-term in patients who undergo colon interposition as compared to gastric pull-up.[39]

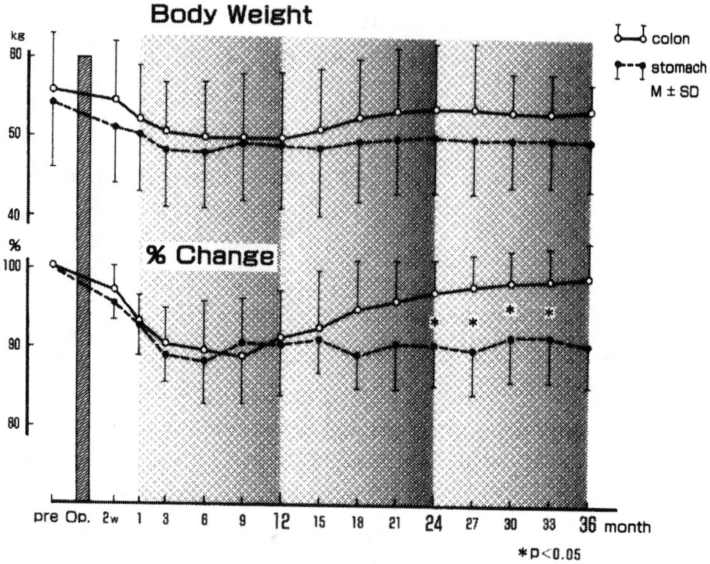

Figure 7-6. Relative weight over time of patients reconstructed with colon or stomach after esophagectomy. From Ando et al.[38]

Other

The long-term function of the reconstructive organ is more important to consider when performing an esophageal reconstruction for benign disease in a young patient than when constructing a replacement for an elderly patient with advanced cancer. Similar considerations regarding the technical difficulties of the actual operation and the resultant short-term complications are appropriate, because it is likely that a substantial short-term investment, consisting of a longer hospital stay or a greater risk of nonfatal complications, may be offset by better long-term results.

Summary

A synthesis of the various factors that contribute to outcome of esophageal replacement is summarized in Table 7-3. The factors include anatomic properties, functional characteristics, technical issues, and long-term outcome as assessed by weight maintenance and quality of life measurements. There are no published data on some of the categories for some of the replacement types, and these cells were filled by extrapolating from what is known about the function of other types of esophageal replacements. This table should not be used as a rigid guide for determining which type of reconstruction is optimal overall, because there are many

Table 7-3.
Scores for Short and Long Segment Esophageal Replacements.

	Valcular supply	Mortility	Gastric reservoir capacity	Size match	Length	Operative time	Technical difficulty	Acid/alkali	Emptying	Weight maintenance	Total score
Long Segment											
Whole Stomach	2	0	–2	1	2	2	2	1	0	1	9
Gastric Tube	2	0	–2	2	2	2	1	1	1	1	10
Reverse gastric tube	0	–1	–1	2	0	0	–2	1	0	1	0
Jejunum	–1	2	2	1	–2	–2	–2	2	1	2	3
Left + Transverse colon	0	0	2	0	1	0	0	2	1	2	8
Right + Transverse colon	–1	0	2	–1	1	0	0	2	1	2	6
Ileocolic segment	–1	0	2	0	1	0	0	2	1	2	7
Antiperistaltic left + transverse colon	0	–2	2	–1	1	0	0	2	–1	1	2
Short Segment											
Whole stomach	2	0	–1	1	2	2	2	–1	0	1	8
Gastric tube	2	0	–1	2	2	2	1	–1	1	1	9
Free jejunal graft	–2	2	2	2	0	–2	–2	0	1	2	3
Pedicled jejunal graft	0	2	2	1	1	0	–1	0	1	2	8
Left colon	1	0	2	0	2	0	0	0	1	2	8
Transverse colon	0	0	2	0	2	0	0	0	1	2	7
Right colon	0	0	2	–1	2	0	0	0	1	2	6

other variables that should enter into the decision-making process for an individual patient. In addition, differences of 1 or 2 points between weighted scores are unlikely to be significant. The table is of value, however, in assisting the surgeon in assessing the factors that should be considered when selecting an esophageal substitute, and the scores give an approximate ranking of desirability of each type of replacement.

For long segment replacements the gastric tube and whole stomach achieved the highest overall scores, followed closely by combined left and transverse colon and by the ileocolic segment. For short segment replacements the scores were more closely grouped, being led by gastric tube, whole stomach, pedicled jejunal graft, and left colon. These scores reflect two aspects of esophageal replacement that must be carefully balanced by the surgeon. The high scores for stomach used as a replacement are primarily based on its reliable blood supply and ease of use. The scores for colon and jejunal grafts are based more on maintenance of gastric reservoir capacity, relative resistance to gastric acid, and long-term maintenance of weight. Much of the selection among these possibilities remains dependent on the training and experience of the individual surgeon, characteristics for which there is no substitute.

References

1. Gavriliu D. The replacement of the oesophagus by a gastric tube. In **Surgery of the Oesophagus**. Jamieson GG (ed): Churchill Livingstone, New York, 1998, pp 65-775.
2. Tera H, Aberg C. Tissue holding power to a single suture in different parts of the alimentary tract. *Acta Chir Scand* 1976;142:343-348.
3. Furst H, Hartl WH, Lohe F, et al. Colon interposition for esophageal replacement. *Ann Surg* 2000;231:173-178.
4. Wilkins EW Jr. Long-segment colon substitution for the esophagus. *Ann Surg* 1980;192:722-725.
5. Cerfolio RJ, Allen MS, Deschamps C, et al. Esophageal replacement by colon interposition. *Ann Thorac Surg* 1995;59:1382-1384.
6. Read NW, Houghton LA. Physiology of gastric emptying and pathophysiology of gastroparesis. *Gastroenterol Clin N Am* 1989;18:359-373.
7. Keinke O, Ehrlein H-J. Effect of oleic acid on canine gastroduodenal motility, pyloric diameter and gastric emptying. *Q J Exp Physiol* 1983;68:675-686.
8. Little AG, Scott WJ, Ferguson MK, et al. Functional evaluation of organ interposition for esophageal replacement. In **Diseases of the Esophagus**. Siewert JR, Holscher AH (eds): Springer-Verlag, New York, 1988, pp 664-667.
9. Catrambone GN, Iurilli L, Parodi A, et al. A morphologic and functional study of the gastric tube as an esophageal substitute after esophagectomy for cancer. *Res Surg* 1989;1:136-141.
10. Bonavina L, Anselmino M, Ruol A, et al. Functional evaluation of the intrathoracic stomach as an oesophageal substitute. *Br J Surg* 1992;79:529-532.

11. Okada N, Sakurai T, Tsuchihashi S, et al. Gastric functions in patients with the intrathoracic stomach after esophageal surgery. *Ann Surg* 1986;204:114-121.
12. Holscher AH, Voit H, Siewert JR, et al. Function of the intrathoracic stomach. In **Diseases of the Esophagus**. Siewert JR, Holscher AH (eds): Springer-Verlag, New York, 1988, pp 660-663.
13. Morton KA, Karwande SV, Davis RK, et al. Gastric emptying after gastric interposition for cancer of the esophagus or hypopharynx. *Ann Thorac Surg* 1991;51:759-763.
14. Bemelman WA, Taat CW, Slors JFM, et al. Delayed postoperative emptying after esophageal resection is dependent on the size of the gastric substitute. *J Am Coll Surg* 1995;180:461-464.
15. Collard J-M, Romagnoli R, Otte J-B, et al. The denervated stomach as an esophageal substitute is a contractile organ. *Ann Surg* 1998;227:33-39.
16. Coral RP, Constant-Neto M, Velho AV, et al. Scintigraphic analysis of gastric emptying after esophagogastroanastomosis: Comparison of the anterior and posterior mediastinal approaches. *Dis Esoph* 1995;8:61-63.
17. Sarna SK. Physiology and pathophysiology of colonic motor activity. *Dig Dis Sci* 1991;36:827-862.
18. Sarna SK. Colonic motor activity. *Surg Clin N Am* 1993;73:1201-1223.
19. Corazziari E, Mineo TC, Anzini F, et al. Functional evaluation of colon transplants used in esophageal reconstruction. *Dig Dis* 1977;22:7-12.
20. Moreno Gonzalez E, Calleja Kempin IJ, Landa Garcia JI, et al. Functional study of ileocolic interposition after esophagectomy and total esophagogastrectomy. In: **Diseases of the Esophagus**. Siewert JR, Holscher AH (eds). Springer-Verlag, New York, 1988, pp 668-673.
21. Jones EL, Skinner DB, DeMeester TR, et al. Response of the interposed human colonic segment to an acid challenge. *Ann Surg* 1973;177:75-78.
22. Benages A, Moreno-Ossett E, Paris F, et al. Motor activity after colon replacement of esophagus. *J Thorac Cardiovasc Surg* 1981;82:335-340.
23. Neville WE, Najem AZ. Colon replacement of the esophagus for congenital and benign disease. *Ann Thor Surg* 1983;36:626-633.
24. Isolauri J, Koskinen MO, Markkula H. Radionuclide transit in patients with colon interposition. *J Thorac Cardiovasc Surg* 1987;94:521-525.
25. Kao C-H, Wang S-J, Chen C-Y, et al. The motility of interposition in patients with esophageal carcinoma after reconstructive esophageal surgery. *Clin Nucl Med* 1993;18:782-785.
26. DeMeester TR, Johansson K-E, Franze I, et al. Indications, surgical technique, and long-term functional results of colon interposition or bypass. *Ann Surg* 1988;208:460-474.
27. Sarna SK. Cyclic motor activity; migrating motor complex: 1985. *Gastroenterology* 1985;89:894-913.
28. Sarna SK, Soergel KH, Harig JM, et al. Spatial and temporal patterns of human jejunal contractions. *Am J Physiol* 1989;257:G423-G432.
29. Johnson CP, Sarna SK, Cowles VE, et al. Motor activity and transit in the autonomically denervated jejunum. *Am J Surg* 1994;167:80-88.
30. Gaissert HA, Mathisen DJ, Grillo HC, et al. Short-segment intestinal interposition of the distal esophagus. J Thorac Cardiovasc Surg 1993;106:860-867.

31. Nishihira T, Oe H, Sugawara K, et al. Reconstruction of the thoracic esophagus with jejunal pedicled segments for cancer of the thoracic esophagus. *Dis Esoph* 1995;8:30-39.
32. Wright C, Cuschieri A. Jejunal interposition for benign esophageal disease. *Ann Surg* 1987;205:54-60.
33. Hashimoto M, Imamura M, Shimada Y, et al. Twenty-four hour monitoring of pH in the gastric tube replacing the resected esophagus. *J Am Coll Surg* 1995;180:666-672.
34. Nishimura O, Naito Y, Yokoi H, et al. Radionuclide studies of the substituted stomach after esophageal surgery. *Dis Esoph* 1989;2:105-111.
35. Johansson J, Johnsson F, Groshen S, et al. Pharyngeal reflux after gastric pull-up esophagectomy with neck and chest anastomoses. *J Thorac Cardiovasc Surg* 1999;118:1078-1083.
36. Isolauri J, Helin H, Markkula H. Colon interposition for esophageal disease: Histologic findings of colonic mucosa after a follow-up of 5 months to 15 years. *Am J Gastroenterol* 1991;86:277-280.
37. Ando N, Ikehata Y, Ohmori T, et al. Prospective studies on postoperative nutritional status in patients with esophageal carcinoma as evaluated from various substitutes for reconstruction: Gastric tube versus colon interposition. In **Diseases of the Esophagus**. Siewert JR, Holscher AH (eds): Springer-Verlag, New York, 1988, pp 674-678.
38. Ando N, Shinozawa Y, Ikehata Y, et al. Postoperative nutritional status in patients with esophageal carcinoma. In **Diseases of the Esophagus, Volume I: Malignant Diseases**. Ferguson MK, Little AG, Skinner DB (eds): Futura Publishing Co., New York, 1990, pp 261-269.
39. Watson TJ, DeMeester TR, Kauer WKH, et al. Esophageal replacement for end-stage benign esophageal disease. *J Thorac Cardiovasc Surg* 1998;115:1241-1249.

Chapter 8

Routes for Esophageal Replacement

One of the important decisions that helps to determine the outcome after esophageal replacement surgery is the appropriate route for passage of the replacement organ or tissues. Although in some cases only one route is available for reconstruction, in most situations the surgeon can select from at least two options. The factors governing such decisions are outlined in this chapter.

Available Routes

Posterior Mediastinum

Among the options available as routes for esophageal reconstruction, the one most commonly used, particularly in the adult population, is the posterior mediastinal route, or the bed of the resected esophagus (Figure 8-1; Table 8-1). It is highly favored for a number of reasons. This route requires no specific preparation after esophagectomy, provides the straightest connection between the cervical esophagus or pharynx and the abdomen, and thus is the shortest of all available routes. Anatomic studies demonstrate that, in cadavers, this orthotopic route is 1.9 cm shorter than the substernal route and 3.7 cm shorter than the subcutaneous route.[1] The thoracic outlet is widest posteriorly, maximizing the space available for passage of the reconstructive organ (Figure 8-2). Placement of a reconstructive organ through this route minimizes cardiopulmonary compromise that can accompany use of the substernal route (see below). Long-term swallowing function is better in patients in whom an orthotopic route is used than in those with a substernal or antesternal reconstruc-

From Ferguson MK: *Reconstructive Surgery of the Esophagus* Armonk, NY: Futura Publishing Company, Inc., © 2002.

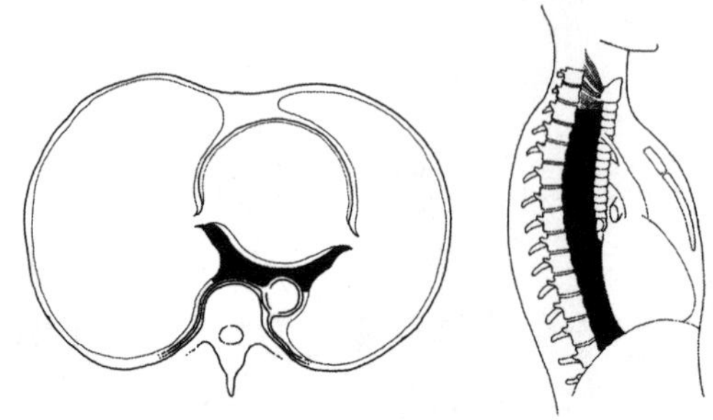

Figure 8-1. The posterior mediastinal route for esophageal reconstruction.

Table 8-1.
Routes for Esophageal Reconstruction.

Orthotopic	
	Posterior mediastinum (bed of resected esophagus)
Heterotopic	
	Retrosternal (substernal)
	Subcutaneous (antesternal)
	Right pleural space
	Left pleural space
Extra-anatomic	

tion.[2] Finally, use of the orthotopic route permits an anastomosis to be constructed at any level within the thorax or neck.

The posterior mediastinal route is not appropriate for reconstruction under certain circumstances. If an esophageal bypass is being performed and no esophagectomy has taken place, the route is not available for use. In some instances there is excess contamination or inflammation of the space, such as after urgent esophagectomy for perforation or caustic ingestion, which precludes safe use of the orthotopic route. In patients in whom a staged reconstruction is to be performed after esophagectomy, the posterior mediastinum will usually be too scarred and contracted to permit its development as a reconstructive route.

Substernal Space

The next most commonly used pathway for reconstruction is the substernal, or retrosternal, route (Figure 8-3). This is favored among many pediatric surgeons and by some adult surgeons for specific indications. Its primary perceived advantage in the pediatric population is greater potential space for the reconstructive organ than is available in the poste-

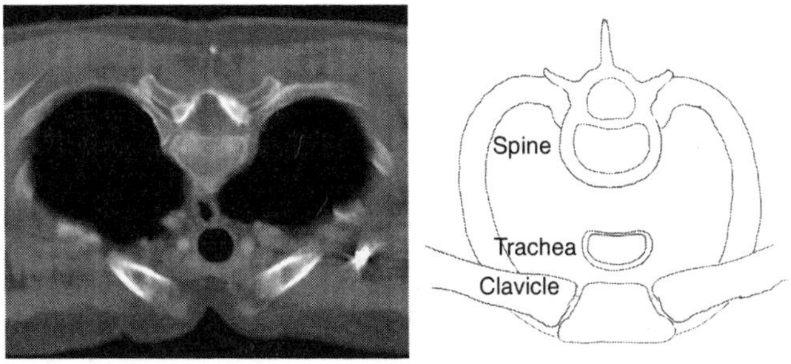

Figure 8-2. The thoracic inlet is widest posteriorly, and becomes relatively narrow in its anterior portion.

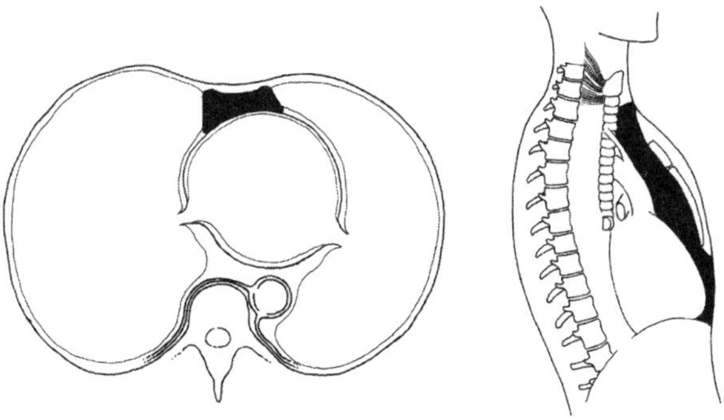

Figure 8-3. The substernal route for esophageal reconstruction.

rior mediastinum. In the adult population, the main advantages attend esophagectomy for malignancy. Since local recurrence rates are in excess of 30% in some series, there is a reasonable likelihood that such recurrences could compromise the function of the reconstructive organ, producing dysphagia.[3] In addition, there is concern that the postoperative administration of external beam radiotherapy could adversely affect motility and circulation of a reconstructive organ if it is placed orthotopically. Finally, fistula formation between the reconstructive organ and airway can sometimes form as a result of recurrent disease or benign ulceration. Positioning the reconstructive organ in the substernal route obviates these risks.

Drawbacks to use of the substernal route are numerous. When this route is used, the vast majority of patients will undergo a cervical anastomosis, which requires the reconstructive organ to traverse a longer distance to reach the cervical esophagus than when the orthotopic route is used.[1] Some authors report that emptying of a gastric pull-up is slower when it is in the retrosternal position than when it is in the orthotopic position, although there is not general agreement on this.[4-6] These factors help explain why the substernal route is associated with a higher incidence of anastomotic leak and operative mortality compared to the orthotopic route.[7,8]

There is a higher incidence of dysphagia in patients with retrosternal reconstructions compared to those with orthotopic reconstructions.[9] This is related to a 60% incidence of a manometrically-identified high pressure zone distal to the cricopharyngeus and may be due to angulation of the conduit as it passes from the posterior cervical space to the retrosternal space or to the somewhat restrictive size of the thoracic inlet anteriorly. This angulation may also make it difficult to perform dilations in the intermediate postoperative period if an anastomotic stricture should develop. In some patients, it is necessary to resect a portion of the manubrium and the left clavicular head to provide sufficient space for passage of the reconstructive organ. Angulation also occurs across the transition from the retrosternal space to the abdomen, which is another potential site for delayed passage of ingested material.[6] Potential sites for the anastomosis are generally limited to the cervical esophagus or pharynx, although intrathoracic anastomoses can be performed through a sternotomy when necessary.

Cardiopulmonary function is compromised by a substernal interposition during the early postoperative period to a much greater extent than is evident after orthotopic reconstruction. Patients with a substernal interposition experience significantly decreased stroke volume and cardiac indices and increased intrapulmonary shunt during the first two postoperative days compared to patients with a posterior mediastinal reconstruction. This is associated with a longer intensive care unit stay for patients with a retrosternal reconstruction and is also a likely factor influencing the increased mortality rate in these patients.[8] Blood flow to the substernal interposition may be adversely affected by positive pressure ventilation in patients who routinely are left intubated postoperatively or who require ventilatory support for respiratory insufficiency.[10]

Subcutaneous (Antesternal) Space

Although this route has been used extensively in the past for esophageal reconstruction, there are few indications for its current use (Figure 8-4). There are a few potential advantages provided by this pathway. No entry into the thorax is necessary for reconstruction, which may benefit patients with severe underlying pulmonary disease, extensive intrathoracic adhesions, or widespread inflammation from causes such as esophageal perforation. Because there is no intrathoracic reconstructive organ, there is no pressure on intrathoracic organs causing cardiopulmonary compromise. Use of this route is associated with a lower incidence of prolonged postoperative ventilation than occurs after reconstruction using the posterior mediastinal or substernal routes.[11] In patients in whom a substantial length of esophagus is available proximal to the anastomosis,

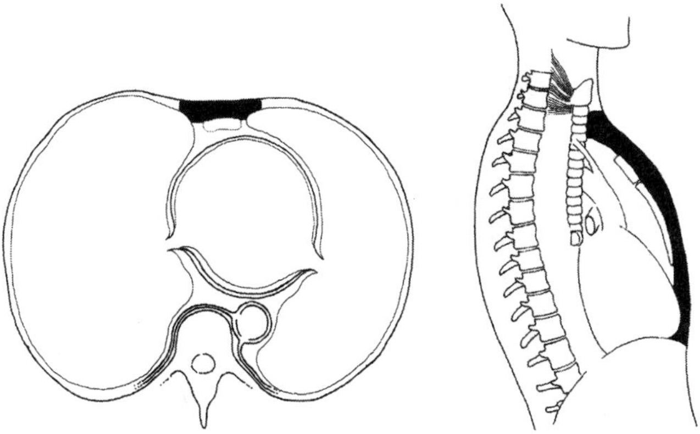

Figure 8-4. The subcutaneous, or antesternal, route for esophageal reconstruction.

and in whom the posterior mediastinal route cannot be used, or in patients in whom a complex reconstruction is necessary, the antesternal route permits the creation of an anastomosis at any level by opening the overlying skin flap. Finally, the subcutaneous route provides easy access to the reconstructive organ for assessment of its viability, drainage of anastomotic leaks, or other ancillary surgical procedures.

There are many drawbacks to the use of the antesternal route. This is the longest of all pathways for reconstruction and therefore requires a greater length of reconstructive organ. This fact also engenders more tension on the anastomosis, possibly leading to a higher incidence of anastomotic leak. The acute angulation necessary for the reconstructive organ or esophagus to pass from the prevertebral cervical space to the antesternal space is greater than for any other route, and creates a relative obstruction to the passage of ingested material. This angulation also makes it difficult to perform dilation in the intermediate postoperative period if an anastomotic stricture develops. Angulation is also present across the transition between the subcutaneous space to the abdomen, and this is often a site of delayed passage of ingested material. The potential space in which the reconstructive organ is situated is almost unlimited, creating the opportunity for substantial dilatation and/or redundancy of reconstructive organs such as colon interpositions (Figure 8-5). The cosmetic drawbacks of this route are self-evident.

Other

A variety of other routes have been used for reconstruction sporadically but are generally impractical for routine use. The pleural spaces may be used for the reconstructive organ, although they necessitate a

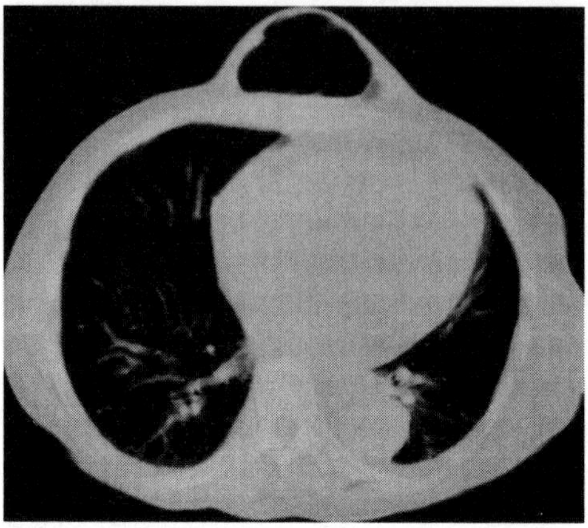

Figure 8-5. The subcutaneous pathway is associated with a large potential space, which may permit dilatation and redundancy in reconstructive organs over long periods of time.

longer length of reconstructive organ than is necessary for any of the other routes. Use of this pathway is relegated almost entirely to highly selected patients in the pediatric population. There has been interest in creating an artificial esophagus since the first successful esophagectomy was performed. Modern-day counterparts to the rubber tubes that were initially used to connect the cervical esophagus to the stomach have been devised from silicone and other materials. Such devices have always been placed in an extra-anatomic location to avoid foreign body reaction and erosion into surrounding structures that would almost certainly accompany their passage through any of the normal anatomic routes (see Chapter 13).

Influence of Reconstructive Organs

It is important to recognize that some organs used for reconstruction of the esophagus are not suitable for use through all reconstructive routes. For example, the jejunum and ileum have a segmental blood supply which permits replacement of a short esophageal segment in the posterior mediastinum with ease, whereas longer segment replacements are usually technically difficult to prepare. This prohibits use of the substernal or antesternal routes for an intestinal interposition, except under special circumstances and in the most experienced of hands. Similar caveats pertain to use of the colon, although the blood supply to the colon is more reliable and long grafts are much easier to prepare. Because the stomach has the potential to easily reach to the neck under most circumstances, its use as an esophageal replacement is most common. The stomach can usually be adapted to all the potential routes for reconstruction.

Influence of Anastomotic Level

Although most esophageal anastomoses for reconstruction are performed in the neck, under a variety of circumstances alternative routes or techniques need to be considered. When using the stomach as a reconstructive organ, if the patient has already undergone a partial gastrectomy, or if a greater extent of gastric resection is necessitated by the extent of the disease process leading to esophageal reconstruction, the surgeon may be required to perform an anastomosis other than in the neck. Similarly, if a partial colectomy has been performed, or the blood supply to a segment of colon to be used for interposition is compromised, one option is to use a shorter segment of colon and perform the anastomosis at a lower level.

The posterior mediastinal route permits creation of an anastomosis at any level. The long-term consequences of an intrathoracic anastomosis compared to a cervical anastomosis are indistinguishable.[12] The surgical approach to the posterior mediastinum is important, however, since not all of the esophagus can be easily reached through a single incision. For patients undergoing a right thoracotomy, the most distal esophagus, just above the diaphragmatic hiatus, is difficult to visualize. Similarly, for patients undergoing a left thoracotomy, the esophagus at and above the level of the aortic arch is generally inaccessible for purposes of performing an anastomosis.

The retrosternal route permits an anastomosis only in the cervical region under most circumstances. It is feasible to do a partial or complete sternotomy to provide access to a substernal reconstructive organ for purposes of creating an anastomosis, but this exposes the patient to the risk of a sternal wound infection. In general, this approach should be avoided if an alternate technique for creating an intrathoracic anastomosis can be used.

The antesternal route provides easy access to the cervical region for an anastomosis. Alternatively, anastomoses may be created inferior to this by incising the skin over the subcutaneous tunnel.

Techniques for Creating Routes for Reconstruction

Posterior Mediastinal Route

After an esophagectomy has been completed, no additional surgery is usually necessary to further prepare the posterior mediastinal route to accept a reconstructive organ. However, there are a few considerations which may facilitate performance of the reconstruction or improve postoperative function. In some patients it is difficult to judge with accuracy the appropriate length of reconstructive organ to leave in the thorax. Excess length is not usually a problem when a transhiatal operation is performed and both pleura are left intact, since the pleura confine the reconstructive organ to the mediastinum. However, when the operation is performed transthoracically, the reconstructive organ tends to migrate into the hemithorax through which the operation was done. The aortic arch forms a natural boundary on the left which prevents migration into the left hemithorax at that level. A similar effect can be achieved by preserving the azygos arch during esophagectomy, which prevents migration of the reconstructive organ into the upper right hemithorax. The more distal intrathoracic portion of a reconstructive organ may be similarly confined to the mediastinum by closure of the overlying pleura, although this is often not possible after esophagectomy for cancer, which typically includes removal of large segments of the parietal pleura.

Substernal Route

Creation of a retrosternal route for esophageal reconstruction is performed with the patient in the supine position. The fascia underlying the xiphoid process is opened sharply, exposing the substernal space. Ultimately, this opening must be wide enough to permit passage of the surgeon's entire hand. The surgeon's fingers are positioned in a wedge shape centered on the posterior aspect of the sternum and the soft tissues are bluntly dissected from the sternum (Figure 8-6). Care should be taken not to extend the tunnel too far laterally, since there is risk of damage to the internal thoracic vessels which could cause bleeding necessitating a sternotomy to gain control.

A low cervical incision is performed either transversely or along the border of the sternocleidomastoid muscle. Most surgeons prefer to do this in the left neck. A left neck anastomosis is technically easier to perform because the esophagus presents more to the left at this level and the risk of recurrent laryngeal nerve injury may be less than if the reconstruction was performed in the right neck.[13] After completing the esophageal dissection, it is often useful to divide the strap muscles which are attached to the manubrium (sternothyroid, sternohyoid) to open the substernal space at this level. The blunt dissection is then continued upwards from below until the surgeon is able to pass at least three fingers into the cervical wound. This maneuver should be performed expeditiously, since the surgeon's forearm is likely to cause compression of the heart. An umbilical tape is grasped in the surgeon's exposed fingers and is drawn back down the completed route for purposes of reconstruction. The hiatus is closed

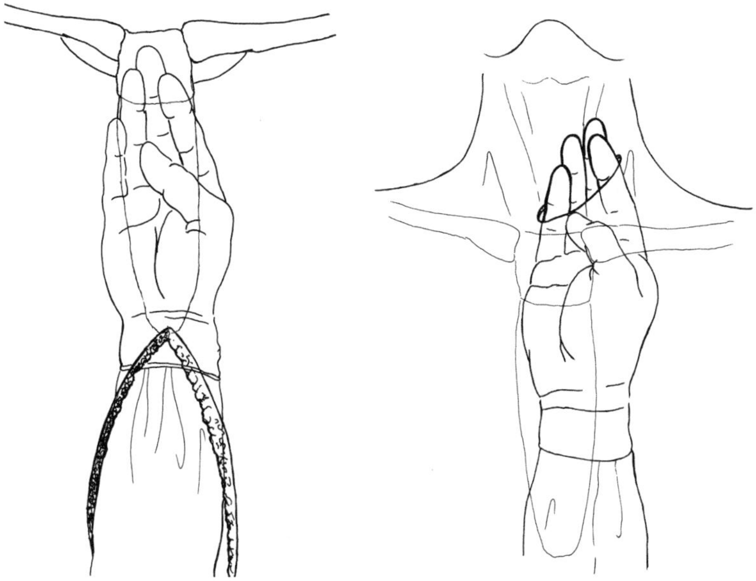

Figure 8-6. Creation of a retrosternal route for esophageal reconstruction is done easily with the tips of the fingers of the surgeon's open hand (left). It is important to ensure an adequate passageway through the thoracic inlet. One way to do this is for the surgeon to pass at least three fingers through this space from below (right).

with interrupted sutures to prevent herniation of abdominal contents into the posterior mediastinum.

If there is inadequate space for the surgeon to pass several fingers into the cervical wound, the thoracic inlet may be too narrow and would compromise the reconstructive organ. In this situation, it is useful to consider resecting a portion of the manubrium and the head of the left clavicle to open the thoracic inlet further. After mobilizing the clavicle circumferentially at the junction of its medial and middle thirds, the bone is divided with a Gigli saw. The upper outer portion of the manubrium is resected en bloc with the clavicular head using a sternal saw or a Lebschke knife while preserving the subclavian vessels and the articulation between the manubrium and the first rib (Figure 8-7).[14]

Antesternal Route

Creation of a subcutaneous route for esophageal reconstruction is straightforward. A subcutaneous tunnel is started at the level of the xiphoid process, making the opening large enough to accommodate the surgeon's entire hand. Blunt and sharp dissection are used to develop the space superiorly. Care is taken not to develop the tunnel too far laterally,

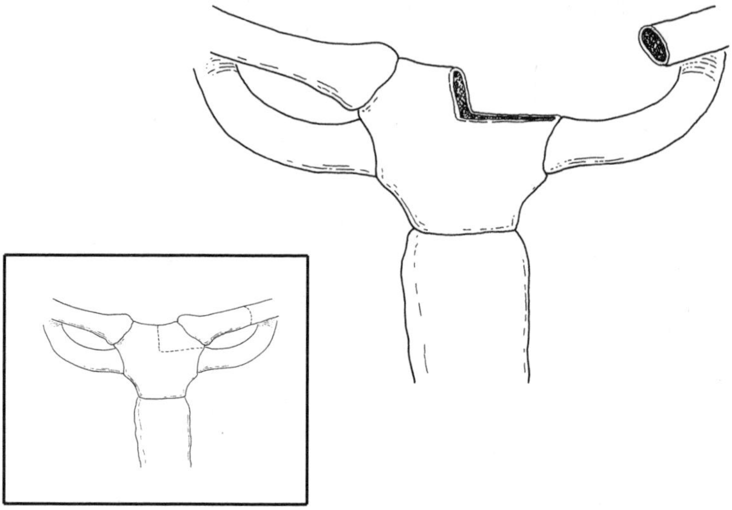

Figure 8-7. Resection of the clavicular head and a portion of the manubrium sometimes is necessary to provide sufficient space at the thoracic inlet for passage of a reconstructive organ through a substernal route.

which may result in injury to perforating vessels from the pectoralis muscles. A lighted blade retractor facilitates this dissection. A cervical incision is made. It is usually necessary to divide the sternocleidomastoid muscle to provide an adequate space for the esophagus and reconstructive organ to pass from the posterior cervical region to the subcutaneous plane. The surgeon's hand is passed into the cervical wound to ensure that an adequate cross-sectional area has been prepared. An umbilical tape is grasped by the surgeon's exposed fingers and is drawn back down the completed route for purposes of reconstruction. The hiatus is closed with interrupted sutures to prevent herniation of abdominal contents into the posterior mediastinum.

References

1. Ngan SY, Wong J. Lengths of different routes for esophageal replacement. *J Thorac Cardiovasc Surg* 1986;91:790-792.
2. Kuwano H, Ikebe M, Baba K, et al. Operative procedures of reconstruction with resection of esophageal cancer and the postoperative quality of life. *World J Surg* 1993;17:773-776.
3. van Lanschot JJB, Hop WCJ, Voormolen MHJ, et al. Quality of palliation and possible benefit of extra-anatomic reconstruction in recurrent dysphagia after resection of carcinoma of the esophagus. *J Am Coll Surg* 1994;179:705-713.

4. Gawad KA, Hosch SB, Bumann D, et al. How important is the route of reconstruction after esophagectomy: A prospective randomized study. *Am J Gastroenterol* 1999;94:1490-1496.
5. Imada T, Ozawa Y, Minamide J, et al. Gastric emptying after gastric interposition for esophageal carcinoma: Comparison between the anterior and posterior mediastinal approaches. *Hepato-gastroenterol* 1998;45:2224-2227.
6. Coral RP, Constant-Neto M, Velho AV, et al. Scintigraphic analysis of gastric emptying after esophagogastroanastomosis: Comparison of the anterior and posterior mediastinal approaches. *Dis Esoph* 1995;8:61-63.
7. Hirai T, Iwata T, Yamashita Y, et al. Investigation of suitability of devascularized upper half of the whole stomach as replacement for the esophagus. *Hiroshima J Med Sci* 1992;41:25-30.
8. Bartels H, Thorban S, Siewert JR. Anterior versus posterior reconstruction after transhiatal oesophagectomy: A randomized controlled trial. *Br J Surg* 1993;80:1141-1144.
9. Shiraha S, Matsumoto H, Terada M, et al. Motility studies of the cervical esophagus with intrathoracic gastric conduit after esophagectomy. *Scand J Thorac Cardiovasc Surg* 1992;26:119-123.
10. Jacob L, Boudaoud S, Rabary O, et al. Decreased mesenteric blood flow supplying retrosternal esophageal ileocoloplastic grafts during positive-pressure breathing. *J Thorac Cardiovasc Surg* 1994;107:68-73.
11. Tsutsui S, Moriguchi S, Morita M, et al. Multivariate analysis of postoperative complications after esophageal resection. *Ann Thorac Surg* 1992;53:1052-1056.
12. Ribet M, Debrueres B, Lecomte-Houcke M. Resection for advanced cancer of the thoracic esophagus: Cervical or thoracic anastomosis? *J Thorac Cardiovasc Surg* 1992;103:784-789.
13. Liebermann-Meffert DMI, Walbrun B, Hiebert CA, et al. Recurrent and superior laryngeal nerves: A new look with implications for the esophageal surgeon. *Ann Thorac Surg* 1999;67:217-223.
14. Orringer MB, Sloan H. Substernal gastric bypass of the excluded thoracic esophagus for palliation of esophageal carcinoma. *J Thorac Cardiovasc Surg* 1975;70:836-851.

Chapter 9

The Stomach as a Reconstructive Organ

The stomach is the organ most commonly used for replacing the esophagus. Its advantages are numerous and include ready availability, technical ease of use, a reliable blood supply, and good postoperative function. There are a number of different techniques that are currently in use for preparing the stomach, which dictate to some extent the postoperative function of the reconstruction. This chapter summarizes important anatomic and technical details related to use of the stomach for esophageal reconstruction.

Anatomy

The stomach is a hollow seromuscular organ that extends from the esophagogastric junction to the pylorus. Grossly, it is made up of the cardia, the fundus, the body (corpus), and the antrum (Figure 9-1). There are no well-defined anatomic boundaries that permit clear recognition of these regions.[1] The dimensions of the stomach vary depending in part on the sex and race of the patient. Even though Asians are, on average, shorter than their Caucasian counterparts, they have a longer greater curvature (45 cm compared to 40 cm) but have a shorter lesser curvature (17 cm compared to 23 cm).[2,3] Interestingly, the pylorus is much more mobile in the Japanese population than in the Caucasian population, frequently being able to reach above the level of the hiatus after complete mobilization.

Beneath the serosa the smooth muscle is comprised of three layers: outer longitudinal, middle circular, and inner oblique. The inner oblique layer is absent along the lesser curvature. For practical purposes, the

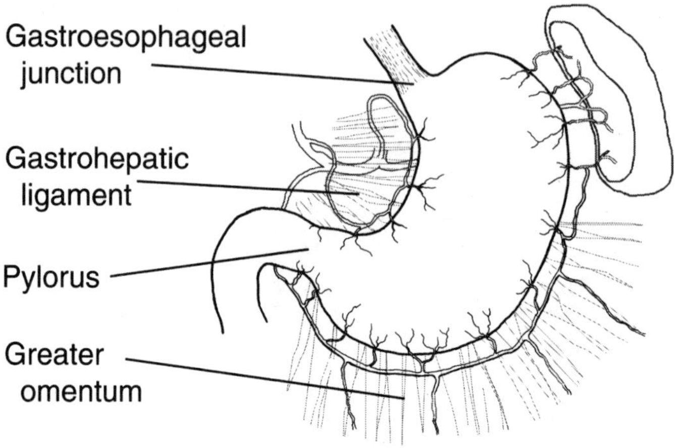

Figure 9-1. The external anatomy of the stomach.

muscle layers are fused. The gastric body usually contains rugal folds which flatten and disappear in the antrum.

There are two types of gastric mucosa: parietal and antral. Parietal mucosa, which is found in the body and fundus, contains parietal and chief cells which secrete acid and pepsin, respectively, and the mucosal surface is acidic. Antral mucosa contains mucous cells and the G cells that secrete gastrin, and there are few parietal and chief cells, resulting in a neutral or slightly alkaline mucosal surface.

The sympathetic innervation of the stomach originates from the preganglionic efferent fibers (fifth or sixth to ninth or tenth thoracic segments) which join the greater splanchnic nerves and ultimately reach the celiac ganglia. There they synapse with postglanglionic fibers that reach the stomach. The afferent system consists of a single neuron that returns along the same pathway and serves as the pathway for sensation of visceral pain. Parasympathetic innervation is supplied solely by the vagus nerves.[4] Preganglionic efferent vagal fibers reach the foregut directly via the right and left vagus nerves which form an esophageal plexus, from which emerge the anterior and posterior vagal trunks. The anterior trunk gives rise to an anterior gastric division (nerve of Latarjet) and an hepatic division, whereas the posterior trunk gives rise to a posterior gastric division and a celiac division.

The arterial blood supply to the stomach arises from four sources: the left gastric artery, the short gastric arteries and left gastroepiploic system, the right gastroepiploic artery, and the right gastric artery (Figure 9-2). There is an extensive submucosal plexus of vessels that provides communication between the major arteries supplying the greater and lesser curves of the stomach.[5,6] Gastric mobilization for reconstruction

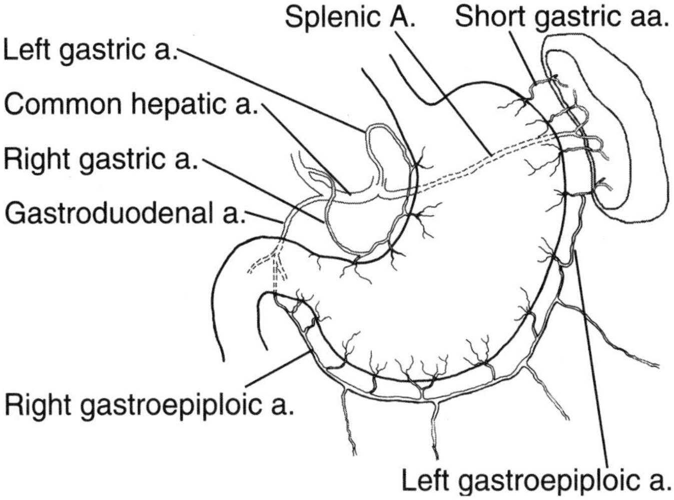

Figure 9-2. The arterial blood supply to the stomach.

often requires division of the left gastric artery. When this is done, the majority of blood flow to the stomach comes from the right gastroepiploic artery, which gets flow equally from the gastroduodenal artery (via the celiac axis through the common hepatic artery) and from the superior mesenteric artery through the pancreaticoduodenal vessels.[3,7] There is sometimes a small communication between the right and left gastroepiploic vessels, although this is often located intramurally and is completely absent in about two-thirds of patients.[8] The right gastric artery contributes little to blood flow in the mobilized stomach. It is important to note that the left gastric artery gives rise to an aberrant left hepatic artery in nearly 10% of patients.[9,10] Division of the left gastric artery in such patients proximal to the take off of the aberrant left hepatic artery may result in necrosis of the left lobe of the liver. Arteriosclerosis of the gastric arterial supply is very uncommon, even among patients with coronary artery atherosclerosis.[11,12] The venous drainage parallels the arterial supply and has few major variations.

Types of Gastric Preparations for Esophageal Replacement

A host of techniques for preparing the stomach as an esophageal substitute have been described, although only two are in common use. The most common stomach preparation used in western medicine is the gastric tube, which is constructed from the greater curvature of the stom-

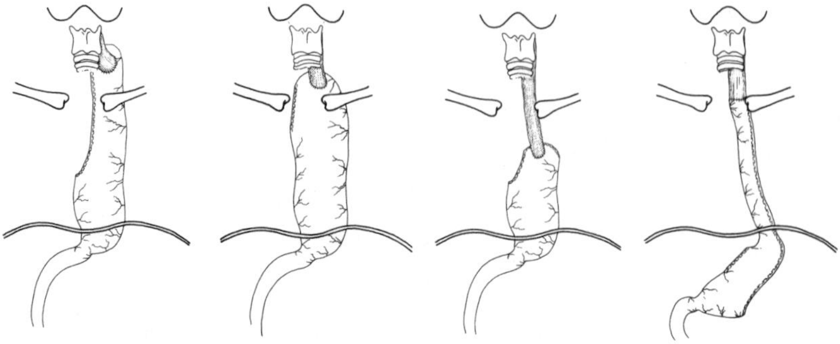

Figure 9-3. Types of stomach preparations used for esophageal replacement.

ach (Figure 9-3). Alternatively, the whole stomach may be used as an esophageal substitute. The advantages of these types of substitutes are ease of preparation, good long-term function, motility patterns which progress in an aboral direction when present, and, most importantly, a reliable blood supply (Table 9-1).

Alternate forms of tubularized stomach have been described but are not in common use. These include the historically important reversed gastric tube, as well as a variety of techniques for use of the greater curvature to create isoperistaltic tubes for esophageal reconstruction. One potential advantage of these tubes is increased length compared to standard gastric tubes, although for some preparations this is not the case. In addition, resection of a large portion of the gastric body may eliminate areas of potential ischemia. Use of the reversed gastric tube may also preserve the gastric reservoir capacity, minimizing the risk of dumping symptoms in some patients. The drawbacks to use of these types of gastric tube preparations include increased technical difficulties, unnecessary resection of large portions of the gastric body in some cases, a long suture/staple line that is at increased risk for leakage (especially in the reversed gastric tube preparation), and a more tenuous blood supply due to loss of portions of the submucosal plexus that feed the gastric fundus. In general, these drawbacks outweigh most potential advantages for use of the more exotic gastric tubes except under special circumstances.

Postoperative Function of Gastric Conduits

Performance of a vagotomy has important effects on gastric blood flow and function. In animals, vagotomy results in an immediate decrease

Table 9-1.
Scores for Advantages and Disadvantages of Different Types of Gastric Preparations for Esophageal Reconstruction.

	Length	Technical Ease	Vascular Supply	Gastric Reservoir	Aboral Motility
Standard tube	2	2	1	0	1
Whole stomach	2	3	1	1	1
Reversed tube	0	–1	0	2	0
Greater curve tube	–1	–1	–1	2	1
Extended greater curve tube	1	–1	–1	1	0

in blood flow of over 35%, a value which persists for many weeks after vagotomy.[13] There is normally basal gastric tone which is under vagal control.[14] The enterogastric reflex in which duodenal distention results in relaxation of normal gastric tone is under vagal control and is abolished by vagotomy.[15,16] Nutrients within the small bowel (fats in the proximal jejunum, carbohydrates and protein in the distal small intestine) also cause a reflex relaxation of gastric tone which is vagally mediated and presumably is lost after vagotomy.[17,18] Gastric fundic distension causes inhibition of migrating motor complexes in the gastric antrum, duodenum, and proximal jejunum which is vagally mediated and is abolished by vagotomy.[19] Thus, vagotomy disrupts not only enterogastric reflexes, but gastroenteral reflexes as well. However, it should be noted that the denervated stomach is also able to coordinate activity with the small intestine through hormonal factors such as motilin, and that intrinsic gastric relaxation in response to food may be due to release of nitric oxide in addition to direct neural stimulation.[20-22]

The combination of vagotomy and resection of a substantial portion of acid producing gastric mucosa in order to create a gastric tube for esophageal reconstruction does not result in increased levels of intragastric pH. Long-term monitoring demonstrates that pH within a gastric tube is consistently below 3, and often achieves levels sufficient to optimize pepsin activity.[23-25] Gastric acid secretion is sometimes reduced but appears to return to normal more than 3 years postoperatively. Similarly, serum gastrin levels are initially increased but gradually return towards normal several years postoperatively.[26]

The relationship between gastric and biliary tract activity is disrupted after esophageal reconstruction with a gastric tube. Regardless of whether a pyloroplasty is performed, there is evidence for duodenogastric reflux of bile which is associated with postprandial discomfort and bilious eructation.[23,27,28] In addition, there is delayed release of bile into the small intestine after excretion of food from the stomach, regardless of the time interval after the operation.[26,29,30]

Gastric intrinsic factor production remains normal after esophageal resection and reconstruction with stomach. Vitamin B_{12} absorption is usually satisfactory, but in some patients may be abnormally low, possibly owing to reasons other than surgical reconstruction.[26,31]

Gastric emptying after esophageal reconstruction with the stomach is dependent on a number of different factors, including the size of the stomach, the route used for reconstruction, and possibly whether an emptying procedure is performed (see Chapter 14). Patients who have undergone esophagectomy and reconstruction with stomach have emptying patterns in the semi-upright position that are preserved compared to their preoperative patterns.[24] However, compared to normal people, gastric emptying after esophageal reconstruction with the stomach is delayed in the supine position and is more rapid in the upright position.[23,32-34] The tubularized stomach empties more readily than does the whole stomach when either is used as an esophageal replacement.[35]

There is some discrepancy among findings regarding the motility of the stomach when it is used as an esophageal substitute. Most authors believe that the stomach behaves as an inert tube, with emptying occurring as a result of gravity, and report little or no spontaneous motor activity at rest or during meals.[23,36,37] These findings have been disputed by others who contend that the denervated stomach is dynamic and exhibits denervation supersensitivity to prokinetic agents.[38] Gastric reservoir capacity is greater when the whole stomach is used, and the whole stomach appears more likely to regain motor activity several years postoperatively than is a gastric tube.[39,40]

Long-term (1 or more years post-operatively), the quality of life experienced by patients who have undergone esophageal reconstruction with stomach is good. In one study, 86% of patients reported excellent or very good functional results.[41] Ninety percent of patients had a stable weight, fewer than 5% had postprandial fullness or dumping symptoms, and fewer than 10% had diarrhea. However, almost 15% reported dysphagia, and over 20% had heartburn or regurgitation. In patients evaluated 3 years postoperatively, the average symptom rating was 7 out of a possible 10 compared to quality of life prior to the onset of disease.[42] After a 5-year postoperative interval, quality of life in other groups of patients was similar to the national norm.[43,44] However, over 50% of patients had symptoms of reflux and dumping, more than 25% had dysphagia, and fewer than 20% were asymptomatic. After 10 years, the chronic nature of the continuing digestive symptoms may become more apparent, with one-third of patients being dissatisfied with their amount of food intake, nearly half experiencing reflux symptoms, and a large percentage dying of pneumonia or malnutrition.[45]

Operative Techniques

Most operations for esophageal reconstruction are currently performed using open techniques. In the future, however, it is likely that such operations will be performed routinely using minimally invasive techniques, including laparoscopy and thoracoscopy. The techniques described herein refer primarily to the anatomic preparation of the stomach as a reconstructive organ and do not refer to specific surgical techniques. Thus, the general principles can be applied easily to either open or minimally invasive approaches, depending on the skill and experience of the surgeon.

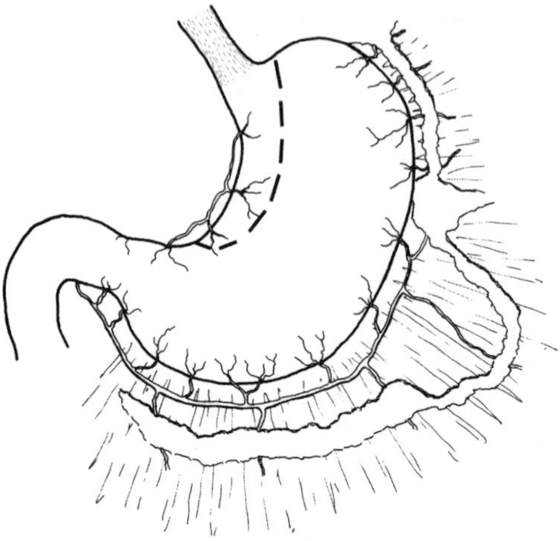

Figure 9-4. Mobilization of the greater curve of the stomach entails dividing the omentum from the stomach while preserving the right gastroepiploic vessels. A pedicle of omentum may be preserved near the terminal end of the right gastroepiploic vessels for use in wrapping the anastomosis.

Standard gastric tube

The stomach is mobilized by first dividing the omentum from the stomach along the greater curve, taking care to preserve the right gastroepiploic artery. The dissection is begun several centimeters from the region of the pylorus and is continued to the patient's left. This can be performed with a mechanical ligating and stapling device, using electrocautery for most of the tissues and ligating larger vessels, or with the harmonic scalpel. Whether the omentum should be resected from the colon as well is a matter of some dispute. Some surgeons recommend that it be discarded due to concerns about its viability and because it may harbor metastatic disease when esophagectomy is being performed for malignancy. However, most surgeons leave the omentum in situ, wherein it may provide tissue to buttress suture lines if necessary. A small pedicle of omentum may be preserved near the terminal end of the right gastroepiploic vessels for use in wrapping the esophagogastric anastomosis (Figure 9-4). A search for suitable communicating vessels between the right and left gastroepiploic arteries is appropriate, but from a practical standpoint there is rarely such a vessel that is worth preserving. Thus, the dissection of the omentum from the stomach usually terminates on a bare area of the stomach between the distribution of these two arcades, which is at a point roughly two-thirds of the way along the greater curvature as measured from the pylorus.

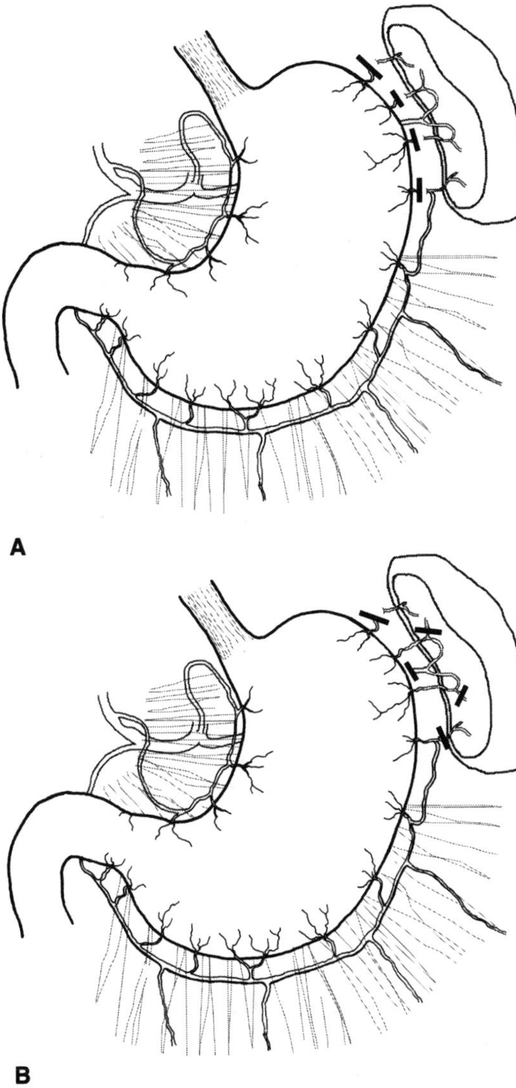

Figure 9-5. Division of the left gastroepiploic and short gastric vessels close to the stomach (**A**). Preservation of these vessels for vascular reconstruction requires sacrifice of the spleen (**B**).

The left gastroepiploic vessels and the short gastric arteries are routinely divided close to the gastric serosa to prevent injury to the spleen. On occasion, these vessels may be divided close to the splenic hilum to preserve communications amongst them, which necessitates splenectomy (Figure 9-5). Alternatively, most of the length of one or two of the short gastric vessels can be preserved without sacrifice of the spleen. These techniques permit the anastomosis of the short gastric vessels to internal mammary vessels or neck vessels after the stomach is brought up for reconstruction in order to optimize the blood supply to the proximal stomach.[46-49]

The lesser curve of the stomach is mobilized by dividing the gastrohepatic omentum close to the liver. Careful inspection of this structure is necessary as the diaphragm is approached because there often is a large inferior diaphragmatic artery present which ascends from the left gastric artery and must be ligated. Palpation may also reveal the presence of an aberrant left hepatic artery, the management of which is detailed below.

The stomach is elevated, exposing the pedicle containing the left gastric artery and coronary vein. The celiac axis is palpated, and the course of the splenic, hepatic, and left gastric arteries is outlined. The coronary vein and left gastric artery are each divided near the origin of the left gastric artery. If an aberrant left hepatic artery is found arising from the left gastric artery, the left gastric artery is divided distal to this to preserve blood supply to the left lobe of the liver. Retroperitoneal attachments are divided to the level of the crura, completing the mobilization of the stomach.

A Kocher maneuver is usually performed unless reconstruction is planned for replacement of only the distal esophagus. Care is taken to avoid injury to the portal structures. This usually provides sufficient mobility that the pylorus can reach to near the esophageal hiatus. If additional length of stomach is necessary, the right gastric artery is also divided.

The lesser curve of the stomach is resected to create the gastric tube (Figure 9-6). The proximal limit of the line of the resection is based in part on the amount of stomach that must be removed to treat malignancy if this is the reason necessitating the esophagectomy. A minimum distal margin of 5 cm from the gross extent of tumor is usually sufficient, although some authors who advocate a radical resection of the esophagus recommend a 10-cm margin.[50-52] The fundus is usually left untouched since it is the most proximal part of the stomach and its preservation ensures that the maximum length of gastric tube will be available. The width of the gastric tube that is created measures 8 to 10 cm, and this dictates the direction of the line of resection distally. Creation of a narrower tube risks injury to the extensive intramural vascular network and may compromise the blood supply to the gastric fundus.[53,54] A point on the lesser curve is selected between vessels entering the serosa, and this is cleared of surrounding tissue. This point is dictated in most instances by the need to clear lesser curvature lymph nodes as part of a cancer operation. If a point is selected just distal to the fifth branch of the left gastric artery along the lesser curve, over 90% of the potentially involved lesser curvature nodes will be resected.[55] Additional length may be gained by incising the seromuscular layer before applying the linear-cutting stapler (Figure 9-7).[56,57] The resection line is most easily created with a

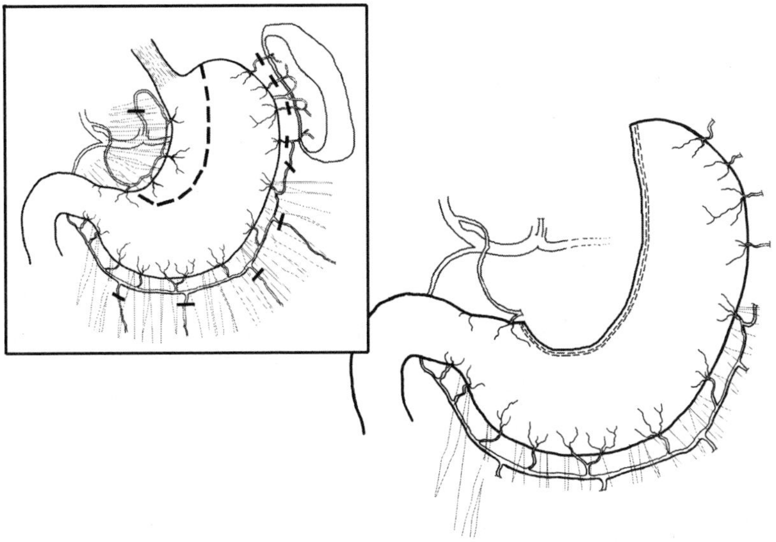

Figure 9-6. Creation of a standard tube from the greater curvature of the stomach.

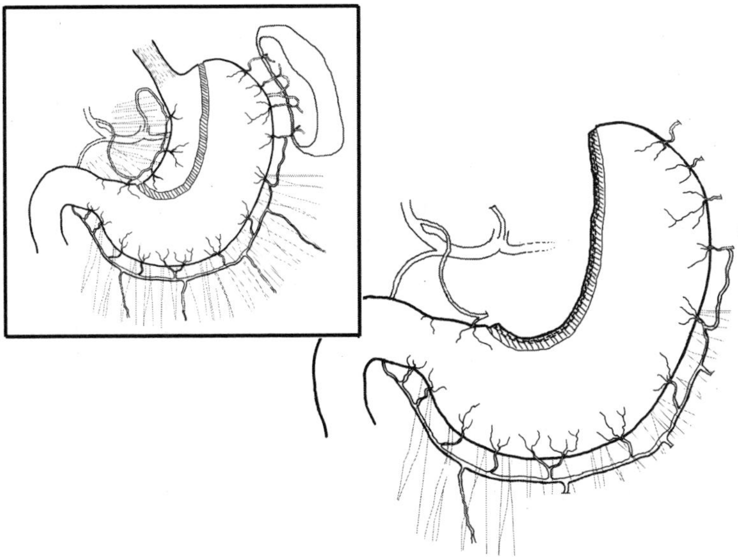

Figure 9-7. Lengthening of a standard gastric tube may be accomplished by dividing the seromuscular layer, which adds an additional 5 cm of length to the preparation in experimental studies.

linear-cutting stapler, although resection along clamps with subsequent suture closure is also sometimes performed. The staple line is imbricated with a running suture to reinforce it and to help prevent adhesions from forming to the raw surface of the staple line.

Whole Stomach

Whole stomach preparations are used most appropriately for reconstruction after resection of tumors of the mid-thoracic, upper-thoracic, and cervical esophagus, after pharyngectomy for management of head and neck cancer, and after resection for benign disease. In these situations there is no issue about the adequacy of the distal margin of resection.

The stomach is mobilized from the omentum while preserving the right gastroepiploic arcade as described above. The remainder of the greater curvature is also mobilized as for a standard gastric tube. The gastrohepatic ligament is divided close to the liver, taking note of any aberrant left hepatic artery that may be present. The left gastric artery and coronary vein are dissected and divided as described above.

The primary issue regarding preparation of the whole stomach as an esophageal replacement is how to manage the tissues along the lesser curvature. For patients with an esophageal malignancy in whom a potentially curative resection is being performed, removal of the lesser curvature lymph nodes is important for appropriate staging as well as possibly for improved survival. This is accomplished by skeletonizing the lesser curvature.[58] The terminal branches of the gastric vessels along the lesser curve are divided flush with the gastric serosa beginning just distal to the fourth or fifth branch of the left gastric artery and progressing proximally (Figure 9-8). The accompanying fat pad, vagal nerve branches, and lymph nodes are removed en bloc to the level of the cardia. One potential advantage of the skeletonization technique is that the whole stomach is lengthened as a result. For benign disease or for some patients who are undergoing only a palliative procedure, these tissues can be left in situ. If additional length is still required, the seromuscular layer may be incised transversely from the lesser curvature to the greater curvature, which provides and additional 1 to 2 centimeters of length.[59]

The stomach is divided from the esophagus at the cardia, taking care to ensure that all of the squamous mucosa is removed with the esophageal specimen. The division is easily performed with a linear cutting stapler, but manual resection with closure by hand is also permissible.

Reversed Gastric Tube

The blood supply for the reversed gastric tube is based on the left gastroepiploic artery, which arises from the splenic artery or its terminal

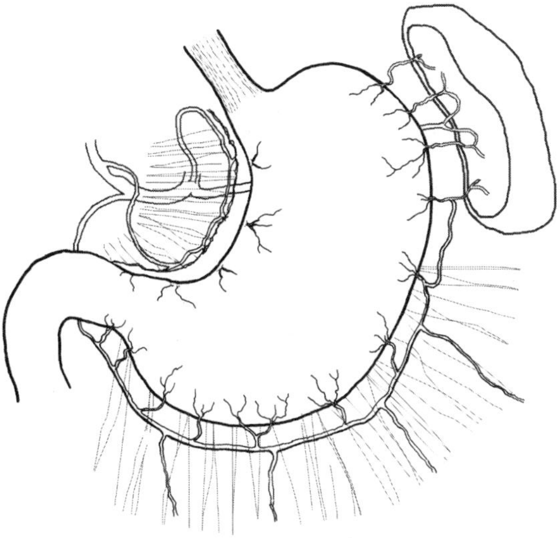

Figure 9-8. Technique for denudation of the lesser curve during preparation of the whole stomach as an esophageal substitute.

branches and passes close to the tail of the pancreas.[60,61] Preparation of a reversed gastric tube necessitates splenectomy, with preservation of the left gastroepiploic arcade and its communicating branches to the right gastroepiploic artery, as well as mobilization of the distal pancreas.

The operation is begun by entering the lesser sac. The distal pancreas is mobilized and a splenectomy is performed. An omental flap is created by dividing the greater omentum at a point 8 to 10 cm from the greater curvature, preserving the right and left gastroepiploic arteries. The right gastroepiploic artery is divided 3 to 4 cm from the pylorus. The stomach is incised at right angles to the greater curve at about this point, which will become the proximal end of the reversed gastric tube. A bougie or other large rubber tube is inserted through the gastrotomy and is positioned along the greater curvature to serve as a guide for creating the actual tube. The stomach is incised using a linear cutting stapler placed adjacent to the bougie until the fundus is reached (Figure 9-9). The length of the tube is maintained by keeping a constant stretch on the stomach as the stapler is applied. The staple lines are reinforced with running suture. The portion of the original gastrotomy that remains on the stomach is closed. The newly created gastric tube is wrapped in the omental flap, which is tacked to the tube with interrupted sutures.

If greater length is necessary, a modification of the standard tube can be created using the pylorus and first part of the duodenum, which is referred to as an extended gastric tube. The pylorus is mobilized, preserving the small feeding branches from the right gastroepiploic artery.

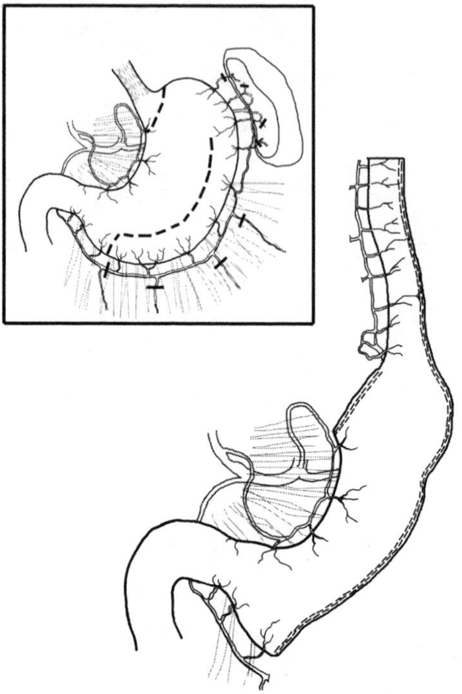

Figure 9-9. Technique for creating a reversed gastric tube.

The first portion of the duodenum is divided just proximal to the common bile duct, taking care not to injure the head of the pancreas and the portal triad. The right gastroepiploic artery is divided near its origin from the gastroduodenal artery. The bougie that is used as a guide for fashioning the gastric tube is passed through the open duodenum and along the greater curvature. The staple line for the gastric tube is begun through the antrum from the lesser curve side, and is then continued parallel to the greater curvature as described above (Figure 9-10). The distal end of the transected duodenum is oversewn, as is the gastric staple line. Emptying of the remaining gastric pouch is achieved by creating a gastrojejunostomy. This preparation adds 6 to 10 cm of length compared to the standard reversed gastric tube.

Other Preparations

A variety of other types of gastric tubes have been described, a few of which will be mentioned only briefly, either because they have not achieved popularity or because their use entails additional extra hazard or is limited to special circumstances. A free isoperistaltic gastric tube may

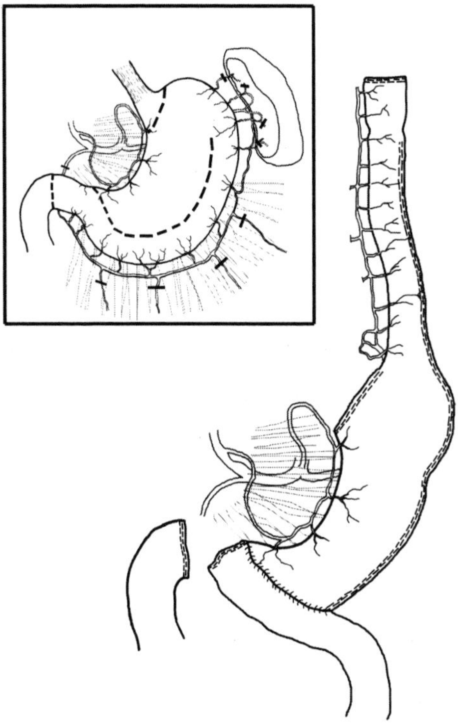

Figure 9-10. Technique for preparing an extended reversed gastric tube.

be created from the greater curvature with its blood supply based on the right gastroepiploic artery (Figure 9-11).[62] In another technique, the whole stomach may be inverted for use as a reversed gastric graft after adequate mobilization (Figure 9-11).[63] Potential advantages of this technique are that there is no need for dissection in the region of the cardia and, because there is no interruption of the continuity between the esophagus and the stomach, no esophageal drainage is required. A gastrojejunostomy is necessary for gastric drainage, however. The fundus alone may also be used as an isoperistaltic tube for reconstruction of short esophageal segments. After division of the esophagus from the stomach at the cardia, the stomach is incised across the lesser curvature, creating a gastric tube from the greater curvature beginning proximally and extending distally for one-third to one-half the length of the greater curvature.[64] This fundus rotation gastroplasty preserves most of the gastric reservoir capacity and only requires a single anastomosis (Figure 9-11).

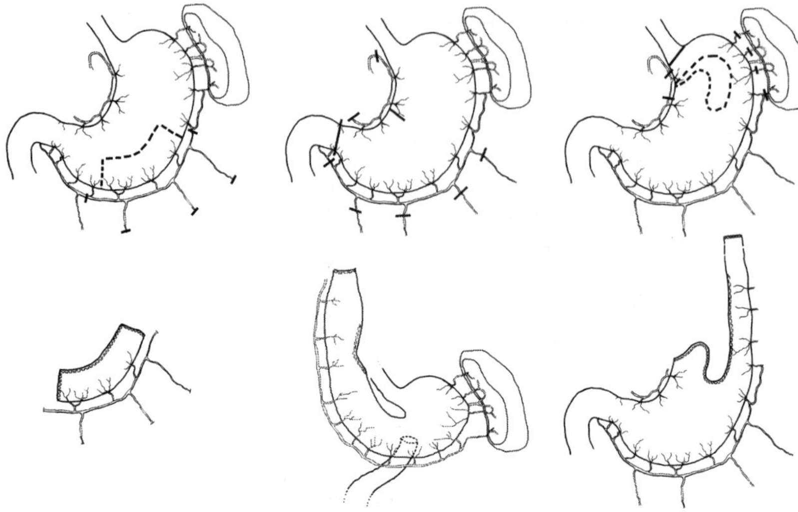

Figure 9-11. Alternative techniques for use of the stomach as an esophageal substitute, including the free isoperistaltic gastric tube (left), the reversed whole stomach (center) and the fundus rotation gastroplasty (right).

Transposing the Stomach

Positioning the stomach through the reconstructive route is simple to accomplish manipulating the preparation by hand when the reconstruction route is completely exposed as it normally is during a thoracotomy with posterior mediastinal reconstruction. In other instances, such as during a transhiatal resection with reconstruction or during any transposition of the stomach through a substernal route, it is necessary to push or pull the stomach through the route. A variety of techniques have been described to accomplish this task that minimize trauma to the stomach and help eliminate any risk of torsion of the stomach during transposition. Some methods involve attaching the stomach to a malleable retractor which is used as a sled to pull on the stomach, while others involve passing a long clamp through the reconstructive route which is then used to grasp sutures placed through the stomach to help maintain its orientation. A popular and effective method utilizes a long and narrow plastic bag and a Foley catheter (Figure 9-12). The catheter is passed through the reconstructive route and the stomach is placed within the bag. The catheter tip is positioned within the closed end of the bag through a small hole and the balloon is inflated. Suction is applied to the catheter, which creates negative pressure within the bag, producing evenly-distributed tension on all surfaces of the stomach. Gentle traction on the catheter is

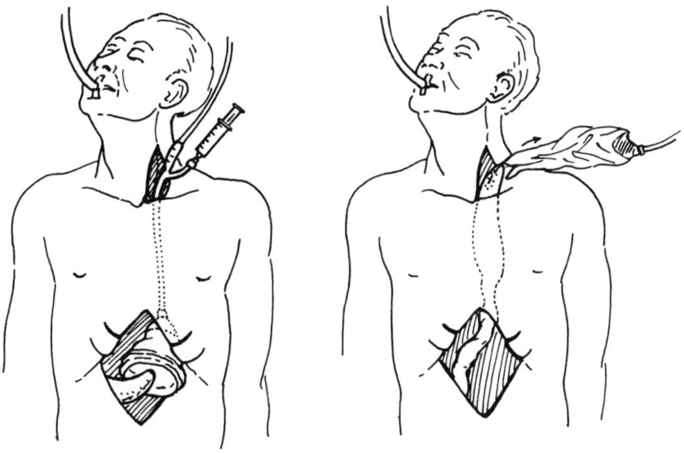

Figure 9-12. A technique for pulling the prepared stomach through the reconstructive route without damage involves placing the stomach into a long, narrow bag to which suction is applied through use of a Foley catheter (left). Traction is then placed on the catheter, enabling the stomach to be pulled with the tension distributed evenly, avoiding damage to the stomach wall and vasculature (right). Reprinted with permission from the Society of Thoracic Surgeons, Annals of Thoracic Surgery, 1988;45:451-452.

used to pull the bag containing the stomach through the reconstructive route.[65]

Other Considerations

There is considerable difference of opinion as to the need for a routine Kocher maneuver. Even the accuracy of the eponym attached to dissection of the second (retrocolic or retroperitoneal) portion of the duodenum off of the underlying tissues has been called into question.[66] In many instances, the duodenum is sufficiently mobile that the pylorus can be elevated to a location near the esophageal hiatus, making the Kocher maneuver unnecessary. The fact that this situation is more common in the Asian population was discussed earlier in this chapter. Similarly, if the stomach is long enough to use as an esophageal substitute without mobilizing the duodenum, there is little advantage in performing a Kocher maneuver. However, when an anastomosis between the cervical esophagus or pharynx and the stomach is necessary, addtional mobilization of the gastric tube is occasionally required. In such instances, the performance of a Kocher maneuver will provide an extra 5 cm or more of length, which is often sufficient to prevent undue tension on the anastomosis. Since the risk of performing a Kocher maneuver is minimal, its use as an adjunct to gastric pull-up for esophageal replacement by a gastric tube is frequently indicated.

Despite the dependability of the blood supply to the stomach when it is used as an esophageal substitute, vascular compromise is occasionally a life-threatening problem. In addition, the relatively high rate of anastomotic leakage suggests that the blood supply to the region of the anastomosis is often suboptimal. A variety of techniques have been used to try to assess the adequacy of the gastric blood supply intraoperatively. Laser Doppler scanning of blood flow demonstrates that flow decreases by an average of up to 41% after formation of a standard gastric tube, and that flow in the fundus decreases by an average of up to 72%.[67,68] Patients who develop an anastomotic leak have a greater decrease in flow in the region of the anastomosis than do patients without evidence for an anastomotic leak. Using a similar technique, others have demonstrated that mean blood flow is much lower in patients who develop an anastomotic leak than in those without evidence for a leak.[69] In contrast, it also has been reported that, although laser Doppler measurement of flow in gastric tubes does not predict anastomotic leak, it can predict the likelihood of anastomotic stricture.[70]

It was suggested in 1990 that pulse oximetry could be used to identify areas of relative ischemia in the stomach and other abdominal viscera.[71] This technique was applied experimentally to gastric tubes in dogs and severe ischemia of the fundus was demonstrated.[72] In humans, oxygen tension has been shown to decrease dramatically after formation of a standard gastric tube, but no further decrease occurs when the gastric tube is placed in the mediastinum for reconstruction.[73] This finding has been used to select patients in whom the tip of the fundus is resected rather than used as a site for an anastomosis in an effort to limit the incidence of anastomotic leak.[74] At present, the use of Doppler flow measurements and oximetry remains investigational, given the lack of important correlation between specific measurements and the risk of anastomotic leak.

To prevent the ischemic consequences of gastric devascularization during preparation of an esophageal replacement, some physicians have theorized that ischemic conditioning of the stomach may decrease the risk of anastomotic leakage and other surgical complications. In experimental models, ischemic conditioning increases blood flow after gastric devascularization and improves wound healing compared to acutely ischemic stomachs.[75-77] In humans, ischemic conditioning has been accomplished using catheter-guided embolization of the right gastric, left gastric, and splenic arteries.[78,79] Flow measured before and after gastric tube formation using a laser Doppler device was compared in patients who underwent preoperative embolization therapy and those in a nonrandomized control group who did not. Patients who underwent embolization had a decrease in blood flow to the stomach of 23% to 28%, compared to a 65% to 69% decrease in patients without embolization. It has been suggested that ischemic conditioning might also be performed by laparoscopic devascularization of the stomach (preserving the right gastroepiploic arcade) 2 to 3 weeks prior to esophagectomy.[80]

If gastric ischemia is a concern at the time of operation, as an alternative to resection of the ischemic portion or delaying completion of the anastomosis, one consideration may be revascularization. Microvascular anastomoses have been suggested for providing additional blood supply in patients with very long gastric tubes used for esophageal reconstruction.[81] Even in patients in whom a standard gastric tube is created, revascularization of the gastric fundus via the short gastric vessels provides additional important blood supply.[49] A venous anastomosis alone increases blood flow by over one third, and the combination of a venous and an arterial anastomosis increases blood flow by more than 100%. Improved blood flow is associated with a decrease in the incidence of anastomotic leakage. Alternatively, an intravenous infusion of prostaglandin E_1 improves flow to the fundus after creation of a gastric tube, and no important side effects of infusion have been noted.[82]

Complications Related to Gastric Pull-Up

It is sometimes difficult to identify complications that arise from a complex operation such as esophagectomy and stomach pull-up which can be attributed specifically to the type of esophageal reconstruction that is performed. The acute and long-term complications that are primarily related to the organ used for reconstruction are detailed here.

Anastomotic Leak

The most common acute complication specifically related to the organ used for esophageal reconstruction is the anastomotic leak. This is believed to result from a variety of causes including excessive tension on the anastomosis, a relative lack of perfusion to the region of the stomach used to construct the anastomosis, and possibly to the fact that the anastomosis is bathed in gastric juices throughout its early healing phase. The risk of anastomotic leak is related in part to whether it is located in the thorax or in the neck, factors which help determine the degrees of anastomotic tension and organ perfusion. Intrathoracic anastomoses are associated with a leak rate of about 5%, whereas cervical anastomoses have a leak rate that is three times greater (Table 9-2).[83-94] Both intrathoracic and cervical anastomotic leaks are associated with an increased

Table 9-2.
The Incidence of Anastomotic Leak after Esophageal Replacement with Stomach.

Author	Year	Total patients	Total leaks	Intrathoracic anastomoses	Intrathoracic leaks	Cervical anastomoses	Cervical leaks
Peracchia et al.[83]	1988	242	14	242	14	0	0
Lozac'h et al.[84]	1991	100	7	100	7	0	0
Dewar et al.[85]	1992	165	28	0	0	165	28
Lam et al.[86]	1992	331	12	240	8	91	4
Patil et al.[87]	1992	617	39	598	34	19	5
Wang et al.[88]	1992	368	47	58	6	310	41
Pac et al.[89]	1993	238	11	120	6	118	5
Vigneswaran et al.[90]	1993	131	32	0	0	131	32
Iannettoni et al.[91]	1995	842	88	0	0	842	88
Honkoop et al.[92]	1996	281	68	0	0	281	68
Ellis et al.[93]	1997	404	25	279	3	125	22
McManus et al.[94]	1999	174	15	108	10	66	5
Totals		3893	386 (9.9%)	1745	88 (5.0%)	2148	298 (13.9%)

Table 9-3.
The Incidence of Anastomotic Stricture after Esophageal Replacement with Stomach.

Author	Year	Patients	Strictures
Dewar et al.[85]	1992	159	50
Wang et al.[88]	1992	267	67
Pac et al.[89]	1993	117	8
Honkoop et al.[92]	1996	269	114
Totals		812	239 (29.4%)

rate of operative mortality. A detailed discussion of the diagnosis and management of esophagogastric anastomotic leaks can be found in Chapters 15 and 16.

Anastomotic Stricture

Anastomotic strictures often develop in the early postoperative period after esophagectomy and gastric pull-up. The relatively high incidence of anastomotic leaks, particularly in cervical esophagogastric anastomoses, predisposes patients to the development of anastomotic stricture. Strictures are documented to occur more often than are anastomotic leaks, which is likely due to a number of factors (Table 9-3). Some leaks may be subclinical, and routine evaluation of patients in the acute postoperative period does not reveal their presence. In some patients there may be subacute ischemia of the stomach which leads to the development of an anastomotic stricture over time. The fact that esophagogastric anastomoses are routinely exposed to a highly acidic environment may also create continuing inflammation resulting in an anastomotic stricture. The management of esophagogastric anastomotic stricture is detailed in Chapter 15.

Gastric Necrosis

The blood supply to the stomach is normally sufficiently redundant that necrosis of the entire stomach after a gastric pull-up has been performed is fortunately rare. When this catastrophic event occurs, the only recourse is rapid intervention to remove the stomach and drain the reconstructive route. The esophagus is exteriorized as an end esophagostomy, and a percutaneous tube is placed for enteral alimentation. Staged reconstruction is performed when the patient has recovered.

Partial necrosis of a gastric pull-up is also relatively rare but poses technical challenges in management. Necrosis of the gastric fundus, the region in which most anastomoses are performed, leads to symptoms compatible with a severe anastomotic leak. The likely etiology of this complication is the fact that the gastric fundus is extremely vulnerable to pressure and tension due to its relatively poor perfusion compared to the rest of the stomach.[3,83,90-92,95,96] Partial gastric necrosis may be implicated as a causative factor in as many as 10% of esophagogastric anastomotic leaks and is the likely cause of disruption of esophagogastric anastomoses.

Management of partial necrosis of a gastric pull-up must be highly individualized. In many instances there is residual gastric length which may permit resection of the necrotic region and re-anastomosis. The redo anastomosis can be performed under the same anesthetic if the patient is otherwise healthy and if there has no undue contamination of the region. Alternatively, the stomach is closed and the re-anastomosis is performed at a later date. This is most often possible when the anastomosis was initially performed in the cervical region, in which case the oversewn body of the stomach is sutured to the side of the cervical esophagus or to the sternocleidomastoid muscle to prevent it from retracting into the mediastinum. If the remaining stomach does not reach to the neck, or if the original anastomosis was intrathoracic, the issues become more complex. The stomach remnant can easily be closed and left in its intrathoracic location, but in this setting decompression of the esophageal stump is problematic and a third thoracotomy is then necessary to complete the reconstruction. It is usually advisable in this situation to transpose the residual stomach back to the abdomen, bring the esophagus out as an end cervical ostomy, and perform the reconstruction at a later date.

Gastric Torsion

Torsion of the stomach will almost always lead to gastric necrosis if the twist is more than 90° to 180°. Torsion initially causes venous congestion, which precedes the development of vascular thrombosis. Substantial congestion is often evident when a gastric tube is pulled through a neck incision in preparation for creating a cervical anastomosis. One way to be certain that torsion has not occurred is to be careful to transpose the stomach without rotating it. If concern remains that gastric torsion has occurred, a careful examination of the proximal and distal ends of the stomach should be sufficient to provide reassurance as to the position of the stomach. If torsion is recognized intraoperatively, urgent reduction of the torsion will usually be sufficient to restore normal circulation to the stomach. If there is delayed recognition of torsion, gastric necrosis usually will have ensued and gastrectomy is necessary.

References

1. Griffith CA. Anatomy of the stomach and duodenum. In Wastell CA, Nyhus LM, Donahue PR (eds): **Surgery of the Esophagus, Stomach, and Small Intestine**. Boston, Little, Brown and Company, 1995, pp 388-416.
2. Goldsmith HS, Akiyama H. A comparative study of Japanese and American gastric dimensions. *Ann Surg* 1979;190:690-693.
3. Liebermann-Meffert DMI, Meier R, Siewert JR. Vascular anatomy of the gastric tube used for esophageal reconstruction. *Ann Thorac Surg* 1992;54:1110-1115.
4. Mitchell GAG. A macroscopic study of the nerve supply of the stomach. *J Anat* 1940;75:50-63.
5. Barlow TE, Bentley FH, Walder DN. Arteries, veins, and arteriovenous anastomoses in the human stomach. *Surg Gynecol Obstet* 1951;93:657-671.
6. Brown JR, Derr JW. Arterial blood supply of human stomach. *Arch Surg* 1952;64:616-621.
7. Thomas DM, Langford RM, Russell RCG, et al. The anatomical basis for gastric mobilization in total oesophagectomy. *Br J Surg* 1979;66:230-233.
8. Yamato T, Hamanaka Y, Hirata S, et al. Esophagoplasty with an autogenous tubed gastric flap. *Am J Surg* 1979;137:597-602.
9. Michels NA. Collateral arterial pathways to the liver after ligation of the hepatic artery and removal of the celiac axis. *Cancer* 1953;6:708-724.
10. Hemming AW, Finley RJ, Evans KG, et al. Esophagogastrectomy and the variant left hepatic artery. *Ann Thorac Surg* 1992;54:166-168.
11. Larsen E, Johansen A, Andersen D. Gastric arteriosclerosis in elderly people. *Scand J Gastroenterol* 1969;4:387-389.
12. Suma H, Takanashi R. Arteriosclerosis of the gastroepiploic and internal thoracic arteries. *Ann Thorac Surg* 1990;50:413-416.
13. Mackie DB, Turner MD. Vagotomy and submucosal blood flow. *Arch Surg* 1971;102:626-629.
14. Azpiroz F, Malagelada J-R. Importance of vagal input in maintaining gastric tone in the dog. *J Physiol* 1987;384:511-524.
15. de Ponti F, Azpiroz F, Malagelada J-R. Relaxatory responses of canine proximal stomach to esophageal and duodenal distension. *Dig Dis Sci* 1989;34:873-881.
16. Logeman F, Borm JJ, van Lanschot JJ, et al. Disturbed enterogastric inhibitory reflex after esophageal resection and narrow gastric tube reconstruction. *Dig Surg* 1999;16:186-191.
17. Azpiroz F, Malagelada J-R. Intestinal control of gastric tone. *Am J Physiol* 1985;249:G501-G509.
18. Azpiroz F, Malagelada J-R. Vagally mediated gastric relaxation induced by intestinal nutrients in the dog. *Am J Physiol* 1986;251:G727-G735.
19. Dalton RR, Zinsmeister AR, Sarr MG. Vagus-dependent disruption of interdigestive canine motility by gastric distension. *Am J Physiol* 1992;262:G1097-1103.
20. Van Lier Ribbink JA, Sarr MG, Tanaka M. Neural isolation of the entire stomach in vivo: Effects on motility. *Am J Physiol* 1989;257:G30-G40.

21. Desai KM, Sessa WC, Vane JR. Involvement of nitric oxide in the reflex relaxation of the stomach to accommodate food or fluid. *Nature* 1991;351:477-479.

22. Tomita R, Tanjoh K, Fujisaki S, et al. The role of nitric oxide (NO) in the human pyloric sphincter. *Hepato-gastroenterol* 1999;46:2999-3003.

23. Bonavina L, Anselmino M, Ruol A, et al. Functional evaluation of the intrathoracic stomach as an oesophageal substitute. *Br J Surg* 1992;79:529-532.

24. Nishikawa M, Murakami T, Tangoku A, et al. Functioning of the intrathoracic stomach after esophagectomy. *Arch Surg* 1994;129:837-841.

25. Hashimoto M, Imamura M, Shimada Y, et al. Twenty-four hour monitoring of pH in the gastric tube replacing the resected esophagus. *J Am Coll Surg* 1995;180:666-672.

26. Okada N, Nishimura O, Sakurai T, et al. Gastric functions in patients with the intrathoracic stomach after esophageal surgery. *Ann Surg* 1986;204:114-121.

27. Mannell A, Hinder RA, San-Garde BA. The thoracic stomach: a study of gastric emptying, bile reflux and mucosal change. *Br J Surg* 1984;71:438-441.

28. Chattopadhyay TK, Shad SK, Kumar A. Intragastric bile acid and symptoms in patients with an intrathoracic stomach after oesophagectomy. *Br J Surg* 1993;80:371-373.

29. Baxter JN, Grime JS, Critchley M, et al. Relationship between gastric emptying of a solid meal and emptying of the gall bladder before and after vagotomy. *Gut* 1987;28:855-863.

30. Nishimura O, Naito Y, Yokoi H, et al. Radionuclide studies of the substituted stomach after esophageal surgery. *Dis Esoph* 1989;2:105-111.

31. Hjelms E, Thirup P, Schou L. Gastric intrinsic factor production and vitamin B_{12} absorption after oesophageal resection using stomach as substitute. *Eur J Cardio-Thorac Surg* 1999;16:273-275.

32. Holscher AH, Voit H, Buttermann G, et al. Function of the intrathoracic stomach as esophageal replacement. *World J Surg* 1988;12:835-844.

33. Morton KA, Karwande SV, Davis RK, et al. Gastric emptying after gastric interposition for cancer of the esophagus or hypopharynx. *Ann Thorac Surg* 1991;51:759-763.

34. Kao C-H, Wang S-J, Chen C-Y, et al. The motility of interposition in patients with esophageal carcinoma after reconstructive esophageal surgery. *Clin Nuc Med* 1993;18:782-785.

35. Bemelman WA, Taat CW, Slors JFM, et al. Delayed postoperative emptying after esophageal resection is dependent on the size of the gastric reservoir. *J Am Coll Surg* 1995;180:461-464.

36. Moreno-Osset E, Tomas-Ridocci M, Paris F, et al. Motor activity of esophageal substitute (stomach, jejunal, and colon segments). *Ann Thorac Surg* 1986;41:515-519.

37. Little AG, Scott WJ, Ferguson MK, et al. Functional evaluation of organ interposition for esophageal replacement. In Siewert JR, Holscher AH (eds): **Diseases of the Esophagus**. Berlin, Springer-Verlag, 1988, pp 664-667.

38. Walsh TN, Caldwell MTP, Fallon C, et al. Gastric motility following oesophagectomy. *Br J Surg* 1995;82:91-94.

39. Collard J-M, Tinton N, Malaise J, et al. Esophageal replacement: Gastric tube or whole stomach? *Ann Thorac Surg* 1995;60:261-267.

40. Collard J-M, Romagnoli R, Otte J-B, et al. The denervated stomach as an esophageal substitute is a contractile organ. *Ann Surg* 1998;227:33-39.
41. De Leyn P, Coosemans W, Lerut T. Early and late functional results in patients with intrathoracic gastric replacement after oesophagectomy for carcinoma. *Eur J Cardio-Thorac Surg* 1992;6:79-85.
42. Collard J-M, Otte J-B, Reynaert M, et al. Quality of life three years or more after esophagectomy for cancer. *J Thorac Cardiovasc Surg* 1992;104:391-394.
43. Suzuki H, Abo S, Kitamura M, et al. An evaluation of symptoms and performance status in patients after esophagectomy for esophageal cancer from the viewpoint of the patient. *Am Surg* 1994;60:920-923.
44. McLarty AJ, Deschamps C, Trastek VF, et al. Esophageal resection for cancer of the esophagus: Long-term function and quality of life. *Ann Thorac Surg* 1997;63:1568-1572.
45. Baba M, Aikou T, Natsugoe S, et al. Appraisal of ten-year survival following esophagectomy for carcinoma of the esophagus with emphasis on quality of life. *World J Surg* 1997;21:282-286.
46. Ueo H, Takeuchi H, Arinaga S, et al. A reliable operative procedure for preparing a sufficiently nourished gastric tube for esophageal reconstruction. *Am J Surg* 1993;165:273-276.
47. Petsikas D, Shamji FM. Revascularization of the ischemic gastric tube using the left internal thoracic artery. *Ann Thorac Surg* 1996;62:568-570.
48. Nagawa H, Seto Y, Nakatsuka T, et al. Microvascular anastomosis for additional blood flow in reconstruction after intrathoracic esophageal carcinoma surgery. *Am J Surg* 1997;173:131-133.
49. Murakami M, Sugiyama A, Ikegami T, et al. Revascularization using the short gastric vessels of the gastric tube after subtotal esophagectomy for intrathoracic esophageal carcinoma. *J Am Coll Surg* 2000;190:71-77.
50. Skinner DB, Little AG, Ferguson MK, et al. Selection of operation for esophageal cancer based on staging. *Ann Surg* 1986;204:391-401.
51. Hagen JA, Peters JH, DeMeester TR. Superiority of extended en bloc esophagogastrectomy for carcinoma of the lower esophagus and cardia. *J Thorac Cardiovasc Surg* 1993;106:850-859.
52. Casson AG, Darnton SJ, Subramanian S, et al. What is the optimal distal resection margin for esophageal carcinoma? *Ann Thorac Surg* 2000;69:205-209.
53. Akiyama H, Miyazono H, Tsurumaru M, et al. Use of the stomach as an esophageal substitute. *Ann Surg* 1978;188:606-610.
54. Pierie JP, de Graaf PW, van Vroonhoven TJ, et al. The vascularization of a gastric tube as a substitute for the esophagus is affected by its diameter. *Dis Esoph* 1998;11:231-235.
55. Akiyama H, Tsurumaru M, Kawamura T, et al. Principles of surgical treatment for carcinoma of the esophagus: Analysis of lymph node involvement. *Ann Surg* 1981;194:438-446.
56. Sugimachi K, Yaita A, Ueo H, et al. A safer and more reliable operative technique for esophageal reconstruction using a gastric tube. *Am J Surg* 1980;140:471-474.
57. Chaimoff C, Turani H, Bayer I. Lengthening of the stomach. An experimental study in dogs. *Res Surg* 1992;4:29-31.

58. Collard JM, Otte JB, Jamart J, et al. An original technique for lengthening the stomach as an esophageal substitute after oesophagectomy. Preliminary results. *Dis Esoph* 1989;2:171-174.

59. Perrachia A, Bardini R, Narne S. Resections for pharygo-oesophageal cancer. In: Jamieson GG (ed): **Surgery of the Oesophagus**. Churchill Livingstone, Edinburgh, 1988, pp 689-699.

60. Gavriliu D, Georgescu L. Esofagoplastie viscerala directa. *Chirurgia* 1955;4:104-138.

61. Gavriliu D. The replacement of the esophagus by a gastric tube. In: Jamieson GG (ed): **Surgery of the Oesophagus**. Churchill Livingstone, Edinburgh, 1988, p 765-775.

62. Yamagishi M, Ikeda N, Yonemoto T. An isoperistaltic gastric tube. *Arch Surg* 1970;100:689-692.

63. Giraud RMA, Berzin S. The reversed gastric esophagoplasty in palliation of carcinoma of the esophagus. *Surg Gynecol Obstet* 1987;165:111-115.

64. Buchler MW, Baer HU, Seiler C, et al. A technique for gastroplasty as a substitute for the esophagus: Fundus rotation gastroplasty. *J Am Coll Surg* 1996;182:241-245.

65. Inculet RI, Finley RJ, Cooper JD. A new technique for delivering the stomach or colon to the neck following total esophagectomy. *Ann Thorac Surg* 1988;45:451-452.

66. Madden JL, Kandalaft S, Eghrari M. Mobilization of the duodenum: A surgical maneuver incorrectly credited to Kocher. *Surgery* 1968;63:522-526.

67. Schilling MK, Redaelli C, Maurer C, et al. Gastric microcirculatory changes during gastric tube formation: Assessment with laser Doppler flowmetry. *J Surg Res* 1996;62:125-129.

68. Boyle NH, Pearce A, Hunter D, et al. Intraoperative scanning laser Doppler flowmetry in the assessment of gastric tube perfusion during esophageal resection. *J Am Coll Surg* 1999;188:498-502.

69. Kudo T, Abo S, Itabashi T. Prognosis of esophageal substitute in tissue viability and anastomotic leakage. In Siewert JR, Holscher AH (eds): **Diseases of the Esophagus**. Berlin, Springer-Verlag, 1988, pp 522-525.

70. Pierie JP, de Graaf PW, Poen H, et al. Impaired healing of cervical esophagogastrostomies can be predicted by estimation of gastric serosal blood perfusion by laser Doppler flowmetry. *Eur J Surg* 1994;160:599-603.

71. Sheridan WG, Lowndes RH, Young HL. Intraoperative tissue oximetry in the human gastrointestinal tract. *Am J Surg* 1990;159:314-319.

72. Uribe N, Garcia-Granero E, Belda J, et al. Evaluation of residual vascularization in oesophageal substitution gastroplasty by surface oximetry-capnography and photoplethysmography. *Eur J Surg* 1995;161:569-573.

73. Cooper GJ, Sherry KM, Thorpe JA. Changes in gastric tissue oxygenation during mobilization for oesophageal replacement. *Eur J Cardio-Thorac Surg* 1995;9:158-160.

74. Salo JA, Perhoniemi VJ, Heikkinen LO, et al. Pulse oximetry for the assessment of gastric tube circulation in esophageal replacements. *Am J Surg* 1992;163:446-447.

75. Urschel JD. Ischemic conditioning of the rat stomach: implications for esophageal replacement with stomach. *J Cardiovasc Surg* 1995;36:191-193.

76. Urschel JD, Antkowiak JG, Delacure MD, et al. Ischemic conditioning (delay phenomenon) improves esophagogastric anastomotic wound healing in the rat. *J Surg Oncol* 1997;66:254-256.
77. Urschel JD, Takita H, Antkowiak JG. The effect of ischemic conditioning on gastric wound healing in the rat: implications for esophageal replacement with stomach. *J Cardiovasc Surg* 1997;38:535-538.
78. Akiyama S, Ito S, Sekiguchi H, et al. Preoperative embolization of gastric arteries for esophageal cancer. *Surgery* 1996;120:542-546.
79. Isomura T, Itoh S, Endo T, et al. Efficacy of gastric blood supply redistribution by transarterial embolization: Preoperative procedure to prevent postoperative anastomotic leaks following esophagoplasty for esophageal carcinoma. *Cardiovasc Intervent Radiol* 1999;22:119-123.
80. Urschel JD. Ischemic conditioning of the stomach may reduce the incidence of esophagogastric anastomotic leaks complicating esophagectomy: A hypothesis. *Dis Esoph* 1997;10:217-219.
81. Matsubara T, Ueda M, Nakajima T, et al. Elongated stomach roll with vascular microanastomosis for reconstruction of the esophagus after pharyngolaryngoesophagectomy. *J Am Coll Surg* 1995;180:613-615.
82. Matsuzaki Y, Edagawa E, Maeda M, et al. Beneficial effect of prostaglandin E_1 on blood flow to the gastric tube after esophagectomy. *Ann Thorac Surg* 1999;67:908-910.
83. Peracchia A, Bardini R, Ruol A, et al. Esophagovisceral anastomotic leak. A prospective statistical study of predisposing factors. *J Thorac Cardiovasc Surg* 1988;95:685-691.
84. Lozac'h P, Topart P, Etienne J, Charles JF. Ivor Lewis operation for epidermoid carcinoma of the esophagus. *Ann Thorac Surg* 1991;52:1154-1157.
85. Dewar L, Gelfand G, Finley RJ, et al. Factors affecting cervical anastomotic leak and stricture formation following esophagogastrectomy and gastric tube interposition. *Am J Surg* 1992;163:484-489.
86. Lam TCF, Fok M, Cheng SWK, et al. Anastomotic complications after esophagectomy for cancer. A comparison of neck and chest anastomoses. *J Thorac Cardiovasc Surg* 1992;104:395-400.
87. Patil PK, Patel SG, Mistry RC, et al. Cancer of the esophagus: Esophagogastric anastomotic leak - a retrospective study of predisposing factors. *J Surg Oncol* 1992;49:163-167.
88. Wang L-S, Huang M-H, Huang B-S, et al. Gastric substitution for resectable carcinoma of the esophagus: an analysis of 368 cases. *Ann Thorac Surg* 1992;53:289-294.
89. Pac M, Basoglu A, Kocak H, et al. Transhiatal versus transthoracic esophagectomy for esophageal cancer. *J Thorac Cardiovasc Surg* 1993;106:205-209.
90. Vigneswaran WT, Trastek VF, Pairolero PC, et al. Transhiatal esophagectomy for carcinoma of the esophagus. *Ann Thorac Surg* 1993;56:838-846.
91. Iannettoni MD, Whyte RI, Orringer MB. Catastrophic complications of the cervical esophagogastric anastomosis. *J Thorac Cardiovasc Surg* 1995;110:1493-1501.
92. Honkoop P, Siersema PD, Tilanus HW, et al. Benign anastomotic strictures after transhiatal esophagectomy and cervical esophagogastrostomy: Risk factors and management. *J Thorac Cardiovasc Surg* 1996;111:1141-1148.

93. Ellis FH Jr, Heatley GJ, Krasna MJ, et al. Esophagogastrectomy for carcinoma of the esophagus and cardia: A comparison of findings and results after standard resection in three consecutive eight-year intervals with improved staging criteria. *J Thorac Cardiovasc Surg* 1997;113:836-848.
94. McManus K, Anikin V, McGuigan J. Total thoracic oesophagectomy for oesophageal carcinoma: Has it been worth it? *Eur J Cardio-Thorac Surg* 1999;16:261-265.
95. Liebermann-Meffert D. Surgical anatomy of the esophagus and stomach in relation to stomach pull-through. *Langenbecks Arch Chir Suppl Kongressbd* 1998;115:951-954.
96. Moorehead RJ, Wong J. Gangrene in esophageal substitutes after resection and bypass procedures for carcinoma of the esophagus. *Hepatogastroenterol* 1990;37:364-367.

Chapter 10

The Colon as a Reconstructive Organ

The colon is the second most commonly used organ for esophageal replacement. Its use is particularly popular among pediatric surgeons for management of congenital anomalies and caustic injury of the esophagus. Preparation of a colon interposition is technically more challenging than creation of a gastric tube for esophageal replacement, and the function of a colon interposition is not reliably better than that of a gastric pull-up. Appropriate patient selection for colon interposition is vital.

Anatomy

The colon is a seromuscular tube that extends from the terminal ileum to the rectum. The portion with the greatest diameter, the cecum, lies in the right iliac fossa and is completely intraperitoneal. The ascending (right) colon is fixed to the abdominal wall by overlying peritoneum and measures about 16 cm along its mesenteric border.[1] The hepatic flexure lies over the lower pole of the right kidney and extends medially as far as the second and third portions of the duodenum. The transverse colon is usually quite mobile due to its wide mesentery and is variable in length, averaging 34 cm along its mesenteric border. The splenic flexure lies over the lower pole of the left kidney, often extends to touch the lower pole of the spleen, and is mostly retroperitoneal. The descending colon is fixed to the lateral abdominal wall by the overlying peritoneum and measures about 15 cm along its mesenteric border. The sigmoid colon is entirely intraperitoneal, is variable in length (averaging 11 cm), and is the narrowest part of the colon. It begins just at the pelvic brim and extends to the rectum, which begins at the sacral promontory. The sigmoid colon is also quite mobile due to its wide mesentery.

From Ferguson MK: *Reconstructive Surgery of the Esophagus* Armonk, NY: Futura Publishing Company, Inc., © 2002.

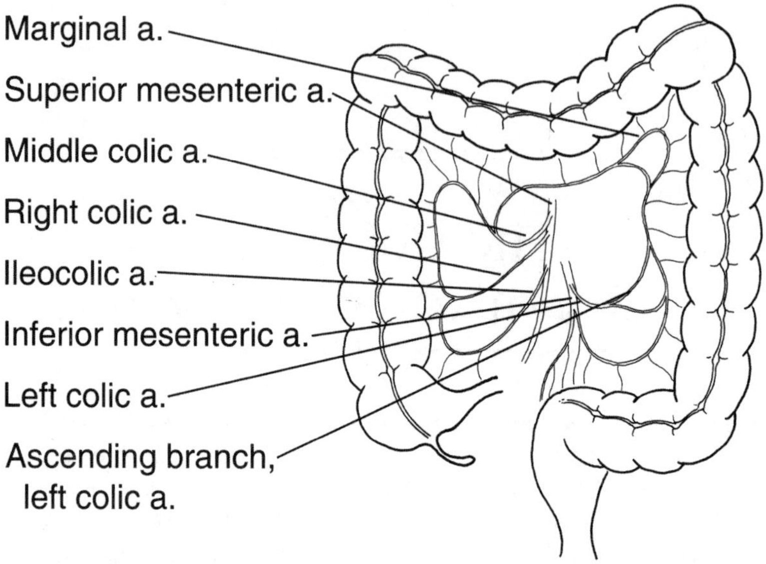

Figure 10-1. The blood supply to the colon.

The colon is comprised of layers including the mucosa, the submucosa, an inner circular muscle layer, an outer longitudinal muscle layer, and the overlying serosa. The longitudinal muscle layer condenses to form three bands (taenia coli) that extend from the base of the appendix to the rectosigmoid junction where they merge. The taenia coli are 15% shorter than the rest of the organ, leading to outpouchings of the colon between them known as haustrations.

The blood supply to the colon comes from the superior and inferior mesenteric arteries (Figure 10-1). The vascular pattern is quite variable, a fact that has an important bearing on the use of the colon for esophageal replacement. The arborization of vessels from the superior mesenteric artery is classically thought to consist of the middle, right, and ileocolic arteries. The middle colic artery is usually single, divides into right and left branches (usually within 3 cm from its origin), and measures nearly 12 cm in length from its origin on the superior mesenteric artery to the colon. The left branch of the middle colic artery is often contiguous with the marginal artery of Drummond (see below). This classic pattern occurs in fewer than 25% of patients.[1] Alternatively, when all three vessels are present and there is only a single middle colic artery, the right colic artery arises from the middle colic artery (22% of total) or the ileocolic artery (23% of total).

In 5% to 10% of patients there is no right colic artery, and in 5% to 15% of patients, the middle colic artery is absent.[1-3] At least one study suggests that the ileocolic artery is often mistaken for the right colic artery, and that the latter vessel is actually present in fewer than 15% of patients.[4] In nearly 10% of patients there are multiple right colic arteries with variable origins from the middle colic, ileocolic, and superior mesenteric arteries. In over 5% of patients multiple middle colic arteries arise from the superior mesenteric artery, or, less commonly, from the right colic artery. Rarely, but occasionally, does the left colic artery arise from the middle colic artery rather than from the inferior mesenteric artery.

The blood supply to the colon from the inferior mesenteric artery is usually more constant. The first branch of the inferior mesenteric artery is the left colic artery, which divides into ascending and descending branches (Figure 10-1). The ascending branch of the left colic artery is present in over 95% of patients.[3] The inferior mesenteric artery gives off subsequent branches to the sigmoid colon and continues inferiorly as the superior hemorrhoidal artery.

The presence of a communicating vessel between the superior and inferior mesenteric blood supply to the colon is vital to its successful use as an esophageal replacement organ. The marginal artery of Drummond provides terminal arteries to the colon, supplying most of the left colon and much of the transverse colon. This communicating arcade theoretically extends from the ileocolic artery to the left sigmoid arteries, but communication between the ileocolic and right colic arteries is absent in about 5% of patients.[5] A communicating vessel between the middle colic and left colic arteries is not visible radiographically in up to 50% of patients and may not be palpable in many patients.[3,6,7] This finding is disputed by others, and personal experience suggests that an adequate marginal artery is present in the vast majority of patients in whom colon interposition is contemplated.[8] In some patients a meandering mesenteric artery of the colon may be found, which runs a tortuous course parallel to the marginal artery along the splenic flexure but is located a substantial distance from the colon.[9] The presence of such an artery, which represents a dilated collateral vessel, suggests the existence of significant arterial occlusion in either the superior or inferior mesenteric systems.

Venous drainage of the colon generally runs parallel to the arterial supply. The inferior and superior mesenteric venous systems drain into the portal system, the inferior mesenteric vein reaching that system via the splenic vein. Thus, the inferior mesenteric vein extends much higher in the abdomen than does the inferior mesenteric artery.

The colon receives sympathetic and parasympathetic innervation.[10] The pattern of innervation follows the arterial supply to some extent and reflects the differing embryologic origins of the right and transverse colon (midgut-derived) versus the left and sigmoid colon (hindgut-derived). Sympathetic fibers for the right and transverse colon arise from T7-T12 and run down the sympathetic trunks to the celiac plexus, from where they course to the superior mesenteric and preaortic plexuses and then to the colon. The parasympathetic supply to these segments of the colon arises from the right (posterior) vagus nerve and passes through the same plexuses as for the sympathetic fibers. The postganglionic fibers synapse with the autonomic plexuses in the bowel wall. The sympathetic innervation to the descending and sigmoid colon arises from L1-L3, traverses the lumbar splanchnic and preaortic plexuses, and reaches the inferior mesenteric plexus before passing into the bowel. The parasympathetic innervation arises from S2-S4, and travels along the presacral nerves to the inferior mesenteric plexus, from where it reaches these segments of the colon.

Postoperative Function of Colon Interpositions

The human colon performs a variety of functions in the healthy state, including absorption of water and electrolytes, secretion of immunoglobulins, acting as a reservoir to permit bacterial metabolism and fermentation, possible participation in complex metabolic processes such as maintenance of nitrogen balance, and storage and evacuation of stool.[11] Many of these functions are undesirable or are no longer possible after interposition of a colon segment as an esophageal substitute. The transit time of the colon segment used as an interposition is normally sufficiently short that no important absorption takes place. Whether immunoglobulin secretion continues in the interposed segment is unknown. Bacterial metabolism and fermentation are undesirable for obvious reasons and fortunately are discouraged by the relatively rapid transit of foodstuffs. The storage function is usually lost, leaving the evacuation function as a possible aid to transit of food through the interposed segment of colon.

The colon also participates in what was once known as the gastrocolic response, which is an increase in motor activity in the colon soon after ingestion of a meal. There are now believed to be two phases to this response: an early postprandial response that occurs prior to entry of digesta into the colon, and a late postprandial response that occurs after entry of digesta into the colon.[12] Whether either response is preserved after colon interposition is not known.

Macroscopic and histologic changes in the mucosa are surprisingly few after colon interposition.[13] More than three-quarters of patients have no visible inflammation. Histologic specimens only rarely demonstrate chronic inflammatory changes or fibrosis.

Transit time through the colon interposition is dependent on the length of the interposition, the route used for esophageal reconstruction, the position of the patient during the evaluation, and possibly whether the interposition is in an isoperistaltic or an antiperistaltic orientation. Some authors have documented anecdotal instances of coordinated orad movement of tracer using scintigraphic techniques in patients with colon interpositions oriented in an antiperistaltic fashion. In general, however, liquid emptying from the colon in the upright position after long-segment interposition is markedly slower than for the normal esophagus and does not appear to depend on whether the interposition is in an iso- or an anti-peristaltic orientation.[14,15] The former finding is dramatically different than after stomach pull-up for esophageal reconstruction, in which case the stomach empties more quickly than the normal esophagus. In contrast, liquid emptying from a long-segment interposition in the supine position is similar for colon and gastric reconstructions, both of which are substantially prolonged compared to the normal esophagus.[16] Solid emptying from a colon interposition in the upright position is similar to that of the normal esophagus for short-segment interpositions, but is markedly prolonged for long-segment interpositions.[17]

The extensive knowledge regarding the motility of the colon in health has stimulated much interest in whether normal motility patterns are retained after a segment of colon is used to replace the esophagus. Some early manometric studies report peristaltic activity at rest in about 25% of patients after colon interposition, although at least one report demonstrated no important contractile activity.[18-22] Acid, and sometimes water instillation in the colon, was found to provoke peristaltic activity in many patients, although there was usually a delay of more than several minutes between instillation and the development of increased activity.[18,20,22] More recent studies report conflicting results. Most suggest that peristaltic activity in the interposed colon is rare, even after stimulation with water or acid.[23-26] In contrast, occasional reports suggest that during acute water instillation or during ambulatory monitoring there is routinely evidence of peristalsis-like activity.[17,27] Currently there is no consensus of opinion regarding this issue, but the majority of investigative and clinical reports suggest that the interposed colon behaves primarily as an inert tube and that passage of material through it is largely dependent upon gravity.

From a nutritional standpoint, colon interposition has no clear advantage over use of the stomach as an esophageal substitute. In adults, body weight in many patients continues to decline for up to 15 months but then stabilizes or increases in the majority of patients.[15,28,29] Serum total protein and albumin levels are lower when measured long-term after colon interposition than after stomach pull-up, whereas lipid levels are similar between the two groups. In the pediatric population, most patients resume normal growth patterns postoperatively despite occasional problems with vitamin B_{12} absorption if a long segment of terminal ileum is included with the interposition.[21,30,31]

Quality of life long-term after colon interposition has been assessed using a variety of techniques. Residual gastrointestinal symptoms are common, and include early satiety in 20% to 75% of patients, regurgitation in 10% to 20%, frequent eructation in over 50%, and postprandial abdominal pain in over 40%.[15,29,32,33] Surprisingly, diarrhea is an uncommon complaint, being present in fewer than 10% of patients during long-term follow-up. Despite these residual symptoms, 75% to 90% of patients rate their level of satisfaction as good or excellent and objective ratings of outcome are similar.[15,32,33]

Types of Colon Preparations for Esophageal Replacement

A variety of different techniques exist for use of the colon as an esophageal replacement. The main controversy in preparation of a colon interposition is whether to use the right or left colon. The choice between the two depends in part on the anatomic findings in an individual patient at the time of surgery but is largely based on personal preferences and training of the surgeon. The left colon is preferred for use in adult patients by most surgeons because it has a more consistent blood supply and a thicker wall, and because its diameter is smaller, providing a better size match for an end-to-end anastomosis. Surgeons for the pediatric age population more often use right colon preparations, a fact that is likely based on tradition and training. The data outlined above detail the fact that variations in the blood supply to the right colon are common, but whether this affects the viability and function of the interposition has not been conclusively determined.

Most colon interpositions involve the use of pedicled grafts, which can be based on the right, middle, or ascending branch of the left colic vessels. One of the vessels most commonly used as a basis for a pedicled graft is the middle colic artery, which can supply a long-segment graft of the right colon in an isoperistaltic orientation or of the left colon in an antiperistaltic orientation. The middle colic artery also provides the ability to create a short-segment graft of the transverse colon which can be placed in either orientation. The ascending branch of the left colic artery permits creation of short- or long-segment interpositions using the descending colon and portions of the transverse colon oriented in an isoperistaltic fashion. The right colic artery sometimes is used as the basis for grafts prepared from the ascending colon. In some instances, a free colon graft can be used if microvascular anastomoses are created to restore the blood supply.

Portions of the colon may be prepared as a short- or long-segment interposition. There are no strict definitions for these terms, although short-segment interpositions typically involve a proximal anastomosis below the level of the aortic arch (often below the level of the inferior pulmonary vein) whereas long-segment interpositions involve a proximal anastomosis high in the thorax or, more commonly, to the cervical esophagus. The categorization of the length of the interposition is not determined by the distance it extends into the abdomen even though this distance can be quite variable. When the stomach is intact the distal anastomosis is frequently made to the body of the stomach. In the absence of a substantially complete stomach, however, an anastomosis between the colon interposition and the first portion of the duodenum sometimes is required, which necessitates extra graft length.

Some surgeons make an effort to provide a valve as part of the reconstruction in the hope of preventing reflux of gastric contents through the colon interposition and into the esophagus. When the right colon is used in an isoperistaltic orientation, this is sometimes accomplished by leaving a segment of the terminal ileum attached, to which the esophagus is anastomosed, which permits the ileocecal valve to serve in an antireflux role. In other instances, an antireflux valve can be constructed using the colon, although this technique is not in widespread use.[34]

The orientation of the interposed segment (iso- versus anti-peristaltic) is not usually elective once the type of interposition has been selected because it is largely based on the anatomy of the interposition, particularly with reference to its blood supply. As described above, some authors have noted the presence of orad sequential contractions or fluid movement in patients in whom an antiperistaltic colon segment has been used for esophageal reconstruction. Most authors agree, however, that the orientation of the colon interposition is not a major determinant of postoperative function.

Operative Techniques

The initial surgical approaches to colon preparations (incisions, etc) will not be detailed because the preparations are not dependent upon them and because they are almost entirely operator-dependent. All colon interpositions can be prepared through an abdominal incision that gives good exposure to the colon, such as upper midline, upper transverse, and chevron incisions. As expertise develops in advanced laparoscopic surgery, it may be feasible to prepare colon interpositions using minimally invasive techniques, although no such procedures were documented prior to 2002. Left colon interpositions can also be prepared through a low left thoracotomy or left thoracoabdominal incision when either incision is used to perform an esophagectomy. With the former incision, access to the upper abdomen is gained through a peripheral incision in the diaphragm. Techniques that are described during preparation of a left colon interposition

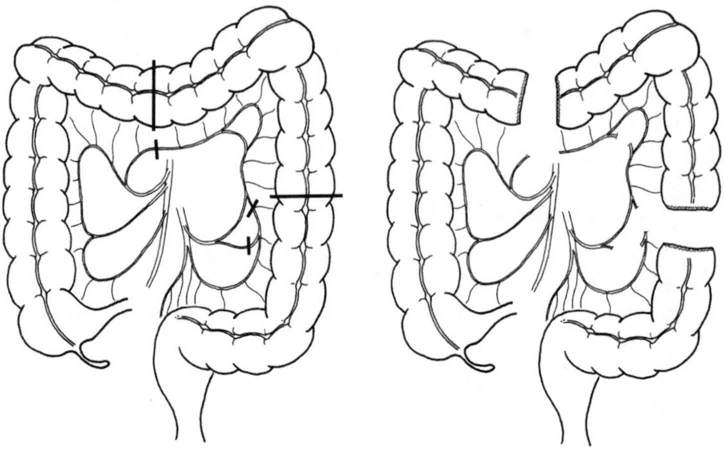

Figure 10-2. Isolation of the ascending branch of the left colic artery and preservation of the marginal artery during mobilization of the transverse and descending colon.

for dissection and trial occlusion of vessels that are to be divided are applicable to the preparation of all colon interpositions.

Isoperistaltic Left Colon Interposition

The omentum is separated from the transverse colon in the avascular plane. It is sometimes useful to leave a pedicle of omentum attached to the region in which the proximal anastomosis will be performed, which can then be used to buttress the anastomosis. The descending colon is mobilized from its lateral peritoneal attachments to the level of the sigmoid colon by dividing the white line of Toldt. Blunt mobilization is used to elevate the descending colon from its retroperitoneal attachments until the origin of the inferior mesenteric artery is identified.

The length of colon necessary for the interposition is estimated by passing a heavy suture or umbilical tape through the planned route of reconstruction. A few extra centimeters are added to the measured length to provide for contraction of the interposition as it is dissected. During preparation of the interposition, the string or tape is placed against the colon on its mesenteric (shorter) border periodically to determine the appropriate extent of mobilization of the vascular arcade.

The ascending branch of the left colic artery as well as the marginal and middle colic arteries are identified visually and by palpation. The mesentery is incised in the avascular windows on either side of the ascending branch of the left colic artery, taking care to leave a substantial amount of tissue on the vessel itself (Figure 10-2). The dissection is carried

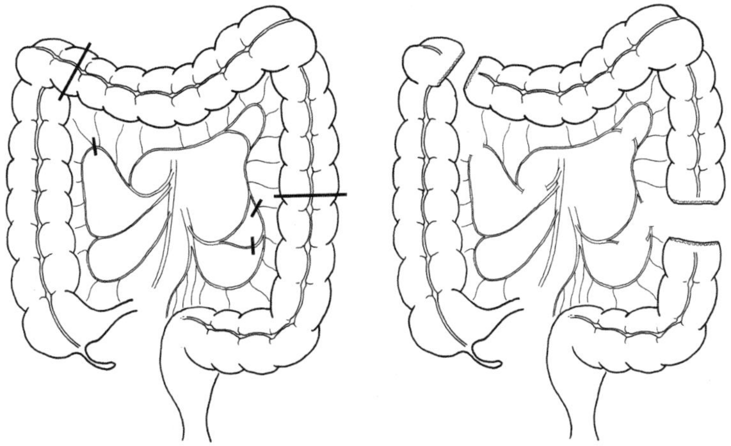

Figure 10-3. Technique for inclusion of the middle colic artery during preparation of a long-segment colon interposition.

proximal from the orad window, taking care to preserve the marginal artery, to a point where the middle colic artery is approached. Transillumination of the mesentery is often helpful for this portion of the procedure. If a short-segment interposition is to be performed, an adequate length of colon is usually available at this point. For long-segment interpositions, it is usually necessary to use the middle colic artery as a portion of the marginal vessel (Figure 10-3). This is sometimes technically challenging if the initial branching of the vessel occurs close to its origin. When this is the case, the origin is dissected out and a partially occluding clamp is placed across its base (Figure 10-4). The origin is oversewn, preserving the communication between the right and left branches, and the superior mesenteric artery is repaired.

The colon just distal to the ascending branch of the left colic artery is skeletonized. The necessary length of colon is again measured along the mesenteric border, and the site selected for proximal division of the colon is also skeletonized, taking care to preserve the marginal artery and the middle colic artery. For a short-segment interposition, the marginal artery is temporarily occluded with an atraumatic clamp so that the only blood supply to the colon comes from the ascending branch of the left colic artery. For a long-segment interposition that requires use of the middle colic artery, this artery and the marginal artery orad to the point of the planned proximal division of the colon are both temporarily occluded with atraumatic clamps and the perfusion of the isolated colon is assessed. Visible and palpable pulsations are usually evident. The arterial supply may sometimes go into spasm during the dissection, and application of topical lidocaine or papaverine may relieve the spasm. If

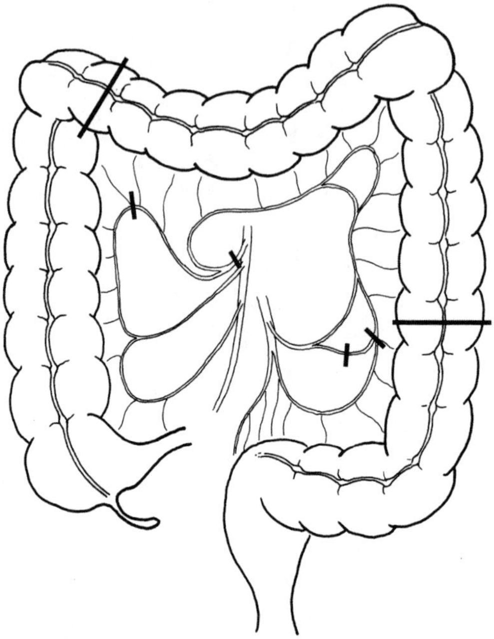

Figure 10-4. Use of a short middle colic artery to maintain the blood supply to the transverse colon during preparation of a long-segment colon interposition.

no adequate pulsations are evident, removing the vascular clamps and waiting for 10 to 20 minutes before reapplying them may clarify the situation. A Doppler flowmeter may be used to assess whether there is flow in the feeding vessels, but if a Doppler signal is the only evidence of flow, serious consideration should be given to use of another graft for esophageal reconstruction.

Once it has been determined that the blood supply is adequate and when the reconstruction route is ready to receive the interposition, the vessels that were temporarily clamped are ligated and divided, and the skeletonized sites are divided using a linear cutting stapler. If the colon is to be placed in the posterior mediastinum, it is brought posterior to the stomach and an anastomosis on the posterior wall of the stomach is performed. For substernal and antesternal routes the colon is brought anterior to the stomach. The proximal anastomosis is performed first, allowing the colon to be drawn back down into the abdomen so that the distal end can be trimmed prior to performing the distal anastomosis (Figure 10-5). This helps to prevent redundancy of the interposition. The remaining ends of the colon are anastomosed in a standard fashion and the mesenteric defect is closed when possible to prevent internal herniation. If a posterior mediastinal route is used, the colon interposition is tacked to

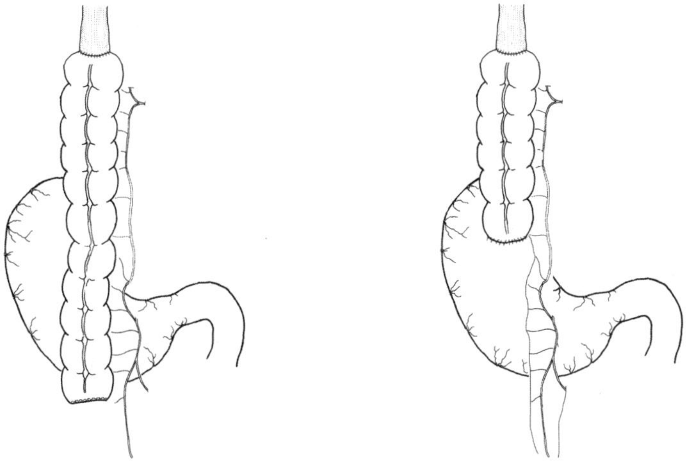

Figure 10-5. Determining the proper length of an interposition, once it has been transposed, is aided by first performing the proximal anastomosis (posterior view, left), then discarding any excess length prior to performing the distal anastomosis (posterior view, right).

the crura at the level of the hiatus to prevent herniation of abdominal contents into the thorax.

Antiperistaltic Left Colon Interposition

This interposition, which is not commonly used, usually is based on the middle colic artery. The left colon is mobilized from its peritoneal attachments and the omentum is divided from the transverse colon. Mesenteric windows on either side of the middle colic vessel are opened, and the transverse and proximal descending colon are dissected, preserving the marginal artery and the ascending branch of the left colic artery. The desired length of colon is measured along the mesenteric border, and short segments of the colon are skeletonized at either end of the measured section. The ascending branch of the left colic artery is temporarily occluded with an atraumatic clamp. When the blood supply is determined to be adequate, the artery is divided, and the segment is freed except for its vascular pedicle by dividing the colon with a linear cutting stapler across the skeletonized segments.

Isoperistaltic Right Colon Interposition

The right colon is mobilized from its peritoneal attachments and the omentum is divided from the transverse colon. If the cecum is to be used as a part of the interposition, the appendix is removed. Mesenteric

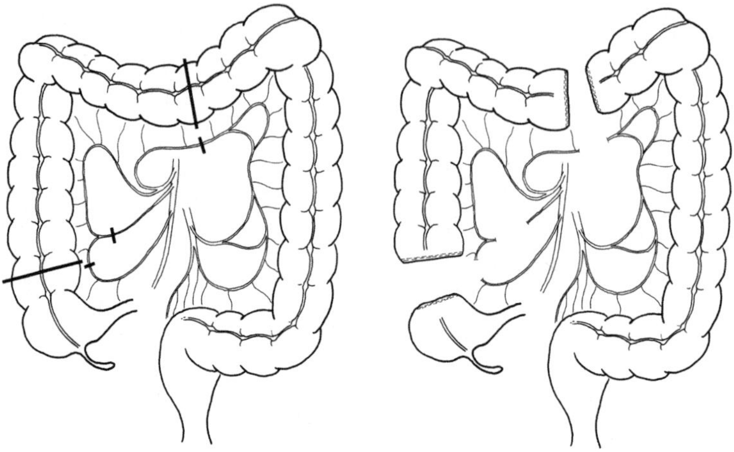

Figure 10-6. Preparation of an isoperistaltic right colon interposition based on the middle colic artery.

windows on either side of the middle colic artery are opened. Alternatively, the graft may be based on the left colic artery, in which case the middle colic artery is eventually divided at its base.[35] The dissection is carried proximally along the colon, taking care to preserve the marginal artery (Figure 10-6). The right colic and ileocolic arteries also are preserved. The desired length of the interposition is determined and is measured along the mesenteric border of the transverse and right colon segments. Short segments of the colon are skeletonized at the margins of the segment selected for use. If the right colic artery is required to serve as part of the marginal vessel, it is temporarily occluded near its origin with an atraumatic clamp to ensure that the blood supply to the segment of the colon most distal from the middle colic artery is sufficient. When the interposition route has been prepared, the right colic artery is divided and the colon segment is isolated by dividing the skeletonized regions with a linear cutting stapler. When creating a short-segment interposition based on the middle colic artery, the cecum and most proximal ascending colon are usually preserved in situ. Long-segment interpositions usually require use of the cecum, which is divided from the ileum at the junction between the two.

Antiperistaltic Right Colon Interposition

The right colon may be prepared as an antiperistaltic interposition based on the right colic artery, but this type of interposition is rarely used. After mobilizing the colon from its peritoneal and omental attachments,

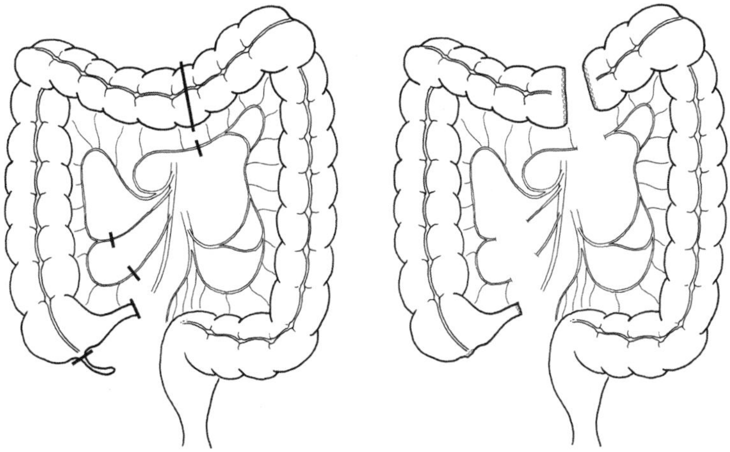

Figure 10-7. Preparation of an ileocolic interposition.

mesenteric windows on either side of the right colic artery are opened. The dissection is carried distally along the ascending and transverse colon, taking care to preserve the marginal and middle colic arteries. The desired length of interposition is marked off and short segments of the colon at each end are skeletonized. If it is necessary to divide the middle colic artery, the vessel is first occluded with an atraumatic clamp to ensure that the remaining blood supply to the colon segment is satisfactory. The remainder of the procedure is performed as described above.

Ileocolic Interposition

Use of an ileal segment attached to a right colon interposition has gained favor among some surgeons because of the good size match between the ileum and the esophagus, and because of the theoretical advantage of having an antireflux valve (the ileocecal valve) positioned between the colon interposition and the esophagus.[36,37] The interposition is based on a pedicle including the middle colic artery as described above for preparation of an isoperistaltic right colon interposition. In addition to dividing the right colic artery near its origin, the ileocolic artery also is divided near its origin (Figure 10-7). The appendix is removed, and a segment of ileum measuring 10 to 15 cm is isolated and left attached to the cecum. The remainder of the procedure is performed as described for preparation of the other types of interposition.

Complications Related to Colon Interposition

It is sometimes difficult to identify complications that arise from a complex operation such as esophagectomy and colon interposition which

Table 10-1.
Acute Complications after Colon Interposition.

	Short-segment interposition	Long-segment interposition
Cervical anastomotic leak	Rare	10%
Gastric anastomotic leak	Rare	5%
Graft necrosis	Rare	5%
Mortality	2%	7%

From references 3,26,32,33,38-41,48,49.

can be attributed specifically to the type of esophageal reconstruction that is performed. The acute and long-term complications that are reconstruction-specific are detailed here.

Graft ischemia or necrosis

Ischemia or necrosis of the graft is the most feared complication of colon interposition and occurs in about 5% of patients (Table 10-1).[3,26,31-33,38-41] This problem may arise regardless of whether adequate perfusion is evident at the time the interposition is prepared, although the risk of vascular compromise is higher when the blood supply is perceived to be marginal. Pulsed Doppler flowmetry may assist in predicting graft viability, in that patients in whom graft necrosis or anastomotic leakage occurs sometimes have evidence for end-systolic or end-diastolic flow reversal.[42] When marginal viability is suspected intraoperatively, microvascular anastomoses can be created in the neck or to the internal mammary vessels to "supercharge" the colon interposition, reducing the risk of graft necrosis and anastomotic leak.[43-46] In some instances, it is apparent prior to transposition of the graft through the reconstructive route that the graft is not viable. In this situation, it may be possible to salvage the colon segment by using it as a free graft and creating microvascular anastomoses in the chest or in the neck. Under most circumstances the segment must be discarded in favor of another reconstructive organ which is prepared either under the same anesthetic or during a subsequent operation.

Ischemia or necrosis of an interposition are not always simple to diagnose in the early postoperative period prior to the onset of frank sepsis, and a high index of suspicion must be maintained. Signs suggestive of colon infarction include tachycardia, supraventricular arrhythmias, unexplained acidosis, leukocytosis, confusion, and hypoxia. The patient may exhibit severe halitosis, or a foul exudate may be found in the nasal tube draining the interposition. Mesenteric arteriography is not of much value in determining whether the colon is viable.[47] Endoscopy may demonstrate ischemic mucosa suggestive of infarction. Aggressive mucosal biopsies that cause no bleeding should raise the suspicion that an ischemic event has occurred. Exploration is often necessary to make a definitive diagnosis of necrosis of the interposition. If a cervical anastomosis has been performed, the neck incision is reopened to enable visualization of the colon. It is usually readily apparent if necrosis has occurred, but if there is any question, one or two partial thickness incisions may be performed to determine if there is still blood flow to the segment. Necrosis of the cephalad portion of the colon is sometimes evident while the caudad segment remains viable, although this is an uncommon occurrence. In such an instance it may be possible to preserve the distal colon for future use in a composite reconstruction. Under most circumstances, however, when graft ischemia develops the entire interposition is infarcted and must be discarded. The organ to which the distal anastomosis was performed is closed, the reconstructive route is drained, and the esophagus is exteriorized as an end-ostomy. Staged reconstruction is considered when the patient has completely recovered.

Anastomotic Leak, Anastomotic Stricture

The incidence of anastomotic leak after colon interposition is about 10%, which is somewhat lower than is documented after gastric pull-up (Table 10-1).[3,26,31-33,38-41,48,49] The lower incidence is most likely a result of less tension on the anastomosis and more selective use of colon grafts, eliminating those that are suspected of having a marginally adequate blood supply. Short-segment interpositions have a lower anastomotic leak rate than do long-segment interpositions. This finding for short-segment interpositions is related to the relative absence of tension on the anastomosis, a more reliable blood supply, and greater caution regarding the use of an intrathoracic anastomosis, which leads to the surgeon being more selective in use of a marginally viable colon segment. Overall management of anastomotic leaks is detailed in Chapters 15 and 16.

The incidence of anastomotic stricture is closely related to the frequency with which anastomotic leaks occur. Some leaks are subclinical, thus the incidence of stricture is usually greater than that of clinically recognized leaks. In addition, chronic ischemia of the colon interposition, which may be due to relative obstruction to venous outflow from the organ, has also been proposed as a cause for anastomotic stricture. The management of anastomotic stricture is discussed in detail in Chapter 15.

Graft Redundancy

Redundancy of the interposed segment of colon is a well-recognized long-term complication of colon interposition. It is most often described

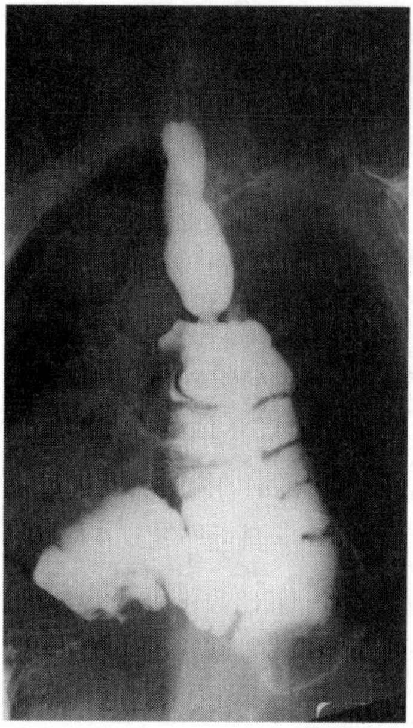

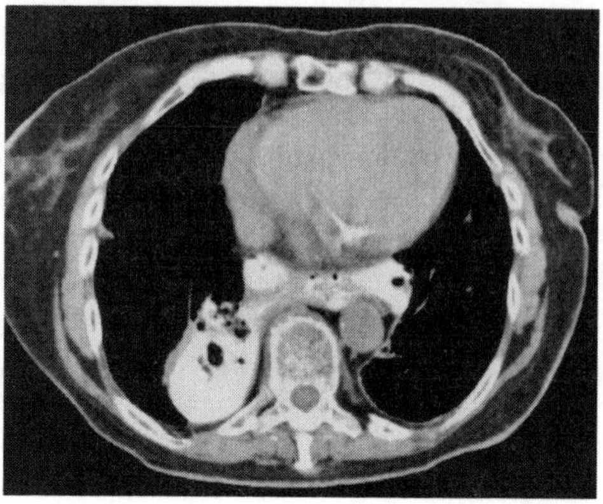

Figure 10-8. Radiographs demonstrating redundancy on barium swallow (left) and computed tomography (right) that can occur if a colon interposition is not trimmed to appropriate length.

in the pediatric population.[36,50,51] Whether this is due to interval growth of the interposition or to the techniques used to perform the esophageal reconstruction is unknown. Redundancy occurs more commonly when there is little restriction to dilatation of the colon interposition, a situation which is most often related to use of a subcutaneous route for reconstruction but may also be present when a transpleural route is used (Figure 10-8).[52,53]

Graft redundancy may lead to dysphagia, obstruction, regurgitation, weight loss, and bacterial overgrowth.[55] Management of clinically important redundancy requires segmental resection of the interposition with preservation of the blood supply. Sometimes this procedure can be performed through an abdominal approach, but often the redundancy resides above the level of the diaphragm.[55-57] Graft revision is straightforward when the colon interposition is in a subcutaneous location. However, except in older or high risk patients, consideration should be given to transposing the colon to a substernal route to create a shorter conduit while eliminating the redundancy. Redundancy of interpositions placed in the substernal or posterior mediastinal routes is technically more difficult to correct, requiring sternotomy or lateral thoracotomy to obtain access. Segmental resection or a side-to-side colocolostomy is then performed.[58]

Chronic Ischemia

It has been theorized that chronic vascular insufficiency of the colon interposition, which is sometimes present from the time of esophageal reconstruction, may lead to the formation of a long stricture. Support for this theory comes from radiographic studies in which morphologic changes in the interposition, including loss of haustrations, thumb printing, and an ill-defined bowel wall border, resemble changes in the chronically ischemic colon in situ.[59-61] Management of this problem depends on the viability of the graft and on the severity of any stricture that has developed. Long-term periodic dilation may suffice for patients with mild to moderate strictures, but loss of viability or the development of a nondilatable stricture necessitates resection of the colon interposition with subsequent reconstruction.

Unusual Complications of Colon Interposition

The interposed colon is subject to the same types of long-term problems for which the in situ colon is at risk.[62,63] There are numerous anecdotal cases of cancer developing in a colon interposition.[58,64-66] Usually these are identified in an early stage and are amenable to resection. Diverticulitis may also develop in a colon interposition, and reports of spontaneous fistula formation between the colon and the pericardium may be a result of such an event.[67,68] Conservative management has sometimes been successful for these patients, although a persistent fistula or sepsis may signal the need for resection and subsequent reconstruction.

References

1. Sonneland J, Anson BJ, Beaton LE. Surgical anatomy of the arterial supply to the colon from the superior mesenteric artery based upon a study of 600 specimens. *Surg Gynecol Obstet* 1958;106:385-398.
2. Sage M, Calmat A, Leguerrier A, et al. Vascularisation du colon transverse. *Bull Assoc Anat* 1977;61:397-406.
3. Peters JH, Kronson JW, Katz M, et al. Arterial anatomic considerations in colon interposition for esophageal replacement. *Arch Surg* 1995;130:858-863.
4. Vandamme JP, Van der Schuren G. Re-evaluation of the colic irrigation from the superior mesenteric artery. *Acta Anat* 1976;95:578-588.
5. Steward JA, Rankin FW. Blood supply to the large intestine. *Arch Surg* 1933;26:843-891.
6. Meyers MA. Griffiths' point: A critical anastomosis at the splenic flexure. Significance in ischemia of the colon. *Am J Roentgenol* 1976;126:77-94.
7. Cheng BC, Gao SZ. Anatomical study on the Riolan's anastomosis arch. *Chin J Surg* 1995;33:232-233.
8. Ventemiglia R, Khalil KG, Frazier OH, et al. The role of preoperative mesenteric arteriography in colon interposition. *J Thorac Cardiovasc Surg* 1977;74:98-104.
9. Fisher DF Jr, Fry WJ. Collateral mesenteric circulation. *Surg Gynecol Obstet* 1987;164:487-492.

10. Mitchell GAG. Nerve supply of the gastrointestinal tract. *Clin Symp* 1959;2:143-169.
11. Moran BJ, Jackson AA. Function of the human colon. *Br J Surg* 1992;79:1132-1137.
12. Sarna SK. Colonic motor activity. *Surg Clin N Am* 1993;73:1201-1223.
13. Isolauri J, Helin H, Markkula H. Colon interposition for esophageal disease: Histologic findings of colonic mucosa after a follow-up of 5 months to 15 years. *Am J Gastroenterol* 1991;86:277-280.
14. Isolauri J, Koskinen MO, Markkula H. Radionuclide transit in patients with colon interposition. *J Thorac Cardiovasc Surg* 1987;94:521-525.
15. DeMeester TR, Johansson K-E, Franze I, et al. Indications, surgical technique, and long-term functional results of colon interposition or bypass. *Ann Surg* 1988;208:460-474.
16. Kao C-H, Wang S-J, Chen C-Y, et al. The motility of interposition in patients with esophageal carcinoma after reconstructive esophageal surgery. *Clin Nuc Med* 1993;18:782-785.
17. Paris F, Tomas-Ridocci M, Galan G, et al. The colon as an oesophageal substitute in non-malignant disease. *Eur J Cardio-Thorac Surg* 1991;5:474-478.
18. Jones EL, Skinner DB, DeMeester TR, et al. Response of the interposed human colonic segment to an acid challenge. *Ann Surg* 1973;177:75-78.
19. Miller H, Lam KH, Ong GB. Observations of pressure waves in stomach, jejunal, and colonic loops used to replace the esophagus. *Surgery* 1975;78:543-551.
20. Corazziari E, Mineo TC, Anzini F, et al. Functional evaluation of colon transplants used in esophageal reconstruction. *Dig Dis* 1977;22:7-12.
21. Rodgers BM, Talbert JL, Moazam F, et al. Functional and metabolic evaluation of colon replacement of the esophagus in children. *J Pediatr Surg* 1978;13:35-39.
22. Benages A, Moreno-Ossett E, Paris F, et al. Motor activity after colon replacement of esophagus. *J Thorac Cardiovasc Surg* 1981;82:335-340.
23. Isolauri J, Reinikainen P, Markkula H. Functional evaluation of interposed colon in esophagus. Manometric and 24-hour pH observations. *Acta Chir Scand* 1987;153:21-24.
24. Little AG, Scott WJ, Ferguson MK, et al. Functional evaluation of organ interposition for esophageal replacement. In Siewert JR, Holscher AH (eds): **Diseases of the Esophagus**. Berlin, Springer-Verlag, 1998, pp 664-667.
25. Moreno Gonzalez E, Calleja Kempin IJ, Landa Garcia JI, et al. Functional study of ileocolic interposition after esophagectomy and total esophagogastrectomy. In Siewert JR, Holscher AH (eds): **Diseases of the Esophagus**. Berlin, Springer-Verlag, 1998, pp 668-673.
26. Gaissert HA, Mathisen DJ, Grillo HC, et al. Short-segment intestinal interposition of the distal esophagus. *J Thorac Cardiovasc Surg* 1993;106:860-867.
27. Peppas G, Payne HR, Jeyasingham K. Ambulatory motility patterns of the transposed short segment colon. *Gut* 1993;34:1572-1575.
28. Ando N, Ikehata Y, Ohmori T, et al. Prospective studies on postoperative nutritional status in patients with esophageal carcinoma as evaluated from various substitutes for reconstruction: Gastric tube versus colon interposition. In Siewart JR, Holscher AH (eds): **Diseases of the Esophagus**. Berlin, Springer-Verlag, 1998, pp 674-678.

29. Collard J-M, Otte J-B, Reynaert M, et al. Quality of life three years or more after esophagectomy for cancer. *J Thorac Cardiovasc Surg* 1992;104:391-394.
30. Kelly JP, Shackelford GD, Roper CL. Esophageal replacement with colon in children: Functional results and long-term growth. *Ann Thorac Surg* 1983;36:634-643.
31. Khan AR, Stiff G, Mohammed AR, et al. Esophageal replacement with colon in children. *Pediatr Surg Int* 1998;13:79-83.
32. Curet-Scott MJ, Ferguson MK, Little AG, et al. Colon interposition for benign esophageal disease. *Surgery* 1987;102:568-574.
33. Cerfolio RJ, Allen MS, Deschamps C, Trastek VF, Pairolero PC. Esophageal replacement by colon interposition. *Ann Thorac Surg* 1995;59:1382-1384.
34. Larsson S, Lycke G, Radberg G. Replacement of the esophagus by a segment of colon provided with an antireflux valve. *Ann Thorac Surg* 1989;48:677-682.
35. Furst H, Hartl WH, Lohe F, et al. Colon interposition for esophageal replacement: An alternative technique based on the use of the right colon. *Ann Surg* 2000;231:173-178.
36. Han M-T. Ileocolic replacement of esophagus in children with esophageal stricture. *J Pediatr Surg* 1991;26:755-757.
37. Touloukian RJ, Tellides G. Retrosternal ileocolic esophageal replacement in children revisited. *J Thorac Cardiovasc Surg* 1994;107:1067-1072.
38. Wilkins EW Jr. Long-segment colon substitution for the esophagus. *Ann Surg* 1980;192:722-725.
39. Huang M-H, Sung C-Y, Hsu H-K, et al. Reconstruction of the esophagus with the left colon. *Ann Thorac Surg* 1989;48:660-664.
40. Lundell L, Olbe L. Colonic interposition for reconstruction after resection of cancer in the esophagus and gastroesophageal junction. *Eur J Surg* 1991;157:189-192.
41. Thomas P, Fuentes P, Giudicelli R, et al. Colon interposition for esophageal replacement: Current and long-term function. *Ann Thorac Surg* 1997;64:757-764.
42. Jacob L, Rabary O, Boudaoud S, et al. Usefulness of perioperative pulsed Doppler flowmetry in predicting postoperative local ischemic complications after ileocolic esophagoplasty. *J Thorac Cardiovasc Surg* 1992;104:385-390.
43. O'Rourke IC, Threlfall GN. Colonic interposition for oesophageal reconstruction with special reference to microvascular reinforcement of graft circulation. *Aust N Z J Surg* 1986;56:767-771.
44. Fujita H, Yamana H, Sueyoshi S, et al. Impact on outcome of additional microvascular anastomosis - supercharge - on colon interposition for esophageal replacement: Comparative and multivariate analysis. *World J Surg* 1997;21:998-1003.
45. Zonta A, Visconti FE, Dionigi P, et al. Internal mammary blood supply for ileo-colon interposition in esophagogastroplasty: A case report. *Microsurgery* 1998;18:472-475.
46. Golshani SD, Lee C, Cass D, et al. Microvascular "supercharged" cervical colon: Minimizing ischemia in esophageal reconstruction. *Ann Plast Surg* 1999;43:533-538.
47. Gossot D, Houlle D, De Longueau M, et al. Coloplasties retrosternales: Apport de l'arteriographie mesenterique post-operatoire. *Gastroenterol Clin Biol* 1988;12:619-623.

48. Cherveniakov A, Cherveniakov P. Colon substitution for radical treatment of cardia and lower third esophageal cancer. *Eur J Cardio-Thoracic Surg* 1993;7:601-605.
49. Cheng B-C, Lu S-Q, Gao S-Z, et al. Colon replacement from esophagus. Clinical experience from 240 cases. *Chin Med J* 1994;107:216-218.
50. Bassiouny I, Bahnassy AF. Transhiatal esophagectomy and colonic interposition for caustic esophageal stricture. *J Pediatr Surg* 1992;27:1091-1096.
51. Ahmad SA, Sylvester KG, Hebra A, et al. Esophageal replacement using the colon: Is it a good choice? *J Pediatr Surg* 1996;31:1026-1031.
52. Stone MM, Fonkalsrud EW, Mahour GH, et al. Esophageal replacement with colon interposition in children. *Ann Surg* 1986;203:346-351.
53. Urschel JD. Late dysphagia after presternal colon interposition. *Dysphagia* 1996;11:75-77.
54. Sterling RP, Kuykendall RC, Carmichael MJ, et al. Unusual sequelae of colon interposition for esophageal reconstruction: Late obstruction requiring reoperation. *Ann Thorac Surg* 1984;38:292-295.
55. Schein M, Conlan AA, Hatchuel MD. Surgical management of the redundant transposed colon. *Am J Surg* 1990;160:529-530.
56. Santos GH. Late volume changes in retrosternal colon bypass. *Ann Thorac Surg* 1991;51:296-298.
57. Jeyasingham K, Lerut T, Belsey RHR. Functional and mechanical sequelae of colon interposition for benign oesophageal disease. *Eur J Cardio-Thorac Surg* 1999;15:327-332.
58. Bonavina L, Chella B, Segalin A, et al. Surgical treatment of the redundant interposed colon after retrosternal esophagoplasty. *Ann Thorac Surg* 1998;65:1446-1448.
59. Isolauri J, Paakkala T, Arajarvi P, et al. Colon interposition. Long-term radiographic results. *Eur J Radiol* 1987;7:248-252.
60. Pye JK, Wong J. Long ischemic stricture of the interposed colon. *Thorax* 1988;43:796-797.
61. Cheng W, Heitmiller RF, Jones B. Subacute ischemia of the colon esophageal interposition. *Ann Thorac Surg* 1994;57:899-903.
62. Kovacs BJ, Griffin RA, Chen YK. Synchronous adenomas in a colonic interposition graft and the native colon. *Am J Gastroenterol* 1997;92:2303-2304.
63. Del Rosario MA, Croffie JM, Rescorla FJ, et al. Juvenile polyp in esophageal colon interposition. *J Pediatr Surg* 1998;33:1418-1419.
64. Haerr RW, Higgins EM, Seymore CH, et al. Adenocarcinoma arising in a colonic interposition following resection of squamous cell esophageal cancer. *Cancer* 1987;60:2304-2307.
65. Houghton AD, Jourdan M, McColl I, et al. Carcinoma after colonic interposition for oesophageal stricture. *Gut* 1989;30:880-881.
66. Lee SJ, Koay CD, Thompson H, et al. Adenocarcinoma arising in an oesophageal colonic interposition graft. *J Laryngol Otol* 1994;108:80-83.
67. Wetstein L, Ergin MA, Griepp RA. Colopericardial fistula: Complication of colon interposition. *Texas Heart J* 1982;9:373.
68. Isolauri J, Markkula H. Recurrent ulceration and colopericardial fistula as late complications of colon interposition. *Ann Thorac Surg* 1987;44:84-85.

Chapter 11

Pedicled Jejunal Grafts

The jejunum is the third most commonly used organ for esophageal replacement. Small bowel usually retains its peristaltic function after interposition, making it an ideal organ for esophageal replacement from a motility standpoint. However, the anatomy of the blood supply to the small bowel is relatively segmental compared to that of the stomach or colon, which increases the risk of ischemia or necrosis, particularly if long segment reconstruction is necessary. Although the jejunum and ileum share similar motility patterns, the jejunum is used almost exclusively for esophageal reconstruction. The jejunum has a larger diameter, its wall is thicker, and its blood supply arises more proximally. In addition, the ileum has unique nutritional functions, such as vitamin B_{12} and bile salt absorption, which would be put at risk if long segments of ileum were used for esophageal reconstruction.

Anatomy

The jejunoileum is a 20- to 35-foot long hollow organ that extends from the duodenojejunal angle (the point where the small bowel transitions through the mesentery of the transverse mesocolon) to the cecum. Its diameter proximally is 20 to 25 mm, and it narrows to 10 to 12 mm at its distal end. Except for its mesenteric attachments, the jejunoileum is unattached to other abdominal structures. Although there is no clear-cut boundary between the jejunum and ileum, the remainder of this description will focus on properties of the proximal portion of the segment, the jejunum. In cross-section the jejunum is comprised of the serosa, the muscularis propria (including an outer longitudinal layer and an inner circular layer), and the submucosa/mucosa. The lumen is lined by folds that run perpendicular to the longitudinal axis called vavulae conniventes.

From Ferguson MK: *Reconstructive Surgery of the Esophagus* Armonk, NY: Futura Publishing Company, Inc., © 2002.

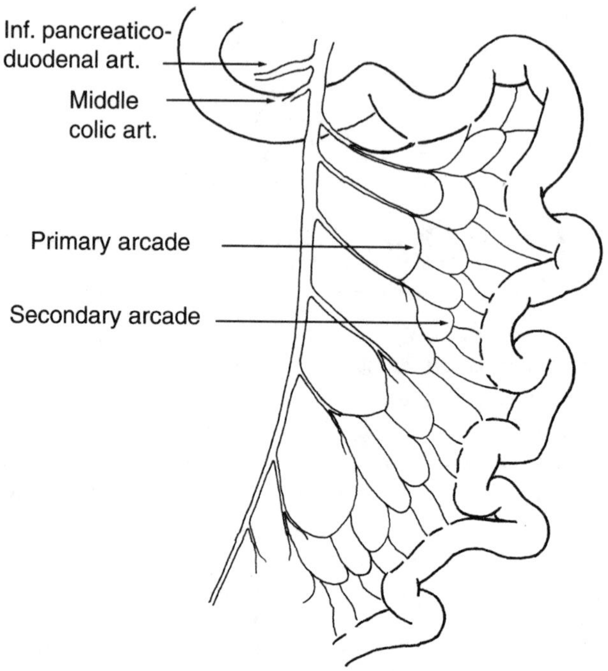

Figure 11-1. Arterial anatomy of the jejunum.

The blood supply to the jejunum arises from the superior mesenteric artery. The right, ileocolic, and middle colic vessels branch from the right side of this artery, whereas the jejunal branches arise from the left side. In the first 60 cm of jejunum there are from one to five jejunal arteries; the average number of arteries for this region is three.[1] The caliber of the jejunal branches diminishes from their origin at the superior mesenteric artery until they reach a series of arches which run parallel to the bowel wall (Figure 11-1). The first arch forms an anastomosis with the inferior pancreaticoduodenal artery over 60% of the time.[1,2] In the proximal jejunum a single primary arcade is usually formed from each vessel, although multiple arches arising from a single vessel are identified 15% of the time.[3] More distally two and sometimes three arches commonly are formed from each branch from the superior mesenteric artery. These arcades usually communicate with the adjacent arcades on either side, but over 15% have weak linkages to arches arising from other arteries. In over 5% of patients there is a complete interruption of the lateral linkages between adjacent jejunal arteries.[3] There are typically two levels of arcades in the proximal jejunum, although as many as four levels may occur. The ultimate arcade gives rise to the vasa recta, which are relatively straight end-vessels that enter the bowel wall. The bases of the ultimate arcade arches are often connected by a marginal artery that runs parallel to the mesenteric border of the jejunum and which may be important in maintaining the viability of the jejunum in the same way that the marginal artery of Drummond protects the colon.

The jejunum is drained by venous branches, which course anterior to the arteries and join the superior mesenteric vein. There is at most one vein per arterial branch and often there is only a single vein per every two or three arterial branches. Some of the proximal venous branches enter the superior mesenteric vein quite high, at the level of the transverse portion of the duodenum.

The innervation of the jejunum is similar to that of the right and transverse colon.[2,4] Sympathetic fibers arise from T7-T12 and run down the sympathetic trunks to the celiac plexus, from where they course to the superior mesenteric and preaortic plexuses and then to the jejunum. The parasympathetic supply arises from the right (posterior) vagus nerve and passes through the same plexuses as for the sympathetic fibers. The postganglionic fibers synapse with the autonomic plexuses in the bowel wall.

Postoperative Function of Jejunal Interpositions

The function of the transposed jejunum has not been studied extensively except for its motility. The important functions of fluid and electrolyte secretion and absorption, digestion, and absorption of nutrients by the transposed jejunum have largely been ignored. The jejunum is primarily responsible for the absorption of calcium, carbohydrates, fats, proteins, fat soluble vitamins, folic acid, magnesium, phosphorus, sodium, vitamin B_1, and water, although the ileum shares somewhat in the ability to absorb these nutrients.[5] In contrast, the ileum is almost exclusively responsible for absorption of ascorbic acid, bile salts, vitamin B_{12}, and zinc. The jejunum also releases gastrointestinal polypeptides that are important for intestinal function including bombesin, cholecystokinin, motilin, and gastric inhibitory peptide, none of which has been studied in the context of the interposed jejunum.

Denervation of the jejunum, as might occur during its preparation for interposition, results in an increase in the frequency with which migrating motor complexes occur. In contrast, there is a decrease in the frequency and amplitude of postprandial contractions, fewer contractions propagate distally, intestinal transit is somewhat slower, and the onset of fed motor activity is delayed. The relatively small magnitude of these changes suggests that motor activity of the jejunum is under primary control of the intrinsic nervous system, and that the extrinsic nerves serve primarily

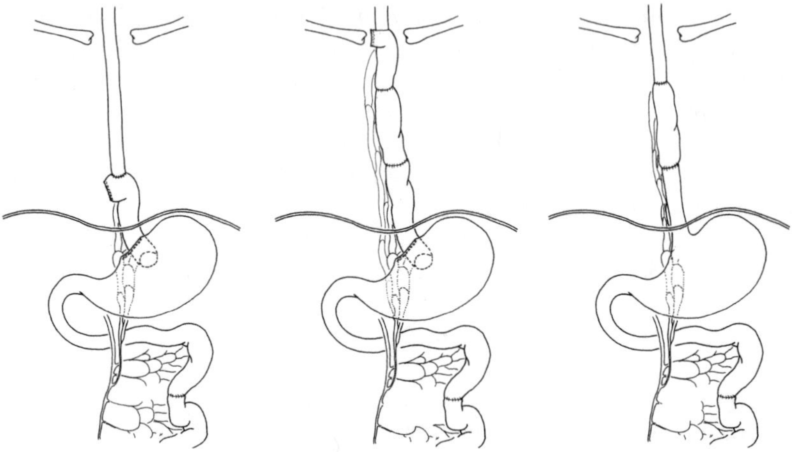

Figure 11-2. Types of jejunal interposition grafts for esophageal replacement include the short-segment graft, the long-segment graft, and a pedicled short-segment graft for use in the thorax.

to modulate this activity.[6] The polarity of this activity in the denervated jejunum is maintained, suggesting that jejunal interpositions should always be oriented in an isoperistaltic direction.[7]

Investigations of motility in the interposed jejunum demonstrate the presence of individual propagated waves during fasting as well as deglutition- and infused fluid bolus-induced propagated waves.[8-12] Hydrochloric acid instillation produces a hyperkinetic response in some patients which is characterized by contractions of high amplitude or long duration.[9] Despite these findings, transit of solids through the interposed jejunal segment is markedly slower than through the normal esophagus.[13]

The clinical status of patients who have undergone jejunal interposition is generally good. Dysphagia, regurgitation, and heartburn are rare, and most patients are able to take an unrestricted diet.[11,13-18] Diarrhea occurs in up to 20% of patients, but body weight is generally well maintained.[12,13]

Types of Pedicled Jejunal Grafts

Pedicled jejunal grafts as esophageal replacements are most often used as short segment interpositions for reconstructing the distal esophagus (Figure 11-2). Longer segments of jejunum can be fashioned to enable replacement of most of the thoracic esophagus as well. Although free jejunal grafts are used most commonly to reconstruct the cervical esophagus, pedicled grafts may also be harvested as segmental replacements for this region. These latter techniques are discussed in detail in Chapter

12. Jejunal segments are always placed in an isoperistaltic orientation because of the frequency with which peristaltic activity is observed after transposition.

Operative Techniques

Adequate operative exposure is necessary to enable the selection of an appropriate segment of jejunum and to permit its harvest. This can be accomplished through any of several standard laparotomy approaches, and left thoracotomy or thoracoabdominal incisions have also been used for this purpose. Recently, laparoscopic techniques have been reported for the harvest of free jejunal grafts (see Chapter 12), but these techniques have not yet been applied to the creation of pedicled jejunal grafts.

Short-Segment Interpositions

Transillumination is used to visualize the pattern of arterial supply to the jejunum. Because the most proximal 15 cm of jejunum is tethered by a relatively short mesentery, a suitable segment of jejunum is sought for beginning in the region of the third jejunal arterial branch from the superior mesenteric artery.[1] The length of jejunum necessary for the interposition is estimated by passing a heavy suture or umbilical tape through the planned route of reconstruction. The mesentery of the jejunum can unexpectedly limit the length of the interposition, and it is appropriate to add an extra 5 to 10 cm to the measured length to provide for this possibility and for contraction of the interposition as it is dissected. During preparation of the interposition, the string or tape is placed against the jejunum on its mesenteric (shorter) border periodically to determine the appropriate extent of mobilization of the vascular arcade. Straightening the segment of bowel to be used while making this measurement will help avoid the catastrophic surprise of an unexpectedly short bowel segment after the preparation is finished.

Depending on the length of the interposition that is required, it may be necessary to harvest a segment of jejunum that normally is supplied by many arterial branches from the superior mesenteric artery. A long pair of vessels (artery and vein) which enters the aboral end of the segment to be used is selected; these will serve as the blood supply. Longer jejunal segments are based on feeding vessels that arise more distally. Care should be taken that all primary and secondary vascular arcades supplying the selected segment have appropriate interconnections, in order to ensure their communication with the root vessels arising from the superior mesenteric vessels. The avascular mesenteric windows between the main

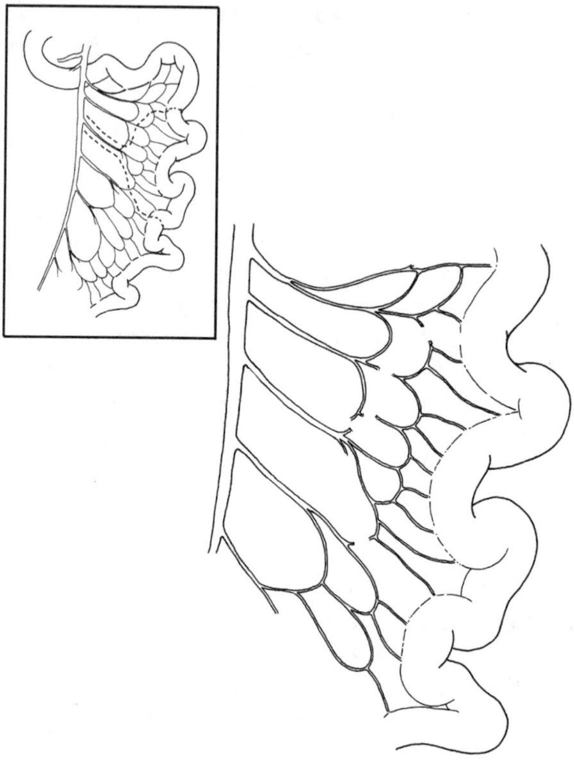

Figure 11-3. Initial preparation of a short-segment graft, during which the jejunal arteries to be divided are dissected and temporarily clamped.

jejunal arteries are divided and the arteries and veins are dissected close to their bases while leaving a substantial amount of tissue on the vessels themselves (Figure 11-3).

Small vascular clamps are used to temporarily occlude the jejunal arteries, leaving the distal blood supply to the segment untouched. The quality of the perfusion is assessed by examining for appropriate color, arterial pulsations, and peristalsis. If the blood supply appears to be adequate, the appropriate length of the segment is again measured and the bowel at each end of the segment is skeletonized. All of the jejunal arteries feeding the segment except the distal artery upon which the segment will be based are again clamped and the perfusion is reassessed. Once it has been determined that the blood supply is adequate, and when the reconstruction route is ready to receive the interposition, the occluded vessels are divided near their bases and the bowel segment is transected at either end using a linear-cutting stapler (Figure 11-4).

If the perfusion does not appear to be adequate, the vascular clamps are removed and the cause for hypoperfusion is sought. The arterial supply

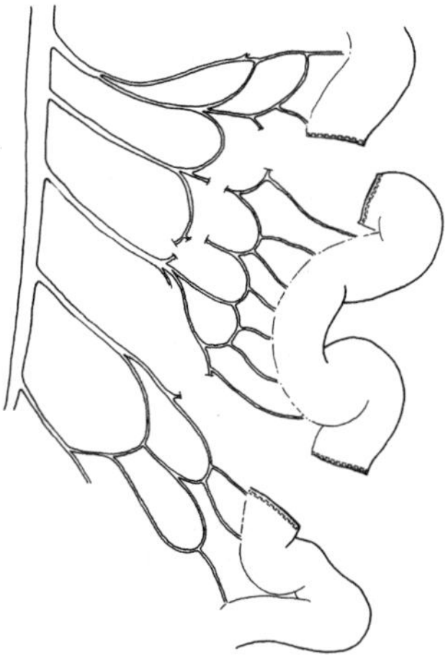

Figure 11-4. Final preparation of a short-segment graft, during which the jejunal arteries are divided and the bowel is transected at either end.

may sometimes go into spasm during the dissection, and application of topical lidocaine or papaverine may relieve the spasm. If no adequate pulsations are evident, removing the vascular clamps and waiting for 10 to 20 minutes before reapplying them may clarify the situation. A Doppler flowmeter may be used to assess whether there is flow in the feeding vessels, but if a Doppler signal is the only evidence of flow, serious consideration should be given to use of another graft for esophageal reconstruction. In some instances, a previously unrecognized interruption between the vascular arcades is evident. In other instances, an injury to the vascular supply may have occurred during preparation of the graft. In either case, preparation of the segment should be abandoned and another means of esophageal reconstruction should be selected.

When preparation of the graft is complete, the segment is placed through a defect created in the transverse mesocolon to permit its passage through as direct a route as possible. This avoids kinking of the graft and the need for additional graft length. The jejunum is brought posterior to the stomach and the proximal anastomosis is performed first, allowing the jejunum to be drawn back down into the abdomen so that the distal end can be trimmed prior to performing the distal anastomosis. This helps prevent redundancy of the interposition. The proximal anastomosis is often created in an end-to-side fashion because of the natural curvature of the jejunum. The remaining ends of the jejunum are anastomosed in a standard fashion and the mesenteric defect is closed when possible to prevent internal herniation. The jejunal interposition is tacked to the crura at the level of the hiatus to prevent herniation of abdominal contents into the thorax.

The distal anastomosis of the graft is performed to the posterior wall of the stomach (Figure 11-5). In patients in whom the stomach has been

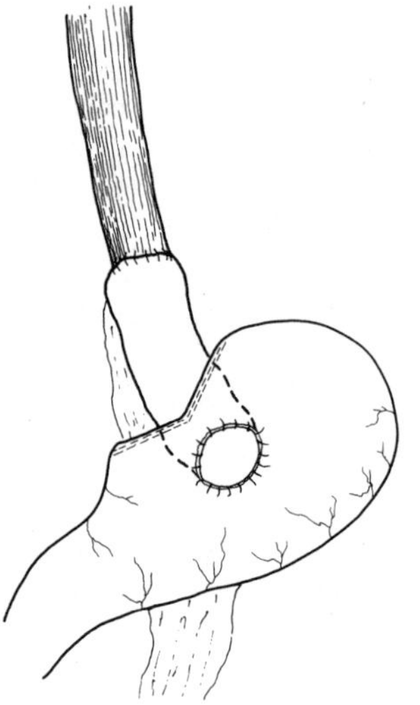

Figure 11-5. For short-segment interpositions, the bowel is brought through the posterior mediastinum to permit an intrathoracic anastomosis to the esophagus, and the distal anastomosis is created to the posterior wall of the stomach.

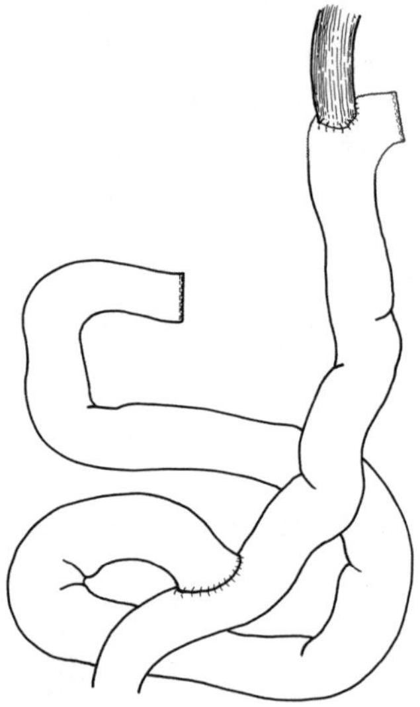

Figure 11-6. Technique for performing a jejunal interposition after total gastrectomy by creating a Roux-en-Y jejunojejunostomy.

resected or in whom gastric continuity will not be restored for other reasons, a long Roux-en-Y limb is created to prevent reflux of bile and pancreatic juices. To accomplish this, the jejunum is transected at the proximal margin of the graft but is left intact distally. The jejunum proximal to the point of transection is anastomosed to the distal jejunum in an end-to-side fashion at least 30 to 45 cm from the point where the jejunum passes into the thorax (Figure 11-6).

Long-Segment and Long-Pedicled Interpositions

The use of longer jejunal segments for total esophageal replacement and longer pedicled segments for high segmental esophageal replacement requires greater technical skill and experience than is required for construction of a short-segment of jejunum for reconstruction. The blood supply to these grafts is more tenuous, good judgment is necessary to determine the appropriate vessel upon which to base the graft, and one or more sleeve resections of the bowel are sometimes necessary to create a straight graft.

Transillumination of the bowel for evaluation of the vascular architecture is performed as was described for the preparation of a short-segment jejunal interposition. The necessary lengths of the bowel and of the mesenteric pedicle need to be carefully assessed. The length of the mesenteric pedicle is the most important factor in determining how the interposition will be developed. In order to determine how long the pedicle ultimately needs to be, it is usually necessary to begin the preparation of the pedicle. The first jejunal arterial branch is identified and preserved, and the second, third, and possibly the fourth branches are divided close to their origin. The arcade between the first and second artery branches is divided. V-shaped mesenteric incisions are created between the major vessels to permit straightening of the graft, leaving redundant tissue along the vessels so that they are not subject to undue stress (Figure 11-7). The length of the graft is assessed periodically by placing it through or along the reconstructive route. Additional jejunal arteries are divided as necessary to create a sufficient length of graft to reach the site for the proximal anastomosis. The graft may appear dusky at this point. Redundant bowel is resected from the oral end and especially from the anal end of the segment that has been mobilized by dividing the vasa recta as close to the bowel wall as possible, leaving all of the mesentery intact. This provides additional blood to the retained bowel and substantially improves the appearance of the bowel.[12,19] In some instances, persistent ischemia may be reversed by supplementing the blood supply through creation of microvascular anastomoses high in the thorax or in the neck, although this technique does not guarantee graft viability.[20] Alternatively, one or two sleeve resections may be necessary to align the bowel on a straight axis (Figure 11-8).

Grafts that have a mesentery that is long enough to reach the upper thoracic or cervical esophagus will frequently have loops of redundant jejunum (Figure 11-9). These redundant loops may develop adhesions between the segments of jejunum leading to obstruction. Food can collect within the stagnant regions leading to early satiety, distension, and halitosis. Redundant loops are aesthetically displeasing in patients in whom a subcutaneous interposition is performed. The redundant loops can also

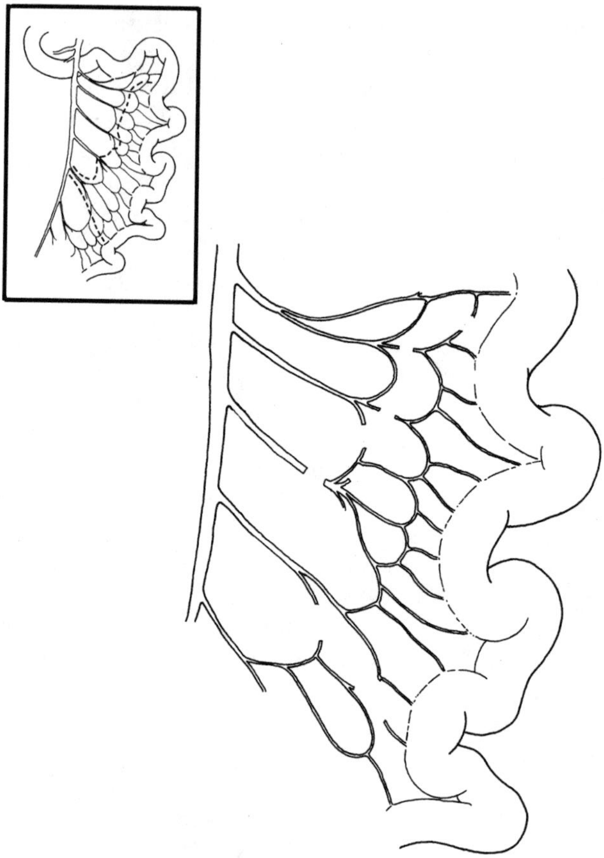

Figure 11-7. Initial mobilization of a long-segment jejunal interposition.

herniate into the pleural space in patients with substernal interpositions, leading to obstructive symptoms.[21] Segmental resection of redundant jejunum with an end-to-end anastomosis is necessary in most instances.

The jejunum is brought posterior to the stomach if it is to be placed in the posterior mediastinum. For substernal and antesternal routes the jejunum is brought anterior to the stomach. The proximal anastomosis is performed first, allowing the jejunum to be drawn back down into the abdomen so that the distal end can be trimmed prior to performing the distal anastomosis. This helps prevent redundancy of the interposition. The proximal anastomosis is often created in an end-to-side fashion because of the natural curvature of the jejunum. The remaining ends of the jejunum are anastomosed in a standard fashion and the mesenteric defect is closed when possible to prevent internal herniation. If a posterior mediastinal route is used, the jejunal interposition is tacked to the crura at

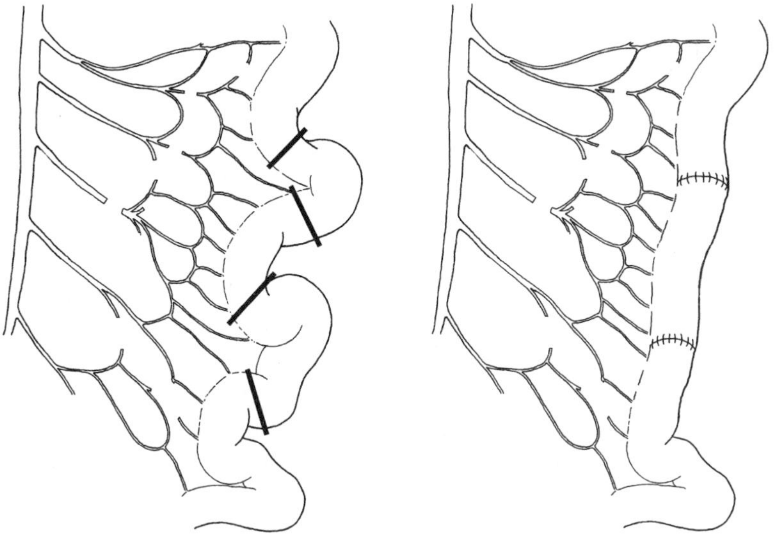

Figure 11-8. Removal of redundant bowel from the jejunal segment to be used, while preserving the entire mesentery, can be accomplished by sleeve resection and end-to-end anastomosis.

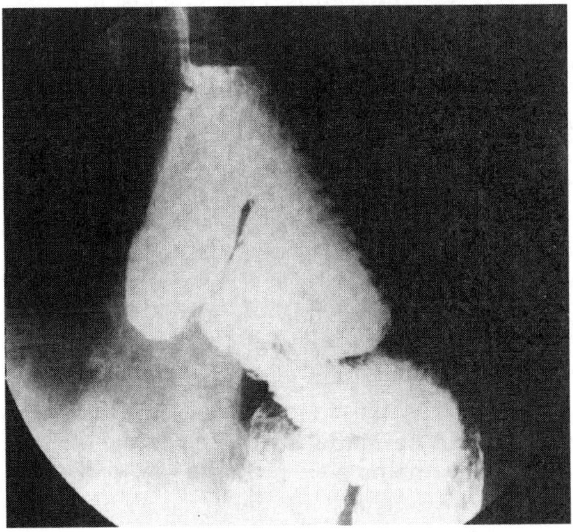

Figure 11-9. A redundant bowel loop that should have been excised prior to transposing a jejunal graft is evident at the level of the anastomosis.

the level of the hiatus to prevent herniation of abdominal contents into the thorax.

The distal anastomosis of the graft is performed to the posterior wall of the stomach for interpositions placed in the posterior mediastinum, whereas grafts brought through other routes are anastomosed to the anterior wall of the stomach. Special care is taken to avoid twisting or kinking the mesentery supplying the graft while transposing it through the reconstructive route.

Complications of Jejunal Interposition

It is sometimes difficult to identify complications that arise from a complex operation such as esophagectomy and jejunal interposition which can be attributed specifically to the type of esophageal reconstruction that is performed. The acute and long-term complications that are reconstruction-specific are detailed here.

Graft Ischemia and Necrosis

Because of the nature of the blood supply to the jejunum, graft ischemia and necrosis occur more often than with colon interpositions or gastric pull-ups. Short-segment interpositions are less likely to develop ischemic problems than are long-segment or long-pedicled interpositions. Arterial insufficiency is usually evident prior to completion of the interposition, in which case the graft is discarded and an alternative reconstructive method is considered. In such instances the loss of the graft is not usually recorded as an operative complication, leading to some inaccuracy in the estimation of the rate of graft loss associated with jejunal interposition. Venous insufficiency can present an insidious clinical picture during the early postoperative period and is a likely cause for late graft failure. The overall incidence of graft necrosis associated with jejunal interposition is reported to be about 2% but has been recorded to be as high as 11%.[11,13,15,16,18,22]

Ischemia and necrosis of a jejunal interposition are not always simple to diagnose postoperatively prior to the onset of frank sepsis, and a high index of suspicion must be maintained. Signs suggestive of jejunal infarction include tachycardia, supraventricular arrhythmias, unexplained acidosis, leukocytosis, confusion, and hypoxia. The patient may exhibit severe halitosis, or a foul exudate may be found in the nasal tube draining the interposition. Endoscopy may demonstrate ischemic mucosa suggestive of infarction. Aggressive mucosal biopsies that cause no bleeding should raise the suspicion that an ischemic event has occurred.

Exploration is often necessary to make a definitive diagnosis of necrosis of the interposition. If a cervical anastomosis has been performed, the neck incision is reopened to enable visualization of the graft. It is usually readily apparent if necrosis has occurred, but if there is any question, one or two partial thickness incisions may be performed to determine if there is still blood flow to the segment. When graft ischemia is identified the entire interposition must be discarded. The organ to which the distal anastomosis was performed is closed, the reconstructive route is drained, and the esophagus is exteriorized as an end-ostomy. Staged reconstruction is considered when the patient has completely recovered.

Anastomotic Leak and Dehiscence

The incidence of anastomotic leak after jejunal interposition is about 5%, which is somewhat lower than is documented after colon interposition and gastric pull-up.[11,13,16,18] As with patients undergoing colon interposition, the lower incidence is a result of minimal tension on the anastomosis and a highly selective use of jejunal grafts in which most grafts that are suspected of having a marginally adequate blood supply are discarded. There are few data regarding the relative incidence of anastomotic leaks related to the length of the interposition, but the data that do exist suggest that short-segment and long-segment interpositions have similar leak rates. Overall management of anastomotic leaks is detailed in Chapters 15 and 16.

Esophagojejunal anastomotic strictures develop in over 10% of patients.[11,13,15,16] The incidence of anastomotic stricture is closely related to the frequency with which anastomotic leaks occur. In a manner similar to that of colon interpositions, chronic ischemia of jejunal interpositions, which may be due to relative obstruction to venous outflow from the organ, has also been proposed as a cause for anastomotic stricture. The management of anastomotic stricture is discussed in detail in Chapter 15.

Chronic Ischemia

Subacute, chronic ischemia of the jejunum has been proposed as a cause of organ dysfunction, bleeding, ulceration, and stenosis.[23,24] In most instances, conservative management leads to complete recovery, and removal of the jejunum with alternative esophageal reconstruction is rarely necessary.

Graft Redundancy

Redundancy of jejunal grafts is a common radiographic finding that rarely requires surgical revision (Figure 11-10). That this complication

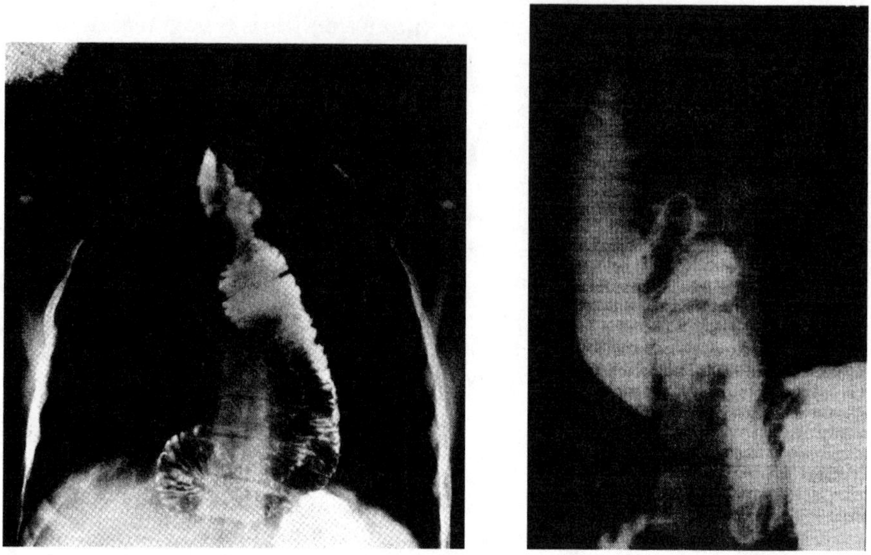

Figure 11-10. Radiographs demonstrating redundant bowel in two patients many years after a long-segment jejunal interposition.

is recognized more frequently after jejunal interposition than after colon interposition is primarily due to the anatomy of the blood supply to the jejunum, which makes creation of a completely straight graft difficult. In addition, many jejunal interpositions are performed in children, and subsequent growth patterns may promote graft redundancy. The frequency of graft redundancy is about 25%, but fewer than 5% of patients require surgical revision for problems of obstruction, regurgitation, or blind-loop syndrome.[11,15,16]

References

1. Michels NA, Siddharth P, Kornblith PL, Parke WW. The variant blood supply to the small and large intestines: Its import in regional resections. *J Int Coll Surg* 1963;39:127-170.
2. Chevrel J-P. Anatomy of the jejunum and ileum. In Wastell C, Nyhus LM, Donahue PE (eds): **Surgery of the Esophagus, Stomach, and Small Intestine**. Boston, Little, Brown and Company, 1995, pp 784-790.
3. Barlow TE. Variations in the blood-supply of the upper jejunum. *Br J Surg* 1955;43:473-475.
4. Mitchell GAG. Nerve supply of the gastrointestinal tract. *Clin Symp* 1959;2:143-169.
5. Thompson JS. The physiology of digestion and absorption. In Wastell C, Nyhus LM, Donahue PE (eds): **Surgery of the Esophagus, Stomach, and Small Intestine**. Boston, Little, Brown and Company, 1995, pp 806-815.

6. Johnson CP, Sarna SK, Cowles VE, et al. Motor activity and transit in the autonomically denervated jejunum. *Am J Surg* 1994;167:80-88.
7. Richards WO, Golzarian J, Wasudev N, et al. Reverse phasic contractions are present in antiperistaltic jejunal limbs up to twenty-one years postoperatively. *J Am Coll Surg* 1994;178:557-563.
8. Miller H, Lam KH, Ong GB. Observation of pressure waves in stomach, jejunal, and colonic loops used to replace the esophagus. *Surgery* 1975;78:543-551.
9. Moreno-Osset E, Tomas-Ridocci M, Paris F, et al. Motor activity in esophageal substitute (stomach, jejunal, and colon segments). *Ann Thorac Surg* 1986;41:515-519.
10. Pandolfo N, Spigno L, Guiddo G, et al. Valutazione funzionale dell'impianto gastrico e digiunale dopo esofagectomia. *Minerva Chirurg* 1991;46(Suppl 1):253-262.
11. Gaissert HA, Mathisen DJ, Grillo HC, et al. Short-segment intestinal interposition of the distal esophagus. *J Thorac Cardiovasc Surg* 1993;106:860-867.
12. Nishihira T, Oe H, Sugawara K, et al. Reconstruction of the thoracic esophagus with jejunal pedicled segments for cancer of the thoracic esophagus. *Dis Esoph* 1995;8:30-39.
13. Wright C, Cuschieri A. Jejunal interposition for benign esophageal disease. *Ann Surg* 1987;205:54-60.
14. Polk HC Jr. Jejunal interposition for reflux esophagitis and esophageal stricture unresponsive to valvuloplasty. *World J Surg* 1980;4:731-736.
15. Ring WS, Varco RL, L'Heureux PR, et al. Esophageal replacement with jejunum in children. *J Thorac Cardiovasc Surg* 1982;83:918-927.
16. Saeki M, Tsuchida Y, Ogata T, et al. Long-term results of jejunal replacement of the esophagus. *J Pediatr Surg* 1988;23:483-489.
17. Keller RJ, Sicular A. Jejunal interposition. *Gastrointest Radiol* 1989;14:9-14.
18. Watson TJ, DeMeester TR, Kauer WKH, et al. Esophageal replacement for end-stage benign esophageal disease. *J Thorac Cardiovasc Surg* 1998;115:1241-1249.
19. Ashizawa I, Nishihira T, Kasai M. Improvement of circulation in pedicled intestinal grafts: Hemodynamics of the intestine after preparation of a sacrificial colonic graft. *J Am Coll Surg* 1997;184:346-352.
20. Cusick EL, Batchelor AA, Spicer RD. Development of a technique for jejunal interposition in long-gap esophageal atresia. *J Pediatr Surg* 1993;28:990-994.
21. Dave KS, Wooler GH, Holden MP, et al. Esophageal replacement with jejunum for nonmalignant lesions: 26 years' experience. *Surgery* 1972;72:466-473.
22. Moorehead RJ, Wong J. Gangrene in esophageal substitutes after resection and bypass procedures for carcinoma of the esophagus. *Hepatogastroenterology* 1990;37:364-367.
23. Subramanyam K, Kolb WG. Upper gastrointestinal hemorrhage from ischemia of an interposed jejunal segment in the esophagus. *Am J Gastroenterol* 1988;83:68-70.
24. Vereczkei A, Rozsos I, Horvath OP. Subacute ischemic lesions in jejunal loops used for esophageal reconstruction. *Dis Esoph* 1998;11:194-197.

Chapter 12

Cervical Esophageal Reconstruction

Reconstruction of the pharyngoesophagus or cervical esophagus is a challenging endeavor due to the complex anatomy, the intensity of the intraoperative effort, and the high rate of postoperative complications. There are many options available for reconstruction, some of which require the expertise of microvascular surgeons, head and neck surgeons, or plastic and reconstructive surgeons. Choosing among the options for reconstruction is difficult and is guided by the immediate and long-term needs of the patient, the availability of reconstructive tissues, and local expertise.

Anatomy

The anatomy of the cervical esophagus and hypopharynx is complex, and only the important highlights will be outlined in this chapter. The hypopharynx is the lowermost of the three segments of the pharynx, which also includes the nasopharynx and oropharynx. The hypopharynx, the longest of these segments, extends as a funnel-shaped muscular tube from the tip of the epiglottis to the cricoid cartilage, where it merges with the cervical esophagus (Figure 12-1). The upper margin of the hypopharynx is at the level of the hyoid bone, and the lower margin is at the level of the sixth cervical vertebra. The outer, circular musculature includes the middle and inferior pharyngeal constrictors, while the inner, longitudinal muscles include the stylopharyngeus and the palatopharyngeus. The inferior pharyngeal constrictor merges with the cricopharyngeus muscle, which constitutes the upper esophageal sphincter. Motor innervation of

From Ferguson MK: *Reconstructive Surgery of the Esophagus* Armonk, NY: Futura Publishing Company, Inc., © 2002.

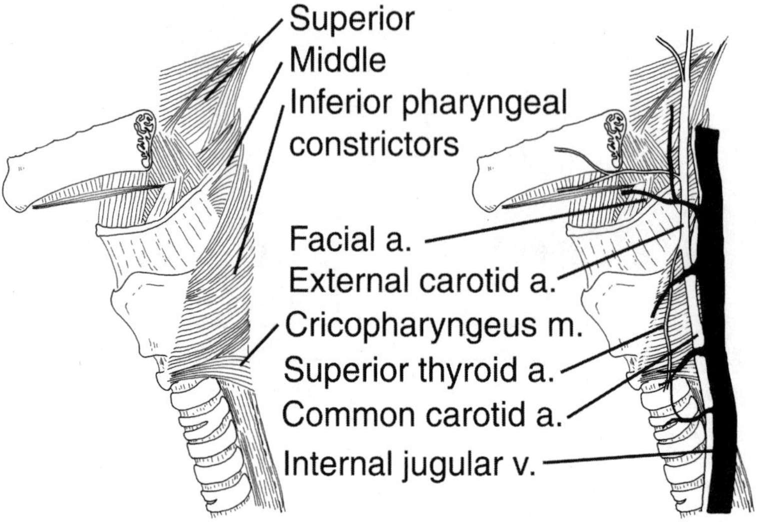

Figure 12-1. Anatomy of the pharyngoesophageal region.

the middle and inferior constrictors is provided by the superior and inferior laryngeal nerves and the pharyngeal plexus (cranial nerves IX, X, and possibly XI). The stylopharyngeus is innervated by the glossopharyngeal nerve (IX). Motor and sensory innervation to all other structures of the hypopharynx is provided by the vagus nerve (X). The outer surfaces of the muscles are contained within buccal fascia. The hypopharynx is lined by stratified squamous mucosa.

The cervical esophagus extends from the cricopharyngeus muscle to the sternal notch. Its length varies depending on an individual's anatomy. The cervical esophagus has an inner circular and an outer longitudinal layer, both of which are composed of striated muscle. The lumen is lined with stratified squamous epithelium.

Postoperative Function After Cervical Esophageal Reconstruction

Function after cervical esophageal or pharyngoesophageal reconstruction is rarely as good as after reconstruction of the thoracic esophagus. There are a number of reasons for this, including deficiencies of the swallowing mechanism, the high rate of long-term complications associated with some types of reconstructions, and the poor physiologic performance of most of the reconstructive organs or tissues.

Under normal circumstances, the glossopharyngeal phase of swallowing propels a food bolus through this region as a result of movement of the tongue, sequential contractions of the pharyngeal constrictors, and the development of negative pressure within the pharyngoesophageal segment distal to the constrictors.[1] Negative pressure arises as a result of anterosuperior displacement of the larynx and due to relaxation of the cricopharyngeal muscle.

Deficiencies of the glossopharyngeal phase of swallowing may be the result of injury to regional nerves or loss of vital structures. The larynx is elevated by the stylopharyngeus muscle, which is innervated by the glossopharyngeal nerve, and by the palatopharyngeus muscle, which is innervated by the glossopharyngeal, vagus, and accessory nerves via the pharyngeal plexus. The pharyngeal plexus, which lies posterior to the pharynx, is subject to injury during pharyngeal dissection. Such an injury may result in incomplete elevation of the larynx and ineffective propulsion of a food bolus. Such an injury might also cause a decrease in pharyngeal constrictor contraction amplitude, resulting in impaired clearance of a food bolus from the hypopharynx.[2] Impairment of tongue function, especially by injury to the glossopharyngeal nerve (which would also affect function of the stylopharyngeus muscle), results in a decrease in the propulsive force of bolus food movement.[3] Laryngectomy usually results in an increase in the propulsive force of the tongue when tongue function is unaltered. This increase is likely a compensation for the absence of the negative pressure that is usually generated by laryngeal elevation during swallowing.[4] The best postoperative results after laryngopharyngectomy are found in patients in whom the anastomosis and the reconstructed segment are widely patent (i.e., the reconstructed segment is nonmotile) and in whom tongue function is not impaired.[5,6]

Long-term complications adversely affect postoperative function and quality of life in patients who have undergone cervical esophageal or pharyngoesophageal reconstruction. These include fistula formation, stricture, and the loss of capacity to produce saliva due to perioperative irradiation. Most of these complications will be discussed in detail at the end of this chapter.

The functional characteristics of specific tissues or organs used in cervical esophageal or pharyngoesophageal reconstruction have an important role in determining postoperative quality of life. Most tissues lack contractile properties and serve as passive conduits for food boluses.[7] These include skin flaps or tubes as well as musculocutaneous flaps or tubed musculocutaneous grafts. As long as there is no stenosis of the reconstructed segment and the anastomoses are widely patent, propulsive forces of the tongue are sufficient to propel a food bolus through the reconstructed segment.

In contrast, jejunal segments used for reconstruction often retain their motor activity. Denervation of the jejunum results in an increase in the frequency with which migrating motor complexes occur. At the same time, there is a decrease in the frequency and amplitude of postprandial contractions, fewer contractions propagate distally, intestinal transit is somewhat slower, and the onset of fed motor activity is delayed. The intrinsic nerves serve primarily to modulate this activity.[8] The polarity of this activity in the denervated jejunum is maintained, suggesting that jejunal interpositions should always be oriented in an isoperistaltic direction.[9]

Investigations of motility in jejunal free grafts demonstrate the presence of individual propagated waves during fasting as well as some deglutition- and bolus-induced propagated waves.[10-12] Introduction of a food bolus directly into the stomach also stimulates contractions in the free jejunal segment, suggesting that there is physiologic hormonal control of this activity.[10] Spontaneous contractile activity is not interrupted by swallows, which suggests the possibility that continued Phase III type contractions may interfere with bolus transport through the free jejunal graft. Experimentally, these conflicting contractile forces are not interrupted by longitudinal myotomy.[13] Transit of solids through the interposed jejunal segment is often slower than through the normal esophagus, with some hang-up evident just proximal to the distal anastomosis.[11]

The mucosa of jejunal free grafts demonstrates a decreased crypt/villi ratio, and there is usually a mild chronic inflammatory infiltrate.[14] Jejunal graft mucosa recovers only about 50% of normal Na+ K+ ATPase activity, possibly indicating a failure of complete adaptation to the chronic trauma of its new position.[15] There is no evidence that jejunal mucosa in this position undergoes metaplastic or dysplastic transformation.

The clinical status of patients who have undergone cervical esophageal reconstruction is generally good. Patients are able to handle their oral secretions, and most are able to take oral nutrition. However, 15% to 20% of patients require additional means of nutritional support such as gastrostomy or jejunostomy tube feedings.[16,17] Regurgitation and heartburn are rare after jejunal interposition. Dysphagia, however, is common and may be related to a variety of problems including discoordinated muscular activity in the graft, graft redundancy, or anastomotic stricture (Table 12-1).[10,16,18-23] The clinical status of patients who have undergone other types of cervical esophageal or pharyngoesophageal reconstruction is less well documented. Part of the reason for this is that many such patients suffer from malignancy, and their life expectancy is short, leading to limited long-term follow-up. Harii and co-authors report that nine of twelve patients who underwent pharyngoesophageal reconstruction with a forearm flap were able to take a regular diet, and that only three patients experienced dysphagia.[24]

Table 12-1.
Functional Status after Free Jejunal Graft Reconstruction of the Cervical Esophagus or Pharyngoesophagus.

Author	Year	Patients	Regular Diet	Dysphagia	Regurgitation	Weight Loss
Meyers et al.[10]	1980	9	9	2	2	0
Gluckman et al.[18]	1985	57	—	7	—	—
Biel et al.[19]	1987	14	12	2	2	2
Salamoun et al.[20]	1987	32	13	6	—	—
Carlson et al.[21]	1992	25	20	5	—	—
Reece et al.[22]	1995	93	57	54	—	2
Urayama et al.[23]	1997	58	—	7	—	—
Totals		288	111 (64%)	83 (29%)	4 (17%)	4 (3%)

Types of Cervical Esophageal Reconstruction

Stomach Pull-Up, Colon or Jejunal Interposition

Methods for use of the stomach or colon to replace the entire esophagus including the cervical portion, or to bypass the esophagus due to abnormalities in the cervical portion, are outlined in detail in Chapters 9 and 10 and are not further described in this chapter. In addition to use of the jejunum as a replacement for the whole esophagus, techniques are available for use of a segment of jejunum that is maintained on its mesenteric vascular as a replacement for the cervical esophagus only.[25] This technique has never been in widespread use, and it has fallen out of favor since the advent of reliable microvascular techniques for composite tissue transfer. Nevertheless, it is appropriate to consider this method among the options for cervical esophageal reconstruction in difficult situations.

Free Jejunal Grafts

The most common technique currently used for cervical esophageal reconstruction is the free jejunal graft. A short segment of jejunum with favorable vascular anatomy is harvested and microvascular anastomoses are performed to revascularize the segment in the neck. Such grafts can be used as an onlay patch to cover a partial defect in the esophagus and/or pharynx or as a tube graft to completely replace a segment of the esophagus. The distal anastomosis is performed either to the remaining esophagus or to another abdominal organ, creating a composite graft. This technique is discussed in more detail below.

Local Flaps—Skin Flaps, Fasciocutaneous Flaps, Musculocutaneous Flaps

In centers without microvascular surgical capability, in patients in whom laparotomy is contraindicated, or as a result of personal preferences of some surgeons, the use of local flaps rather than free grafts is also popular in cervical esophageal reconstruction. Such flaps include skin flaps, fasciocutaneous flaps, and musculocutaneous preparations such as the deltopectoral and pectoralis major flaps. Their use is most common as an onlay patch for reconstruction of partial esophageal defects. However, if the need is present, all of these flaps can be formed into a tube for complete replacement of the cervical esophagus. Creation of local flaps large enough to use for esophageal reconstruction usually requires the application of skin grafts to cover the donor area. The risk of fistula formation is higher with local flaps than with use of free jejunal grafts, due to difficulties in healing of skin to pharyngoesophageal mucosa.

Cervical skin flaps are sometimes used for pharyngoesophageal reconstruction because they are simple to create and are effective for salvage after failure of other reconstructive techniques. However, they are associated with a high incidence of fistula formation and stricture, a long hospital stay is necessary because the procedure is usually staged, and the preoperative administration of local irradiation often precludes their use.

Pectoralis major flaps, and to a lesser extent deltopectoral flaps, can be used as both onlay flaps for partial pharyngoesophageal reconstruction and as tubularized flaps for complete replacement of a segment of the cervical esophagus. The deltopectoral flap is vascularized through the skin pedicle, and thus requires two stages to complete. In contrast, the pectoralis flap is vascularized by the thoraco-acromial artery and vein, and the paddle of skin is transferred as an "island" attached to the muscle and its vascular supply. This permits the reconstruction to be completed in a single stage. One of the drawbacks to use of this flap as a tubularized graft for total replacement of the cervical esophagus is the fact that some individuals have considerable subcutaneous fat overlying the pectoralis muscle, which precludes formation of an effective tube.

Free Flaps

Forearm and Leg Flaps

The absence of adequate local tissues, the need for longer lengths of tissue, and the desire to avoid abdominal surgery have all led to the use of fasciocutaneous free flaps for pharyngoesophageal reconstruction. The most commonly used flap is the radial forearm flap, but use of ulnar flaps has also been described.[26] In addition, tensor fascia lata free flaps have recently been used for pharyngoesophageal reconstruction.[27] Because of its frequent use, the radial forearm free flap is the only fasciocutaneous flap that will be described in this chapter. The radial flap has a complex arterial supply and venous drainage pattern, both of which provide multiple options for revascularization. Partial circumferential defects are easily reconstructed with this flap, whereas complete circumferential defects are more challenging problems. Although the latter situation once was often complicated by anastomotic strictures, the use of Z-plasties has reduced the frequency of this problem. As with local flaps, healing of mucosa to skin is often difficult to achieve initially, leading to a high incidence of fistula formation.

Gastroomental Flap

Free gastroomental grafts have been described for use as onlay patches for defects of the floor of the mouth and hypopharynx and their use might be applicable to reconstruction of partial defects of the pharyngoesophagus.[28] The advantages of this type of reconstruction include a reliable blood supply, the availability of a wide variety of flap sizes, and facilitated healing between oral and gastric mucosal surfaces. The potential disadvantages are the need for a laparotomy for tissue harvest, loss of the stomach as a future reconstructive organ, and the possible presence of acid-producing mucosa in the pharyngoesophageal region.

Composite Grafts

Composite grafts are any grafts that use tissue from more than one source (skin, stomach, colon, jejunum) for purposes of esophageal reconstruction. They are used primarily in situations where standard reconstructive techniques have failed or are not possible due to prior surgical procedures or previous injury. Types of composite reconstruction include a free jejunal graft combined with stomach pull-up or colon interposition, and stomach pull-up or colon interposition combined with local flaps. Operative techniques for these grafts are varied and nonstandard.

Operative Techniques

Jejunal Free Graft

Once the extent of the pharyngoesophageal or esophageal defect is determined, jejunal graft harvest is performed through a laparotomy incision. A two-team approach is often used to reduce operating time. Laparoscopic techniques for harvest have been described and will likely become standard in the future.[29-31]

The anatomy of the jejunum is described in Chapter 11. A segment of jejunum 20 to 30 cm from the ligament of Trietz is identified that has a reliable vascular arcade, usually a segment that is based on the second or third jejunal vessels (Figure 12-2). The length of jejunum to be harvested depends on the size of the defect, and extra length is usually obtained and then trimmed off subsequently. A 20-cm length is sufficient for most purposes. The proximal end is marked with a suture to facilitate placement of the segment in an isoperistaltic orientation. The vascular arcade is isolated at either end of the segment and a wedge of supporting mesentery is divided using meticulous surgical technique to avoid hematoma formation. Magnifying loupes are often helpful in this regard. The vessels

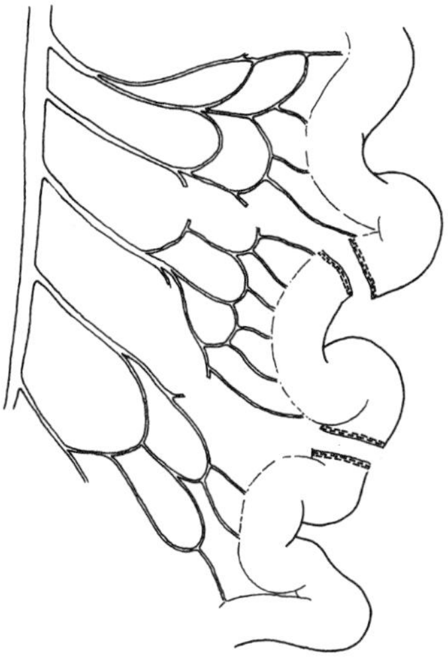

Figure 12-2. Isolation of a segment of jejunum in preparation for performing a jejunal free graft.

that will be supplying the graft are isolated near their junction with the superior mesenteric artery and vein. The branches of the arcade that extend beyond the limits of the graft are divided. The bowel segment is placed back in the abdomen to keep it warm.

The preparation of the recipient site is completed during this stage of the operation. All anatomic dissection and ablative procedures are finished. Vessels are identified and prepared for the venous and arterial anastomoses. Branches of the ipsilateral external carotid or transverse cervical artery are usually used for arterial inflow. A good size match is important when performing an end-to-end anastomosis. If the diameter discrepancy is greater than 1.5 to 1, an end-to-side anastomosis is used. Some surgeons prefer to use the common carotid artery for this purpose. If insufficient length is available, an interposition vein graft may be used to prevent tension or angulation on the arterial anastomosis, although this is rarely necessary. Alternatively, vessels in the contralateral neck may be used. The venous anastomosis is usually performed to the external jugular vein, internal jugular vein, or posterior facial vein. Preoperative irradiation of the recipient field creates increased arterial wall thickness, fibrin deposition, and intimal dehiscence compared to control vessels, changes which apparently have no important effect on operative times or outcomes.[32,33]

The jejunum is divided with a linear cutting stapler at either end of the selected segment, taking care to preserve its orientation, and the segmental vessels are divided near their junction with the superior mesenteric artery and vein. The stumps of the vessels are ligated or oversewn. The second surgical team performs an end-to-end anastomosis of the ends of the jejunum that remain in situ and the mesenteric defect is closed. Abdominal closure is performed after placement of a feeding jejunostomy tube.

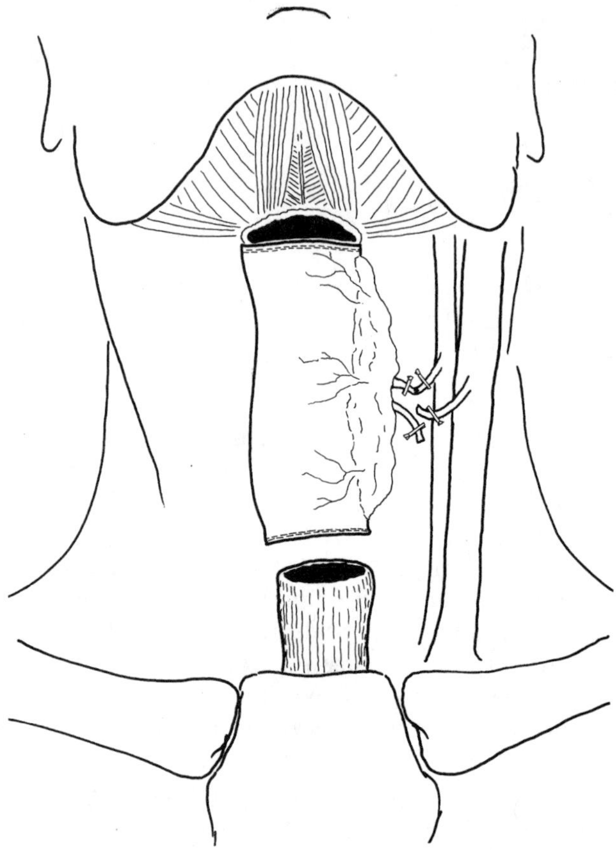

Figure 12-3. Completion of the first microvascular anastomosis for a free jejunal graft.

The graft is immediately placed in its bed in the cervical region in an isoperistaltic orientation. If a high pharyngeal defect exists, the proximal anastomosis is performed first in an end-to-end fashion using interrupted absorbable sutures in a single layer. If the pharyngeal defect is larger than the cross-sectional area of the jejunal lumen, the graft can be opened for a distance along its antimesenteric border to create a better size match. If the proximal defect lies lower, such as in the cervical esophagus, the vascular anastomoses are performed first.

An operating microscope is positioned over the operating field. Some surgeons administer intravenous heparin (1 mg/kg) prior to dividing the vessels in the recipient field. The artery is divided and adequate outflow is assured, after which the end is atraumatically clamped. The vein is similarly divided and clamped. The first vascular anastomosis is performed to the vessel deepest in the field, whether this is the artery or the vein. The more superficial anastomosis is then performed (Figure 12-3).

Anastomoses are performed with interrupted, fine (8-0) monofilament sutures. Clamps are removed, first from the vein, then from the artery, and perfusion should be readily apparent. Peristalsis should be evident within minutes of reestablishing blood flow.

Completion of revascularization within 3 hours is optimal for graft survival.[34] Experimentally, ligation of the vascular pedicle within 1 week of graft placement leads to the loss of every graft. After 2 weeks, local graft neovascularization leads to preserved viability in 60% of grafts, and this percentage gradually increases until all grafts are viable without a vascular pedicle 4 weeks after implant.[35] Placement of a free jejunal graft without revascularization has been performed successfully in the clinical setting, but this technique requires stenting and healing by secondary intention is often necessary.[36] Therefore, revascularization is recommended except under unusual circumstances.

If it has not already been performed, the proximal anastomosis to the jejunal graft is accomplished at this point in the operation. The necessary length of the graft is then checked, and the graft is trimmed to an appropriate size. The distal anastomosis is performed with interrupted absorbable sutures, during which a nasogastric drainage tube is positioned through the jejunal graft (Figure 12-4). Tacking sutures are placed to keep the vessels and bowel in appropriate locations. The residual mesentery is sutured over the carotid artery if possible. There is usually no problem in closing the skin flaps.

Standard clinical monitoring of free jejunal grafts for postoperative viability using observation of the patient's condition and vital signs is unreliable. Loss of graft viability is usually not detected for up to 7 days postoperatively, and graft salvage at that late point in time is not possible.[37] The use of specialized techniques for postoperative monitoring of graft viability has become routine in some centers. Doppler probes implanted along the jejunal vessels can detect loss of flow due to vessel kinking or thrombosis during closure of the skin flaps.[38] Another technique is to exteriorize a pedicled segment of jejunum through a portion of the neck incision. The condition of this segment usually reflects the condition of the buried segment, allowing for early exploration for graft salvage when appropriate.[39,40] Alternatively, a small window in the cervical incision is left open and the serosal surface of the jejunum is sutured to the dermis. Coverage of the jejunum with a split thickness skin graft permits visualization of peristalsis and serosal color.[41]

Musculocutaneous Flaps

The pectoralis major muscle flap is the most frequently used local flap for reconstruction after head and neck surgery and is the only muscu-

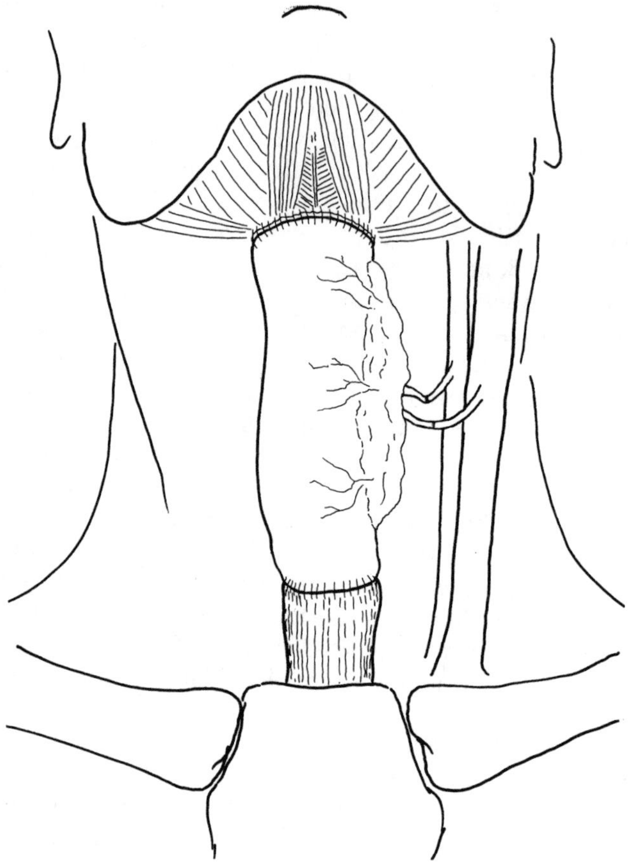

Figure 12-4. A completed jejunal free graft.

locutaneous flap that will be described in this chapter. It is best suited for use in men and in small-breasted women. Use of this flap in large-breasted women creates a substantial cosmetic deformity, and the amount of subcutaneous fat that accompanies the flap may provide more bulk than is suitable for reconstructive purposes. If the pectoralis major flap is deemed unsuitable, other options to consider include the trapezius and latissimus dorsi flaps.[42,43]

The pectoralis major flap is based on the pectoral branch of the thoraco-acromial artery and is sometimes supplemented by the lateral thoracic vessels. After completing the ablative portion of the head and neck operation, the size of the deformity is measured and a suitable skin flap is outlined (Figure 12-5). The skin flap is positioned caudad and medial to the nipple in the region of the sixth rib and extends superiorly and laterally along the axis of the feeding vessels. Skin in the infraclavicular region is

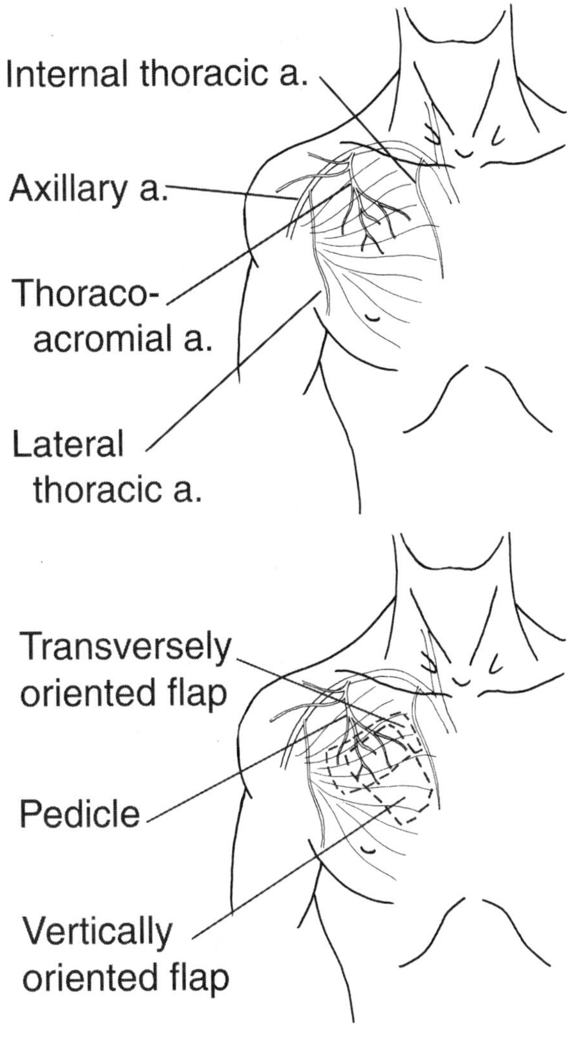

Figure 12-5. Arterial anatomy (top) and possible orientations (bottom) of the pectoralis major musculocutaneous flap.

spared in case a subsequent deltopectoral flap is necessary. The margins of the skin flap are incised to the level of the pectoralis major muscle, and the skin is sutured to the fascia to prevent shearing. The pectoralis major muscle is mobilized by dividing its medial, lateral, and deep attachments, which exposes the ribs and intercostal muscles. The thoraco-acromial artery is identified and preserved while the muscle pedicle is suitably narrowed (Figure 12-6).

A tunnel is created under the skin which permits the flap to be passed over the clavicle into the cervical defect without twisting or constricting

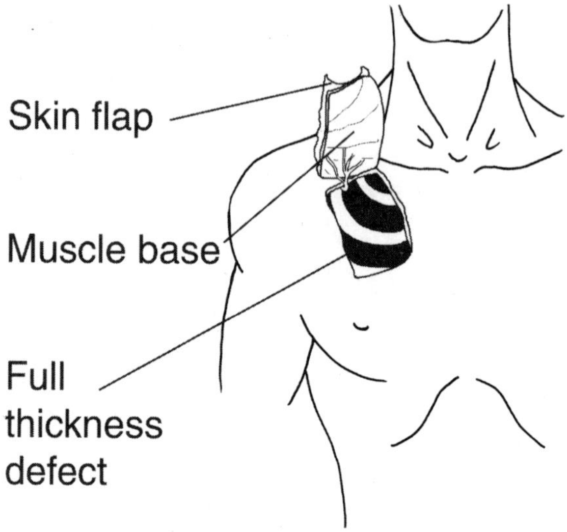

Figure 12-6. A mobilized pectoralis major musculocutaneous flap.

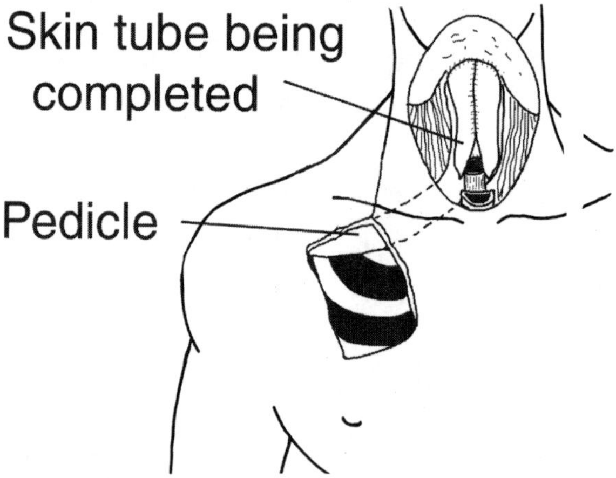

Figure 12-7. Use of a pectoralis major musculocutaneous flap to reconstruct a circumferential defect of the cervical esophagus.

the vascular pedicle. Onlay patch repair of partial defects is easily performed with interrupted absorbable sutures. If a circumferential defect is to be repaired with a tubed graft, the posterior portions of the anastomoses are accomplished first. The graft is then tubed by suturing the opposing skin edges together, permitting the anterior portions of the anastomoses to be completed (Figure 12-7). A second layer of closure of pectoralis muscle over the edges of the skin tube is performed when feasible. A

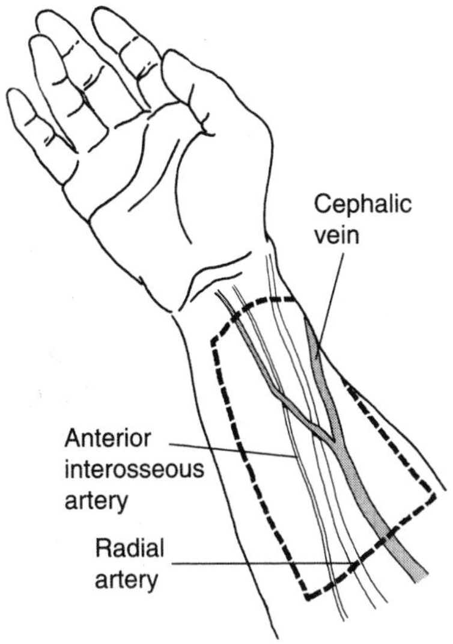

Figure 12-8. Anatomy of a radial forearm flap.

nasogastric tube is placed through the graft for enteral feeding and drains are placed adjacent to the graft because of the high incidence of fistula formation. The skin flaps of the cervical incision are closed. The donor site is usually able to be closed primarily after suitable elevation of the adjacent skin margins.

Radial Forearm Flap

The radial forearm free flap is useful in situations in which a well-vascularized, thin flap of skin is necessary to reconstruct the pharynx or cervical esophagus and the use of a free jejunal flap is contraindicated. This fasciocutaneous flap is based on the radial artery with venous drainage primarily through the cephalic vein, although superficial cutaneous veins and venae comitantes also provide drainage (Figure 12-8). Prior to beginning the operation, an Allen test is performed to ensure the patency of the ulnar artery and the communication between the deep and superficial vascular arches within the hand.

The flap is located either over the radial artery or along the volar surface of the arm. The latter location is more cosmetically appealing, and there is less hair on that surface, which can be important for subsequent function of the graft. After ablative procedures are completed in the head and neck region, the size of the defect to be reconstructed is determined. The flap is outlined on the arm taking these measurements into consideration. When there is a pharyngeal defect, either the base or the tip of the flap is made accordingly wider than the region to be anastomosed to

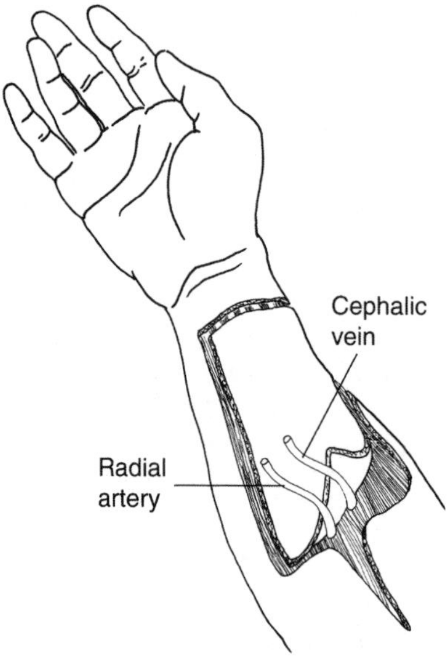

Figure 12-9. The raised radial forearm flap.

the esophagus, depending on where the vascular anastomoses are to be performed. This forms the flap into a trapezoid.

The arm is elevated to encourage exsanguination and a tourniquet is applied. The skin incision is begun along the cephalic vein and is extended along the ulnar margin of the flap. The flap is then raised towards the radial margin superficial to the paratenons of the superficial flexor tendons. The radial margin is also incised, and the flap is raised in a similar plane from this perspective. The superficial radial nerve is preserved. The radial vessels are approached in their bed beneath the brachioradialis and flexor carpi radialis tendons, and the intermuscular septum containing the vessels is carefully preserved. The radial artery and veins are ligated distal to the flap, and the flap is then raised proximally including a vascular pedicle composed of the radial vessels and the cephalic vein (Figure 12-9). The tourniquet is released and the graft is harvested after its viability is confirmed. The donor site is closed with a split thickness skin graft. The flap is tubed or used as an onlay graft as is appropriate to the situation. Vascular anastomoses are performed as described above (Figure 12-10). One or more segments of the flap may be separated and externalized for monitoring, as described for jejunal free flaps.[44,45]

Local Skin and Fasciocutaneous Flaps

Cervical skin flaps have been described for use in esophageal reconstruction, but are no longer employed for this purpose except in unusual

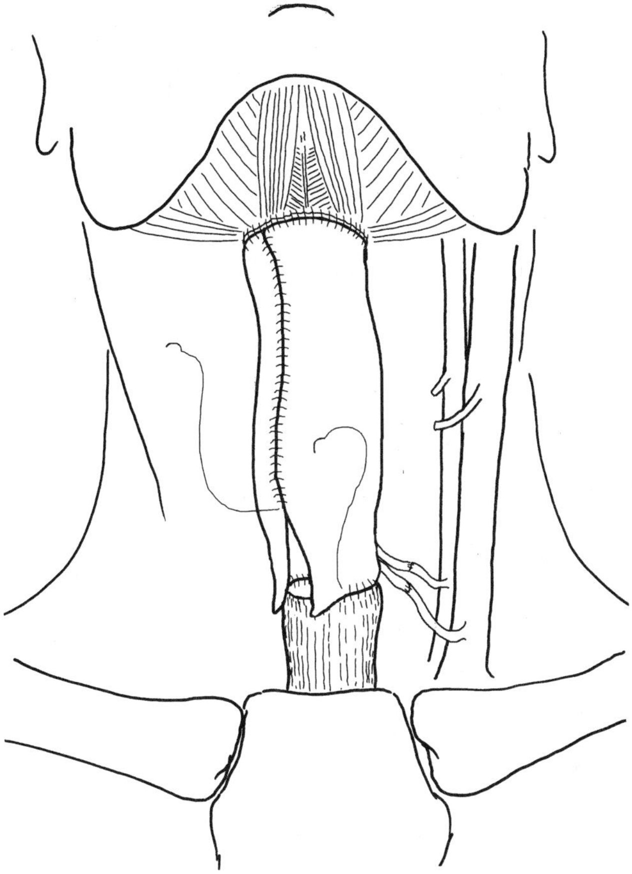

Figure 12-10. Use of a radial forearm flap to reconstruct a circumferential defect of the cervical esophagus.

circumstances. The only local flap that is used frequently for reconstruction of the cervical esophagus and pharyngoesophagus is the deltopectoral flap. This is an axial pattern fasciocutaneous flap, which is based on the first three perforators of the internal mammary artery. The upper border traces the inferior margin of the clavicle, the inferior border parallels the anterior axillary fold, and the flap can extend laterally over the medial portion of the deltoid muscle if that much length is required. After the flap is raised, taking care to preserve the pedicle containing the feeding vessels, it is tubed or placed as an onlay patch. The donor site is covered with a split-thickness skin graft (Figure 12-11). The pedicle is divided in a second stage operation after 4 to 5 weeks.

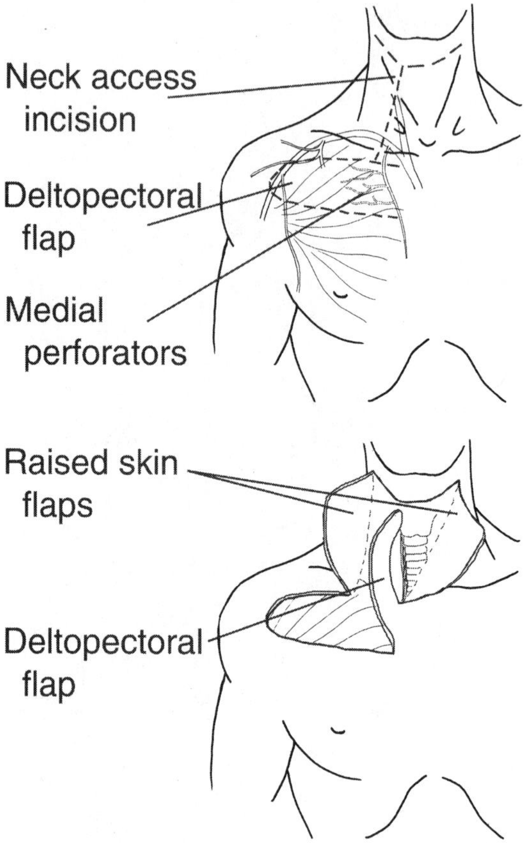

Figure 12-11. Use of the deltopectoral flap, which is based on medial perforators of the internal thoracic artery (top), for patch reconstruction of the cervical esophagus (bottom).

Complications of Cervical Esophageal Reconstruction

It is sometimes difficult to identify complications that arise from a complex operation such as cervical esophageal reconstruction which can be attributed specifically to the type of reconstruction that is performed. The acute and long-term complications that are reconstruction-specific are detailed here.

Graft Ischemia and Necrosis

Because of the nature of the blood supply to the reconstructive tissues, graft ischemia and necrosis occur more often than for more typical reconstructions of the entire esophagus. For free grafts, acute arterial insufficiency is usually evident prior to completion of the reconstruction, in which case the graft is discarded and an alternative reconstructive method is considered. In such instances the loss of the graft is not usually recorded as an operative complication, leading to some inaccuracy in the estimation of the rate of graft loss associated with cervical esophageal reconstruction. The viability of pedicled grafts is not always obvious when no direct monitoring is performed, and free grafts usually are not salvageable because ischemia is not recognized until necrosis has occurred. In contrast, grafts that are directly monitored postoperatively are amenable to appropriate intervention for salvage. Venous insufficiency can present an insidious clinical picture during the early postoperative period and is a common cause for late graft failure.

Ischemia and necrosis of a free flap that is not being directly monitored are not always simple to diagnose postoperatively prior to the onset of frank sepsis, and a high index of suspicion must be maintained. Signs suggestive of infarction include tachycardia, supraventricular arrhythmias, unexplained acidosis, leukocytosis, confusion, and hypoxia. Fistula formation may be evident. Endoscopy may demonstrate ischemic tissue suggestive of infarction. Aggressive biopsies that cause no bleeding should raise the suspicion that an ischemic event has occurred. Exploration is sometimes necessary to make a definitive diagnosis of necrosis. When necrosis has occurred, appropriate intervention is dictated by the overall condition of the patient and by reconstructive options that remain. In patients in good clinical condition, immediate reconstruction is often considered. Delayed reconstruction is appropriate for patients who are septic or are otherwise clinically unstable, and drainage of the pharynx or esophagus, protection of the carotid vessels, and airway protection become the dominant foci for the short term. Staged reconstruction is considered when the patient has completely recovered.

The incidence of loss of free jejunal grafts is about 8% (Table 12-2).[16,18-22,46-53] When a free jejunal flap is lost, another jejunal free flap reconstruction may be attempted immediately if the patient's clinical condition is satisfactory. The success rate of this type of reconstruction is greater than 80%.[16,18-22,48,53] Monitoring of an exteriorized segment of jejunum has led to early intervention for vessel kinking or thrombosis with a success rate for graft salvage of 100% in one small series.[22]

The rate of loss of forearm flaps used for pharyngoesophageal and cervical esophageal reconstruction is less than 2% and is lower than that for jejunal free flaps (Table 12-3).[26,45,46,52,54,55] This low incidence of graft loss may be a result of the small number of patients reported, but the low incidence may also be reflected in the longer vascular pedicle and the larger vessels in this graft that are usually available for anastomosis. The rate of loss of pectoralis major musculocutaneous flaps is less than

Table 12-2.
Complications of Free Jejunal Transfer for Pharyngoesophageal or Cervical Esophageal Reconstruction.

Author	Year	Graft Loss Patients	Graft Loss Incidence	Fistula Patients	Fistula Incidence	Stricture Patients	Stricture Incidence
Gluckman et al.[18]	1985	52	4	52	4	52	6
Biel et al.[19]	1987	17	3	17	6	14	3
Kato et al.[46]	1987	21	0	21	7	21	0
Salamoun et al.[20]	1987	32	2	32	12	—	—
Ferguson et al.[47]	1988	18	1	18	4	17	2
Coleman et al.[48]	1989	101	12	101	33	101	18
Fisher et al.[16]	1990	47	9	47	4	47	8
Steffen et al.[49]	1991	10	0	10	1	10	1
Carlson et al.[21]	1992	26	1	25	5	25	4
Omura et al.[50]	1994	24	0	24	2	—	—
Ancona et al.[51]	1995	28	3	28	1	28	11
Reece et al.[22]	1995	93	3	93	18	93	14
Nakatsuka et al.[52]	1998	70	4	70	3	64	6
Bottger at al.[53]	1999	19	1	19	1	—	—
Totals		558	43 (7.7%)	557	101 (18.1%)	472	73 (15.5%)

Table 12-3.
Complications of Forearm Free Flap Transfer for Pharyngoesophageal or Cervical Esophageal Reconstruction.

Author	Year	Graft Loss Patients	Graft Loss Incidence	Fistula Patients	Fistula Incidence	Stricture Patients	Stricture Incidence
Kato et al.[46]	1987	10	0	10	5	10	0
Anthony et al.[54]	1994	22	0	22	7	22	2
Akin et al.[55]	1997	9	1	9	3	9	0
Cho et al.[45]	1998	23	0	23	4	23	3
Li et al.[26]	1998	19	1	19	3	19	1
Nakatsuka et al.[52]	1998	39	0	39	15	33	13
Totals		122	2 (1.6%)	122	37 (30.3%)	116	19 (16.4%)

3%, a low incidence that is due both to its reliable blood supply and the fact that it is a pedicled flap (Table 12-4).[56-61]

Fistula Formation, Stricture

Fistulas commonly occur after pharyngoesophageal and cervical esophageal reconstruction. They are recognized by the development of sepsis or a wound infection with salivary drainage. A prominent danger of fistula formation is erosion into surrounding structures such as the airway or carotid arteries, either of which may be a fatal event. The development of a fistula may also cause inflammation in the region of the graft resulting in thrombosis of one or both of the vessels in its vascular pedicle, causing graft necrosis.

The likelihood of developing a fistula after cervical esophageal reconstruction is dependent in large part on the type of reconstruction that is performed. Healing of the oral or esophageal mucosa to the mucosa of a jejunal free flap is more likely to occur by primary intention than is healing to the skin of a local or free flap. The position of the graft is also a determinant of the likelihood of fistula formation. There is often a size discrepancy between the graft and the pharyngeal defect, resulting in a higher incidence of fistula formation than when the proximal anastomosis is performed to the cervical esophagus. The rate of fistula formation for jejunal free flaps is 20% (Table 12-2).[16,18-22,46-53] In comparison, other types of soft tissue reconstruction in this region are complicated by fistula formation in 25% to 30% of patients (Tables 12-3, 12-4).[17,26,45,46,52,54, 55, 57-61]

Most fistulas are relatively easy to control, although they often take weeks to close spontaneously. Some fistulas will require reoperation to achieve closure, employing techniques such as skin or muscle flap reinforcement.[48] Further information regarding the management of anastomotic leak and fistula formation is available in Chapter 15.

The development of a fistula and the presence of chronic ischemia are the two major causes of anastomotic stricture formation after pharyngoesophageal or cervical esophageal reconstruction. The use of postoperative irradiation as adjunctive therapy after surgery for head and neck cancer or cervical esophageal malignancies does not appear to increase the risk of anastomotic stricture.[62-65] Strictures develop in up to 20% of patients who undergo jejunal free flap reconstruction and appear to occur more commonly at the distal anastomosis (Table 12-2).[16,18,19,21,22,46,48,49,51,52] About 16% of patients who undergo forearm free flap transfer suffer anastomotic stricture (Table 12-3).[26,45,46,52,54,55] In contrast, just over 5% of patients who undergo reconstruction with a pectoralis major flap develop a stricture (Table 12-4).[59-61] The usual management is dilation, although strictures that encompass relatively large portions of the circumference of an

Table 12-4.
Complications of Pectoralis Major Musculocutaneous Flap Rotation for Pharyngoesophageal or Cervical Esophageal Reconstruction.

Author	Year	Graft Loss		Fistula		Stricture	
		Patients	Incidence	Patients	Incidence	Patients	Incidence
Biller et al.[56]	1981	42	0	—	—	—	—
Mehrhof et al.[57]	1983	67	3	67	12	—	—
Neifeld et al.[58]	1983	5	0	5	2	—	—
Fabian et al.[59]	1988	22	1	22	6	21	1
Cusumano et al.[60]	1989	10	0	10	4	8	1
Ko et al.[61]	1998	6	0	6	3	6	0
Totals		152	4 (2.6%)	110	27 (24.5%)	35	2 (5.7%)

anastomosis sometimes require division and rotation of soft tissue from a local flap for correction. Further information on the management of anastomotic stricture is available in Chapter 15.

Graft Redundancy

Excessive length or angulation of interposition grafts, particularly jejunal free grafts, occasionally has been reported as a cause for postoperative dysphagia in patients undergoing reconstruction of the pharyngoesophagus or cervical esophagus. One problem that has been noted is difficulty swallowing after performing a proximal end-to-side anastomosis to a free jejunal graft. Reasons for the development of dysphagia are unclear, but may be related to angulation of or motor activity within the graft. Redundancy after end-to-end anastomoses of free jejunal grafts is uncommon, but requires revision of the graft if substantial dysphagia is present.

References

1. McConnel FMS, Cerenko D, Jackson RT, et al. Timing of major events of pharyngeal swallowing. *Arch Otolaryngol Head Neck Surg* 1988;114:1413-1418.
2. McConnel FMS, Cerenko D, Mendelsohn MS. Manofluorographic analysis of swallowing. *Otolaryngol Clin N Am* 1988;21:625-635.
3. McConnel FMS. Analysis of pressure generation and bolus transit during pharyngeal swallowing. *Laryngoscope* 1988;98:71-78.
4. McConnel FMS, Cerenko D, Mendelsohn MS. Dysphagia after total laryngectomy. *Otolaryngol Clin N Am* 1988;21:721-726.
5. McConnel FMS, Hester TR, Mendelsohn MS, et al. Manofluorography of deglutition after total laryngopharyngectomy. *Plast Reconstr Surg* 1988;81:346-351.
6. Walther EK. Dysphagia after pharyngolaryngeal cancer surgery. Part I: Pathophysiology of postsurgical deglutition. *Dysphagia* 1995;10:275-278.
7. Okamura H, Inaki S, Mori T. Swallowing function following hypopharyngeal reconstruction with the pectoralis major musculocutaneous flap. *Auris Nasus Larynx* 1991;18:383-389.
8. Johnson CP, Sarna SK, Cowles VE, et al. Motor activity and transit in the autonomically denervated jejunum. *Am J Surg* 1994;167:80-88.
9. Richards WO, Golzarian J, Wasudev N, et al. Reverse phasic contractions are present in antiperistaltic jejunal limbs up to twenty-one years postoperatively. *J Am Coll Surg* 1994;178:557-563.
10. Meyers WC, Seigler HF, Hanks JB, et al. Postoperative function of "free" jejunal transplants for replacement of the cervical esophagus. *Ann Surg* 1980;192:439-450.
11. Kerlin P, McCafferty GJ, Robinson DW, et al. Function of a free jejunal "conduit" graft in the cervical esophagus. *Gastroenterology* 1986;90:1956-1063.

12. Wilson JA, Maran AGD, Pryde A, et al. The function of free jejunal autografts in the pharyngo-esophageal segment. *J R Coll Surg Edinb* 1995;40:363-366.
13. Haughey BH, Forsen JW. Free jejunal graft: Effects of longitudinal myotomy. *Ann Otol Rhinol Laryngol* 1992;101:333-338.
14. Deans JA, Hills J, Bennett M. Histologic changes in free jejunal grafts used in pharyngeal reconstruction. *J Laryngol Otol* 1991;105:556-557.
15. Smith RW, Batten J, Davies DM. The functional recovery of revascularised colon and jejunum replacing the cervical oesophagus. *Scan J Plast Reconstr Surg* 1988;22:117-120.
16. Fisher SR, Cameron R, Hoyt DJ, et al. Free jejunal interposition graft for reconstruction of the esophagus. *Head Neck* 1990;12:126-130.
17. Carlson GW, Coleman JJ III, Jurkiewicz MJ. Reconstruction of the hypopharynx and cervical esophagus. *Curr Probl Surg* 1993;30:427-472.
18. Gluckman JL, McDonough JJ, McCafferty GJ, et al. Complications associated with free jejunal graft reconstruction of the pharyngoesophagus - a multiinstitutional experience with 52 cases. *Head Neck Surg* 1985;7:200-205.
19. Biel MA, Maisel RH. Free jejunal autograft reconstruction of the pharyngoesophagus: Review of a 10-year experience. *Otolaryngol Head Neck Surg* 1987;96:369-375.
20. Salamoun W, Swartz WM, Johnson JT, et al. Free jejunal transfer for reconstruction of the laryngopharynx. *Otolaryngol Head Neck Surg* 1987;96:149-150.
21. Carlson GW, Schusterman MA, Guillamondegui OM. Total reconstruction of the hypopharynx and cervical esophagus: A 20-year experience. *Ann Plast Surg* 1992;29:408-412.
22. Reece GP, Schusterman MA, Miller MJ, et al. Morbidity and functional outcome of free jejunal transfer reconstruction for circumferential defects of the pharynx and cervical esophagus. *Plast Reconstr Surg* 1995;96:1307-1316.
23. Urayama H, Ohtake H, Ohmura K, et al. Pharyngoesophageal reconstruction with the use of vascular anastomoses: Operative modifications and long-term prognosis. *J Thorac Cardiovasc Surg* 1997;113:975-981.
24. Harii K, Ebihara S, Ono I, et al. Pharyngoesophageal reconstruction using a fabricated forearm free flap. *Plast Reconstr Surg* 1985;75:463-474.
25. Kasai M, Nishihira T. Reconstruction using pedicled jejunal segments after resection for carcinoma of the cervical esophagus. *Surg Gynecol Obstet* 1986;163:145-152.
26. Li KK, Salibian AH, Allison GR, et al. Pharyngoesophageal reconstruction with the ulnar forearm flap. *Arch Otolaryngol Head Neck Surg* 1998;124:1146-1151.
27. Endo T, Nakayama Y. Pharyngoesophageal reconstruction: A clinical comparison between free tensor faciae latae and radial forearm flaps. *J Reconstr Microsurg* 1997;13:93-97.
28. Panje WR, Little AG, Moran WJ, et al. Immediate free gastro-omental flap reconstruction of the mouth and throat. *Ann Otol Rhinol Laryngol* 1987;96:15-21.
29. Staley CA, Miller M, King TJ, et al. Laparoscopic harvest of jejunal tissue for autologous transplantation. *Surg Laparosc Endosc* 1994;4:192-195.
30. Rosenberg MH, Sultan MR, Bessler M, et al. Laparoscopic harvesting of jejunal free flaps. *Ann Plast Surg* 1995;34:250-253.

31. Gherardini G, Gurlek A, Staley CA, et al. Laparoscopic harvesting of jejunal free flaps for esophageal reconstruction. *Plast Reconstr Surg* 1998;102:473-477.
32. Guelinckx PJ, Boeckx WD, Fossion E, et al. Scanning electron microscopy of irradiated recipient blood vessels in head and neck free flaps. *Plast Reconstr Surg* 1984;74:217-226.
33. Kiener JL, Hoffman WY, Mathes SJ. Influence of radiotherapy on microvascular reconstruction in the head and neck region. *Am J Surg* 1991;162:404-407.
34. Hikida S, Takeuchi M, Hata H, et al. Free jejunal graft autotransplantation should be revascularized within 3 hours. *Transplant Proc* 1998;30:3446-3448.
35. Cordeiro PG, Santamaria E, Hu QY, et al. The timing and nature of neovascularization of jejunal free flaps: An experimental study in a large animal model. *Plast Reconstr Surg* 1999;103:1893-1901.
36. Panje WR, Hetherington HE. Jejunal graft reconstruction of pharyngoesophageal defects without microvascular anastomoses. *Ann Otol Laryngol* 1994;103:693-698.
37. Disa JJ, Cordeiro PG, Hidalgo DA. Efficacy of conventional monitoring techniques in free tissue transfer: An 11-year experience in 750 consecutive cases. *Plast Reconstr Surg* 1999;104:97-101.
38. Jones NF, Rocke AM, Swartz WM, et al. Experimental and clinical monitoring of free jejunal transfers using an implantable ultrasonic Doppler probe. *Br J Plast Surg* 1989;42:274-280.
39. Katsaros J, Banis JC, Acland RD, et al. Monitoring free vascularized jejunum grafts. *Br J Plast Surg* 1985;38:220-222.
40. Bradford CR, Esclamado RM, Carroll WR. Monitoring of revascularized jejunal autografts. *Arch Otolaryngol Head Neck Surg* 1992;118:1042-1044.
41. Bafitis H, Stallings JO, Ban J. A reliable method for monitoring the microvascular patency of free jejunal transfers in reconstructing the pharynx and cervical esophagus. *Plast Reconstr Surg* 1989;83:896-898.
42. Yamamoto K, Yokota K, Higaki K. Entire pharyngoesophageal reconstruction with latissimus dorsi myocutaneous island flap. *Head Neck Surg* 1985;7:461-464.
43. Koshima I, Moriguchi T, Soeda S, et al. Extended latissimus dorsi musculocutaneous flaps for extremely wide cervical skin defects involving the cervical esophagus. *Ann Plast Surg* 1992;29:149-152.
44. Furuta S, Hataya Y, Ishigaki Y, et al. Monitoring the free radial forearm flap in pharyngo-oesophageal reconstruction. *Br J Plast Surg* 1997;50:40-42.
45. Cho BC, Kim M, Lee JH, et al. Pharyngoesophageal reconstruction with a tubed free radial forearm flap. *J Reconstr Microsurg* 1998;14:535-540.
46. Kato H, Watanabe H, Iizuka T, et al. Primary esophageal reconstruction after resection of the cancer in the hypopharynx or cervical esophagus: Comparison of free forearm skin tube flap, free jejunal transplantation, and pull-through esophagectomy. *Jpn J Clin Oncol* 1987;17:255-261.
47. Ferguson JL, DeSanto LW. Total pharyngolaryngectomy and cervical esophagectomy with jejunal autotransplant reconstruction: Complications and results. *Laryngoscope* 1988;98:911-914.
48. Coleman JJ III, Tan K-C, Searles JM, et al. Jejunal free autograft: Analysis of complications and their resolution. *Plast Reconstr Surg* 1989;84:589-598.

49. Steffen R, Mayer B, Knoop M, et al. Technique of microvascular jejunum transfer for replacement of the cervical esophagus. *Chirurg* 1991;62:332-335.
50. Omura K, Misaki T, Watanabe Y, et al. Reconstruction with free jejunal autograft after pharyngolaryngoesophagectomy. *Ann Thorac Surg* 1994;57:112-118.
51. Ancona E, Pianalto S, Merigliano S, et al. Free jejunal transfer for the reconstruction of the pharyngo-esophagus. *Dis Esoph* 1995;8:40-43.
52. Nakatsuka T, Harii K, Asato H, et al. Comparative evaluation in pharyngo-oesophageal reconstruction: Radial forearm flap compared with jejunal flap. *Scand J Plast Reconstr Surg Hand Surg* 1998;32:307-310.
53. Bottger T, Bumb P, Dutkowski T, et al. Carcinoma of the hypopharynx and the cervical oesophagus: A surgical challenge. *Eur J Surg* 1999;165:940-946.
54. Anthony JP, Singer MI, Deschler DG, et al. Long-term functional results after pharyngoesophageal reconstruction with the radial forearm free flap. *Am J Surg* 1994;168:441-445.
55. Akin I, Torkut A, Ustunsoy E, et al. Results of reconstruction with free forearm flap following laryngopharyngo-oesophageal resection. *J Laryngol Otol* 1997;111:48-53.
56. Biller HF, Baek SM, Lawson W, et al. Pectoralis major myocutaneous island flap in head and neck surgery: Analysis of complications in 42 cases. *Arch Otolarnygol* 1981;107:23-26.
57. Mehrhof AI Jr, Rosenstock A, Neifeld JP, et al. The pectoralis major myocutaneous flap in head and neck reconstruction. Analysis of complications. *Am J Surg* 1983;146:478-482.
58. Neifield JP, Merritt WA, Theogaraj SD, et al. Tubed pectoralis major musculocutaneous flap for cervical esophageal replacement. *Ann Plast Surg* 1983;11:24-30.
59. Fabian RL. Pectoralis major myocutaneous flap reconstruction of the laryngopharynx and cervical esophagus. *Laryngoscope* 1988;98:1227-1231.
60. Cusumano RJ, Silver CE, Brauer RJ, et al. Pectoralis myocutaneous flap for replacement of cervical esophagus. *Head Neck* 1989;11:450-456.
61. Ko JY, Sheen TS. Reconstruction of circumferential pharyngeal defect following cancer surgery with tubed pectoralis major myocutaneous flap and interdigitating anastomosis. *J Formos Med Assoc* 1998;97:360-363.
62. Petruzzelli GJ, Johnson JT, Myers EN, et al. The effect of postoperative radiation therapy on pharyngoesophageal reconstruction with free jejunal interposition. *Arch Otolaryngol Head Neck Surg* 1991;117:1265-1268.
63. Cole CJ, Garden AS, Frankenthaler RA, et al. Postoperative radiation of free jejunal autografts in patients with advanced cancer of the head and neck. *Cancer* 1995;75:2356-2360.
64. Barrett WL, Gluckman JL, Aron BS. Safety of radiating jejunal interposition grafts in head and neck cancer. *Am J Clin Oncol* 1997;20:609-612.
65. Wei WI, Lam LK, Yuen PW, et al. Mucosal changes of the free jejunal graft in response to radiotherapy. *Am J Surg* 1998;175:44-46.

Chapter 13

Artificial Tubes

Efforts to create an artificial esophagus began as early as the beginning of the twentieth century when surgeons such as Torek provided an external tube connecting a cervical esophagostomy to a gastrostomy to restore alimentary tract continuity in patients who had undergone esophagectomy (Figure 1-11). During the subsequent years of the twentieth century, rubber and Silastic tubes were used extracorporeally for this purpose. Beginning in the 1950s, efforts have been directed towards the creation of an internal artificial esophagus, using a variety of materials such as autologous tissues, homologous tissue, wire mesh, plastics, rubber, and polymers.

The satisfactory experience with esophageal reconstruction using autologous tissues since the 1940s has led to a low level of interest in the development of artificial tubes for use as esophageal substitutes. However, the use of autologous tissues is accompanied by complications associated with their harvest and, in some instances, loss of normal function of the harvested tissue. For example, use of the stomach as an esophageal replacement is complicated by loss of gastric reservoir capacity, and use of the colon sometimes results in an increased frequency of bowel movements. In addition, prior disease and prior surgery make reconstruction with autologous tissues virtually impossible in some patients. This has led to a need for the development of an internal artificial tube for esophageal replacement in selected patients.

The search for an artificial substitute for the esophagus has been stimulated by recent advances in artificial organ research including the development of composite constructs that incorporate both biological materials and autologous tissues. Potential advantages of such an approach include primary healing of the anastomosis, lack of stricture formation of the neoesophagus, and the elimination of the risk of erosion of foreign material into surrounding structures. Such advances open the possibility

From Ferguson MK: *Reconstructive Surgery of the Esophagus* Armonk, NY: Futura Publishing Company, Inc., © 2002.

that at some future time an artificial esophagus can be used routinely to replace the esophagus without the need for use of other organs.

History of the Internal Artificial Esophagus

Replacement of the esophagus by something other than autologous tissue has been a goal of surgeons for more than a century. The earliest permanent use of foreign material was for esophageal intubation. This was initially attempted using decalcified ivory tubes in 1845 and was first successfully accomplished in the mid-1880s.[1,2] Since then a variety of rubbers, metals, and plastics have been used both experimentally and clinically to substitute for the full circumference of the esophagus over short distances. Neuhof and Ziegler used rubber tubes to reestablish continuity of the cervical esophagus in dogs in 1922.[3] In a pattern that was to be repeated many times in the future, they discovered that the tubes failed to become incorporated into the surrounding tissues. When the tubes were expelled early, sepsis and death usually resulted. When the tubes were expelled later and the animals survived, a fibrous sheath developed around the indwelling tube and a mucosal lining developed within the fibrous sheath after a period of several months. Stricture formation was the inevitable result.

Tantalum wire mesh was used by Rob and Bateman in the 1940s in four patients after pharyngoesophagectomy to establish a passageway between the pharynx and cervical esophagus. To provide an initial seal the wire mesh was covered by fascia lata, which sloughed within a few weeks. A fibrous tube formed over the tantalum, during which time the wire mesh separated from the esophagus and pharynx and was removed endoscopically. The fibrous tube eventually became lined with a delicate mucosa and, at least in one patient, permitted ingestion of a regular diet.[4] The use of tantalum mesh covered by a split-thickness skin graft rather than fascia lata led to good results in four patients after cervical esophageal resection.[5] Experimental use in dogs of tantalum covered by fascia lata was unsuccessful.[6] Braunwald and Hufnagel used a similar technique experimentally in the canine thoracic esophagus employing stainless steel wire mesh to enable ingrowth of tissue (Figure 13-1). The prostheses were initially stented with a plastic tube which eventually sloughed and was passed through the gastrointestinal tract.[7] In some of the dogs the mediastinal structures created sufficient pressure to collapse the wire mesh, making swallowing difficult. Most of the dogs survived the postoperative period and developed an epithelialized fibrous tube incorporating the wire mesh, which permitted ingestion of regular dog chow.

Plastic tubes of methacrylate and polyethylene were used experimentally in dogs and rabbits in the 1950s (Figure 13-2). They never became

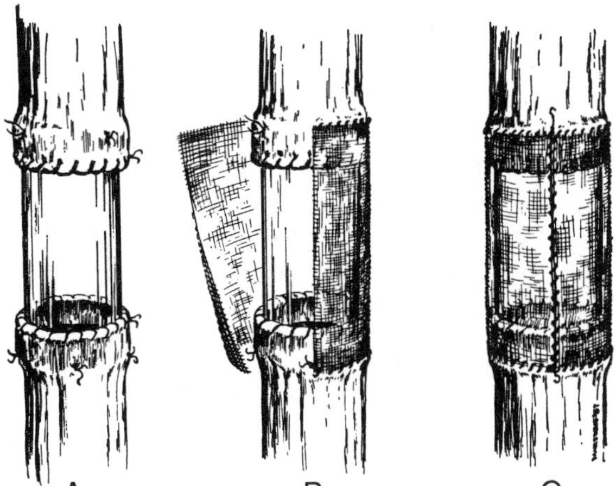

Figure 13-1. Tygon tubing is sutured within the ends of the partially resected esophagus (**A**). The tubing is covered with wire mesh (**B**) which is sutured to the edges of the cut esophagus and to itself to completely encase the Tygon tubing (**C**). Reprinted with permission from: Braunwald NS, Hufnagel CA. Reconstruction of the esophagus with wire mesh prosthesis. *Surgery* 1958;43:600-605.

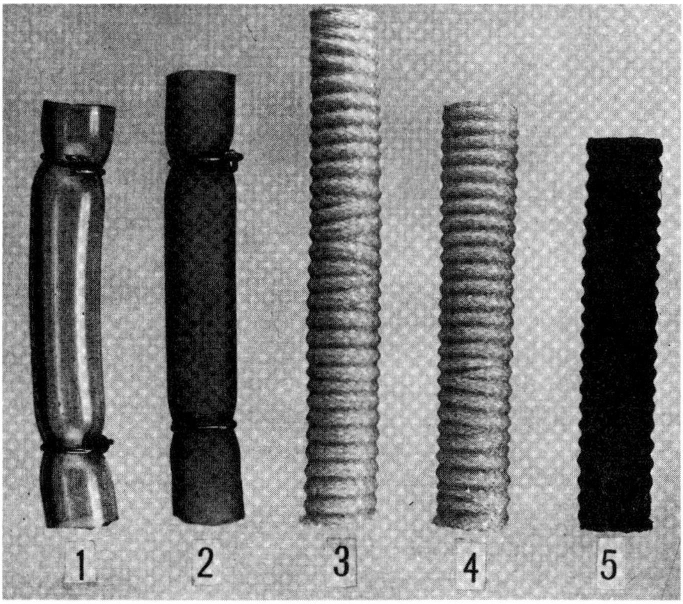

Figure 13-2. Various types of experimental esophageal prostheses, including: 1. Tygon untreated; 2. Tygon treated with dicetyl phosphate; 3. untreated crimped nylon; 4. crimped nylon sprayed with Krylon; 5. crimped nylon sprayed with shellac. Reprinted with permission from: Rubenstein LH. Experiments with substitute esophagus. *J Thorac Surg* 1956;32:691-696.

incorporated into the ends of the esophagus, and when the animals survived, they did so because of the development of a fibrous sheath around the foreign material that took up to 3 months to epithelialize.[6,8-10] Layers of polyethylene film sandwiched between layers of nylon mesh and formed into a tube produced similar results in a dog model.[11] The need for such external support of a film of polyethylene was reinforced by later experimental work, also in dogs.[12] Teflon tubes were used to bridge gaps in the esophagus of dogs in the 1950s with initial good success, some animals surviving for more than 2 years.[13] Corrugated tubing of tightly woven nylon mesh covered with a flap of pleura or platysma in dogs permitted ingrowth of tissue and early partial incorporation of the prosthesis in short-term experiments.[14,15] Silastic tubes also failed to become incorporated into surrounding tissues, although use of Dacron sewing rings attached to each end of the tubes prevented their dislodgment and thus eliminated stricturing as a problem in the few long-term survivors.[16] Reinforcement of polyurethane tubes by an omental flap prevented leakage in dogs and resulted in uniformly successful intermediate-term outcomes in a small group of animals.[17]

The limited success in the experimental use of plastic tubes as segmental replacements for the esophagus does not appear to have prevented their application in patients with esophageal cancer. Shackelford reported that plastic tubes had been used in over 70 patients, with satisfactory results in most instances.[18] In his single case report the patient survived for 6 months and was able to eat a regular diet. The tube had not dislodged, and death was due to bronchopneumonia due to a malignant esophageal-airway fistula. In contrast, Wawro reported the deaths of two patients in whom plastic tubes were used to reconstruct the esophagus.[19] One died of sepsis due to a leak during the first postoperative week, and the other died 5 months after reconstruction due to prosthetic dislodgement and erosion into the aorta.

The lack of flexibility of some of the plastics used for esophageal replacement led to the investigation of siliconized rubber (silicone) for this use. In a series of modifications, one group developed a silicone-reinforced Dacron graft that had a toothed nylon ring at each end to facilitate its attachment to the esophagus.[20] In dog experiments, fewer than 30% of the animals survived for more than 5 weeks free of major complications. Graft separation or erosion was the usual cause of death. Use of this device in a single patient was reported, who was alive and taking a soft diet 6 weeks after surgery. Use of a Dacron-reinforced silicone prosthesis for partial replacement of the porcine esophagus resulted in early incorporation with eventual sloughing of the silicone.[21] Anastomotic leaks were not evident, but stricture formation was the inevitable result after the silicone prosthesis migrated.

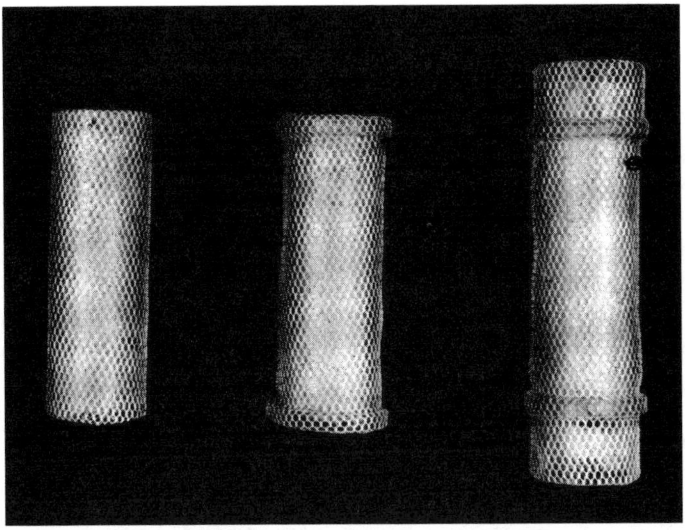

Figure 13-3. Flanged and unflanged silicone rubber prostheses with an outer jacket of Dacron mesh. Reprinted with permission from: Fukushima M, Kako N, Chiba K, Kawaguchi T, Kimura Y, Sato M, Yamauchi M, Koie H. Seven-year follow-up study after the replacement of the esophagus with an artificial esophagus in the dog. *Surgery* 1983;93:70-77.

The perceived need for ingrowth of surrounding tissues into the artificial esophagus led to the use of woven Teflon and Dacron as well as polyethylene (Marlex) mesh as experimental esophageal replacements. These materials possess noncontinuous surfaces that encourage their incorporation into surrounding tissues, permit easier suturing, and provide the possibility of a tight, permanent seal to the esophagus. The results of most of these experiments were as disappointing as were those involving the previous prostheses. An occasional animal survived long-term and at post mortem examination was found to have a fibrous sheath with an epithelial lining, which permitted ingestion of regular chow. Most animals either died in the early postoperative period due to anastomotic leak and empyema, or succumbed to the effects of a high grade esophageal stricture.[22-25] Subsequent application of woven Teflon or Dacron to the outer surface of a methacrylate-based polymer or polyethylene tube permitted some ingrowth of connective tissue around the grafts and made them temporarily water-tight, although most grafts still failed to become incorporated into surrounding tissue and most of the dogs died of disruption or leakage.[26,27] Covering Dacron mesh with Silastic led to the familiar problem of sloughing of the prosthesis, usually prior to the time a complete fibrous sheath had developed.[28] The use of silicone tubes covered with a Dacron mesh resulted in long-term survival in seven of 16 dogs in which reconstruction was performed (Figure 13-3).[29] The prostheses sloughed in a predictable manner, and the stricturing process appeared to progress for up to 6 months but then did not advance further for up to 7 years. This long-term success provided an impetus for continued research into the use of artificial prostheses for esophageal replacement.

This experimental and clinical work helped to define requirements for an artificial esophagus. The ideal replacement must be sufficiently rigid to resist external compression, pliable enough to avoid erosion into surrounding structures, and flexible so that undue tension is not transmitted to the anastomosis by either the motion of surrounding structures or peristalsis of the esophagus. The material must be nonreactive, impervious to microorganisms, and must allow ingrowth of tissue to permit its full incorporation and thus provide a watertight seal at the anastomoses. Even under the best of circumstances, the artificial esophagus is never likely to be able to transmit peristaltic activity and will remain inert.

Advances in Intracorporeal Tubes

Two of the important advances in the design of esophageal prostheses were the use of porous materials to permit more rapid and complete tissue ingrowth and the use of biodegradable materials so that no foreign body was present long-term. A biodegradable graft created from a polyurethane-polylactide mixture that was implanted in rabbits completely degraded over time but was not sufficiently stable to prevent fatal leak or stricture formation.[30] A biodegradable implant made from polymers and co-polymers of polylactic acid and polyglycolic acid prevented anastomotic leakage and permitted long-term survival in several dogs despite the need for continued bougienage for many months after graft placement (Figure 13-4).[31]

The natural fibrotic response to the presence of completely synthetic materials as esophageal replacements led to the introduction of biological materials in recent years. The use of a collagen-silicone copolymer rather than silicone alone reduced the incidence of anastomotic leak and led to survival up to 7 months in dogs.[32] Freeze-dried collagen sponge was used to coat a nylon-reinforced silicone tube to produce a prosthesis that substantially limited anastomotic leakage in dogs and sloughed into the gastrointestinal tract after neoesophageal epithelization was complete (Figures 13-5 and 13-6).[33-35] Strictures did not develop if the silicone tube remained in situ for at least 4 weeks.[36-38] Seeding the prosthesis with cultured autologous oral mucosal cells accelerated both the process of epithelization and the regeneration of mesenchymal tissue around the stent.[39]

Substitution of a mesh made of a copolymer of glycolic acid and lactic acid (Vicryl) for the silicone tube resulted in rapid digestion of the Vicryl

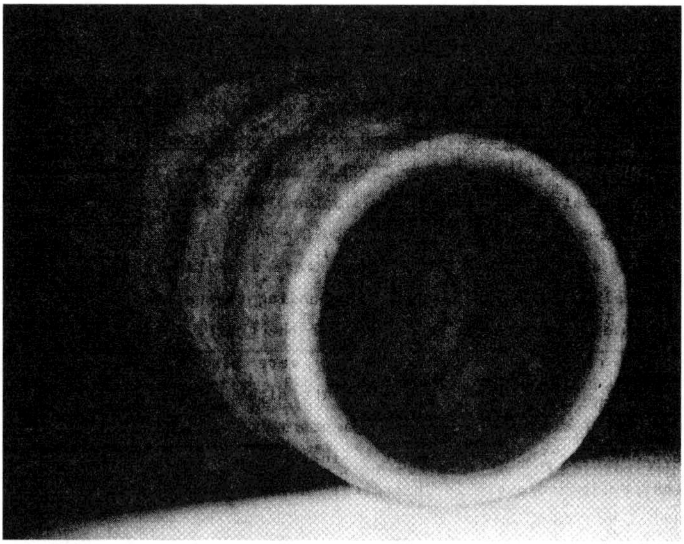

Figure 13-4. A biodegradable prosthesis made of polymers of polylactic and polyglycolic acid. Reprinted with permission from: Grower MF, Russell EA, Cutright DE. Segmental neogenesis of the dog esophagus utilizing a biodegradable polymer framework. *Biomater Artif Cells Artif Organs* 1989;17:291-314.

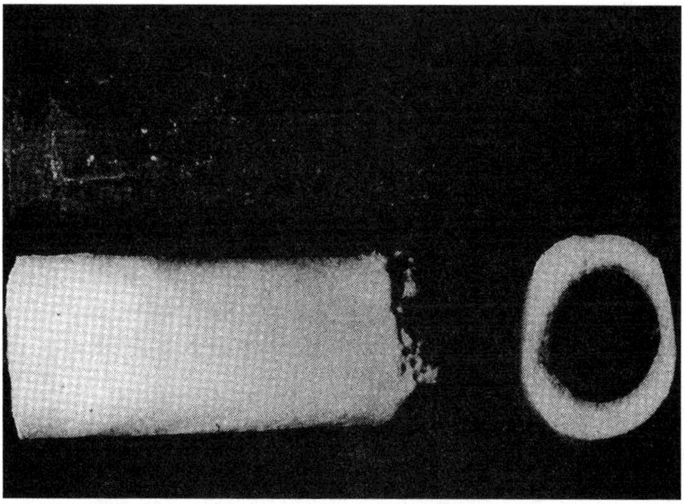

Figure 13-5. A nylon-reinforced silicone tube covered with a 5-mm thick layer of freeze-dried collagen sponge. Reprinted with permission from: Takimoto Y, Teramachi M, Okumura N, Nakamura T, Shimizu Y. Relationship between stenting time and regeneration of neoesophageal submucosal tissue. *ASAIO J* 1994;40:M793-M797.

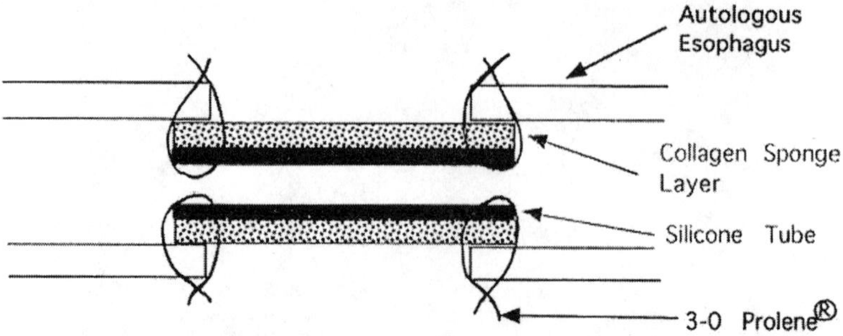

Figure 13-6. Technique for insertion of a composite prosthesis made up of a silicone tube covered with collagen sponge. Reprinted with permission from: Takimoto Y, Nakamura T, Yamamoto Y, Kiyotani T, Teramachi M, Shimizu Y. The experimental replacement of a cervical esophageal segment with an artificial prosthesis with the use of collagen matrix and a silicone stent. *J Thorac Cardiovasc Surg* 1998;116:98-106.

tube when it was exposed to gastric contents that were refluxed into the esophagus.[40] Glutaraldehyde treatment of the Vicryl mesh eliminated the problem of early material breakdown and leakage, but stenosis was still a common development in the intermediate-term. The addition of a layer of cultured human epithelial cells eliminated the fibrotic response that develops during breakdown of polyglycolic acid mesh in vitro.[41,42] Embedding esophageal fibroblasts into the collagen enhanced epithelial cell stratification in vitro, resulting in an epithelial layer similar to that in the human esophagus.[43]

Extracorporeal Tubes

The most modern extracorporeal tubes were initially developed by Akiyama and colleagues in Japan in the late 1960s and are made of siliconized rubber or silicone.[44-46] They consist of separate upper and lower segments with a central connector (Figure 13-7). The upper segment originates in either a small or a large mushroom tip for insertion into a cervical esophagostomy. The central connector is made of clear plastic and contains a port for air evacuation. The lower segment terminates in a mushroom tip for insertion into a gastrostomy. Multiple sizes are available which accommodate patients of varying heights.

Instances in which this type of tube should be used are rare. Most patients are able to undergo some type of formal esophageal reconstruction with autologous tissue. However, some patients are high risk or have no alternative means for reconstruction. Use of the extracorporeal tube permits patients to ingest food who would otherwise be relegated to gastrostomy tube feedings. The use of the extracorporeal tube in this setting has an obvious positive impact on the quality of life in such patients.

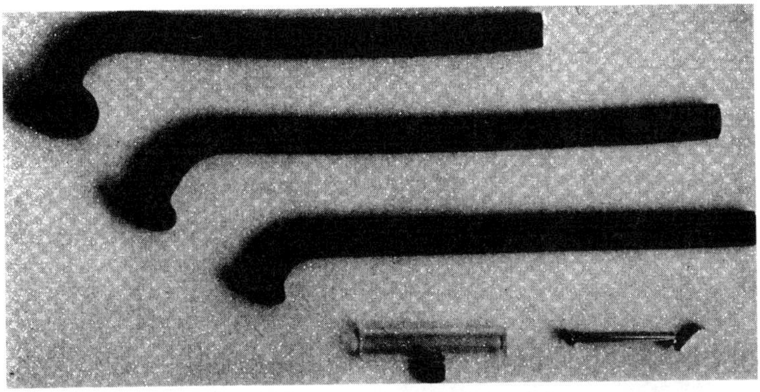

Figure 13-7. Extracorporeal prosthesis set including, from top to bottom, a gastrostomy tube, two esophagostomy tubes, a connector with vent, and a clamp. Reprinted with permission from The Society of Thoracic Surgeons, *Annals of Thoracic Surgery* 1976;22:107-111.

Insertion and use of the tube are straightforward. A cervical esophagostomy and a gastrostomy are created. The cervical portion of the external tube normally is not used until the esophagostomy has matured, which usually requires 2 to 3 weeks. The distal segment may be placed in the gastrostomy at any time in the postoperative period, but it is probably best to use a more traditional gastrostomy tube during the early postoperative period. The standard gastrostomy tubes are easier to use for tube feedings and provide a slightly better seal, thus simplifying their care.

During the first two postoperative weeks the cervical stoma is digitally dilated to prevent its contraction, which would make placement of the extracorporeal tube impossible. When the external conduit is to be used, the smaller of the mushroom tips is initially chosen for insertion into the esophagostomy. After a time, there may be progressive dilation of the cervical stoma necessitating use of a larger tip. Alternative devices such as the "telescope type" prosthesis have been designed that help to avoid this dilatation.[47] Alternatively, the mushroom tip is inserted only during meals, and a stoma bag is applied during all other periods.

The patient must be in an upright position to use the extracorporeal tube because it relies entirely on gravity for movement of foods from the esophagus into the stomach (Figure 13-8). The clamp is removed at the beginning of the meal, and liquids, semisolids, and a wide variety of solid foods comprise the meal. At the end of the meal the valve is opened on the central connector to permit swallowed air to be evacuated from the stomach, after which the clamp is replaced to prevent reflux of gastric contents back into the cervical esophagus.

Use of the extracorporeal tube has been recorded infrequently, and the reported results have been mixed. No new reports of its use have

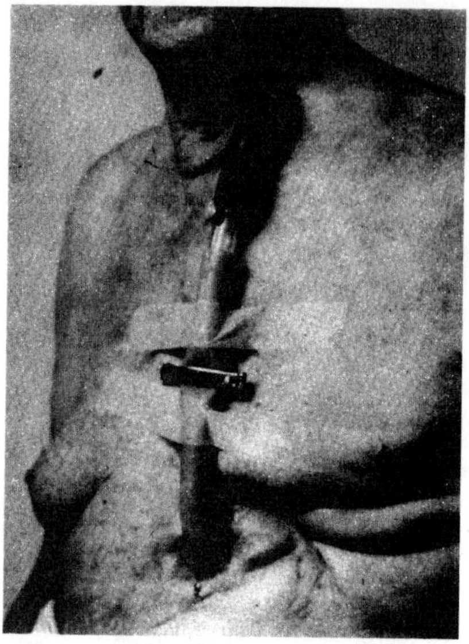

Figure 13-8. The extracorporeal prosthesis assembled and in place. Reprinted with permission from The Society of Thoracic Surgeons, *Annals of Thoracic Surgery* 1976;22:107-111.

been published in the English literature since 1980. The extracorporeal esophagus is able to sustain an acceptable quality of life in selected individuals for more than a decade.[48] Most patients are able to maintain themselves exclusively with use of the extracorporeal tube and eat a regular diet.[47,49-51] However, 10% to 20% of patients are not able to adapt to use of the tube and must resort to intake of all nutrients through the gastrostomy.

Future Directions

With little interest in or need for improvements in extracorporeal tubes, attention will continue to be focused on the development of an intracorporeal tube for esophageal replacement. The basic conditions for a successful artificial tube that are outlined above must still be met. There are a number of important advances underway that may ultimately provide the ability to grow an artificial tube in vitro or in vivo in a heterotopic location that will permit its more routine use for esophageal replacement. Autologous cells placed on a three-dimensional matrix may permit the development of complex tissues, a process which can be performed in vitro or in vivo. Once such a construct has been developed, at the time of implant rapid ingrowth of appropriate structures such as smooth muscle and blood vessels may be stimulated by the presence of specific proteins such as, in the case of blood vessels, angiogenesis factor. The proteins may be made available by incorporating them in polymers that are used to construct the original matrix, or may be added at the time of implant in the form of injectable biodegradable polymers. Instead of using growth factors themselves, genes that encode for these molecules might be used to provide a more durable source of stimulation of tissue formation. Within the first two decades of the twenty-first century it is likely that clinical use of such constructs will be possible. Whether their use for esophageal replacement will become commonplace depends in large part on the ability of surgeons to overcome the problems of anastomotic leakage and long-term fibrosis that have plagued the experimental efforts to date.

References

1. Symonds CJ. The treatment of malignant stricture of the oesophagus by tubage or permanent catheterism. *Br Med J* 1887;1:870-873.
2. Celestin LR. Permanent intubation in inoperable cancer of the oesophagus and cardia. *Ann Royal Coll Surg Engl* 1959;25:165-170.
3. Neuhof H, Ziegler JM. Experimental reconstruction of the oesophagus by granulation tubes. *Surg Gynecol Obstet* 1922;34:767-775.
4. Rob CG, Bateman GH. Reconstruction of the trachea and cervical oesophagus. *Br J Surg* 1949;37:202-205.
5. Edgerton MT. One-stage reconstruction of the cervical esophagus or trachea. *Surgery* 1952;31:239-250.
6. Hawk JC Jr, Jeffords JV. Replacement of esophageal segments: Experimental and clinical observations. *Am Surg* 1955;21:939-949.
7. Braunwald NS, Hufnagel CA. Reconstruction of the esophagus with wire mesh prosthesis. *Surgery* 1958;43:600-605.
8. Berman EF. The experimental replacement of portions of the esophagus by a plastic tube. *Ann Surg* 1952;135:337-343.
9. Moore HD. The replacement of segments of the thoracic esophagus by polythene tubes. *Surg Gynecol Obstet* 1954;98:619-624.
10. Berman EF. Plastic prosthesis in carcinoma of the esophagus. *Surg Clin N Am* 1956;36:883-892.
11. Battersby JS, King H. Esophageal replacement with plastic tubes. *Arch Surg* 1954;69:400-409.
12. Klopp CT, Alford C, Pierpont H. The use of polyethylene film and split-thickness skin graft in reconstruction of cervical esophageal and pharyngeal defects. *Surgery* 1957;29:231-239.
13. Morfit HM, Kramish D. Long-term end results in bridging esophageal defects in human beings with Teflon prostheses. *Am J Surg* 1962;104:756-760.
14. Rubenstein LH. Experiments with substitute esophagus. *J Thorac Surg* 1956;32:691-696.
15. Schobinger R. The use of platysma and nylon tubing in the reconstruction of the cervical esophagus in dogs. *Plast Reconstr Surg* 1959;23:36-48.
16. Watanabe K, Mark JBD. Segmental replacement of the thoracic esophagus with a Silastic prosthesis. *Am J Surg* 1971;121:238-240.

17. Barnes WA, Redo SF, Ogata K. Replacement of portion of canine esophagus with composite prosthesis and greater omentum. *J Thorac Cardiovasc Surg* 1972;64:892-896.
18. Shackelford RT, Sparkuhl K. Palliative resection of the esophagus with use of a plastic tube. *Ann Surg* 1953;138:791-794.
19. Wawro NW. Fatal complications after esophageal replacement with plastic tube. *Surgery* 1954;36:903-905.
20. Fryfogle JD, Cyrowski GA, Rothwell D, et al. Replacement of the middle third of the esophagus with a Silicone rubber prosthesis. *Dis Chest* 1963;43:464-475.
21. Salama FD. Prosthetic replacement of the esophagus. *J Thorac Cardiovasc Surg* 1975;70:739-746.
22. Sheena KS, Ballantyne AJ, Healey JE Jr. Replacement of the cervical esophagus with Marlex mesh. *Surgery* 1962;51:648-651.
23. Mark JBD, Briggs HC. Segmental replacement of the thoracic esophagus with woven Teflon. *J Surg Res* 1964;4:400-402.
24. Lister J, Altman RP, Allison WA. Prosthetic substitution of thoracic esophagus in puppies: Use of Marlex mesh with collagen or anterior rectus sheath. *Ann Surg* 1965;162:812-824.
25. Schuring AG, Ray JW. Experimental use of Dacron as an esophageal prosthesis. *Ann Otol Rhinol Laryngol* 1966;75:202-207.
26. Lyons AS, Beck AR, Lester LJ. Esophageal replacement with prosthesis. *J Surg Res* 1962;2:110-113.
27. LaGuerre JN, Schoenfeld H, Calem W, et al. Prosthetic replacement of esophageal segments. *J Thorac Cardiovasc Surg* 1968;56:674-682.
28. Leininger BJ, Peacock H, Neville WE. Esophageal mucosal regeneration following experimental prosthetic replacement of the esophagus. *Surgery* 1970;67:468-473.
29. Fukushima M, Kako N, Chiba K, et al. Seven-year follow-up study after the replacement of the esophagus with an artificial esophagus in the dog. *Surgery* 1983;93:70-77.
30. Wang F-L, Nieuwenhuis P, Gogolewski S, et al. Oesophageal prosthesis. In Planck H, Egbers G, Syre I (eds): **Polyurethanes in Biomedical Engineering**. Amsterdam, Elsevier Science Publishers B.V., 1984, pp 317-332.
31. Grower MF, Russell EA, Cutright DE. Segmental neogenesis of the dog esophagus utilizing a biodegradable polymer framework. *Biomater Artif Cells Artif Organs* 1989;17:291-314.
32. Kawamura I, Sato H, Ogoshi S, et al. Experimental studies on an artificial esophagus using a collagen-silicone copolymer. *Jpn J Surg* 1983;13:358-367.
33. Ike O, Shimizu Y, Okada T, et al. Experimental studies on an artificial esophagus for the purpose of neoesophageal epithelization using a collagen-coated silicone tube. *ASAIO Trans* 1989;35:226-228.
34. Natsume T, Ike O, Okada T, et al. Porous collagen sponge for esophageal replacement. *J Biomed Mater Res* 1993;27:867-875.
35. Yamamoto Y, Nakamura T, Shimizu Y, et al. Intrathoracic esophageal replacement in the dog with the use of an artificial esophagus composed of a collagen sponge with a double-layered silicone tube. *J Thorac Cardiovasc Surg* 1999;118:276-286.

36. Takimoto Y, Okumura N, Nakamura T, et al. Long-term follow-up of the experimental replacement of the esophagus with a collagen-silicone composite tube. *ASAIO J* 1993;39:M736-M739.
37. Takimoto Y, Teramachi M, Okumura N, et al. Relationship between stenting time and regeneration of neoesophageal submucosal tissue. *ASAIO J* 1994;40:M793-M797.
38. Takimoto Y, Nakamura T, Yamamoto Y, et al. The experimental replacement of a cervical esophageal segment with an artificial prosthesis with the use of collagen matrix and a silicone stent. *J Thorac Cardiovasc Surg* 1998;116:98-106.
39. Natsume T, Ike O, Okada T, et al. Experimental studies of a hybrid esophagus combined with autologous mucosal cells. *ASAIO Trans* 1990;36:M435-M437.
40. Purushotham AD, Carachi R, Gorham SD, et al. Use of a collagen coated Vicryl tube in reconstruction of the porcine esophagus. *Eur J Pediatr Surg* 1991;1:80-84.
41. Sato M, Ando N, Ozawa S, et al. An artificial esophagus consisting of cultured human esophageal epithelial cells, polyglycolic acid mesh, and collagen. *ASAIO J* 1994;40:M389-M392.
42. Nagashima A, Ando N, Sato M, et al. Basic studies on the application of an artificial esophagus using cultured epidermal cells. *Surg Today* 1997;27:915-923.
43. Miki H, Ando N, Ozawa S, et al. An artificial esophagus constructed of cultured human esophageal epithelial cells, fibroblasts, polyglycolic acid mesh, and collagen. *ASAIO J* 1999;45:502-508.
44. Akiyama H, Shima F, Funaki G, et al. External esophageal tube. *Jpn J Surg Soc* 1967;68:110-117.
45. Akiyama H, Hatano S. Esophageal cancer: Palliative treatment. *Jpn J Thor Surg* 1968;21:391-396.
46. Akiyama H, Okuyama T, Kogure T, Satoh Y. Palliative surgery of broncho-esophageal fistula caused by malignant esophageal cancer, with special reference to palliation of the esophagus and cardiostomy. *Shujutsu* 1969;23:418-425.
47. Okamoto Y, Obitsu R. Eight years' experience with an artificial extra-thoracic esophagus. *Jpn J Surg* 1974;4:1-10.
48. Akiyama H, Tsurumaru M. External tubes for oesophageal bypass. In Jamieson GG (ed): **Surgery of the Oesophagus**. Edinburgh, Churchill Livingstone, 1988, pp 777-779.
49. Heimlich HJ. Permanent extracorporeal esophagogastric tube for esophageal replacement. *Ann Thorac Surg* 1976;22:203.
50. Skinner DB, DeMeester TR. Permanent extracorporeal esophagogastric tube for esophageal replacement. *Ann Thorac Surg* 1976;22:107-111.
51. Skinner DB. Esophageal reconstruction. *Am J Surg* 1980;139:810-814.

Chapter 14

Gastric Drainage Procedures

Preparation of the stomach as an esophageal substitute necessitates a bilateral truncal vagotomy. Loss of vagal nerve function may cause a delay in gastric emptying, theoretically resulting in early satiety, weight loss, and the risk of regurgitation and aspiration in patients who undergo gastric pull-up after esophageal reconstruction. Use of a gastric emptying procedure has been standard after truncal vagotomy for peptic ulcer disease since the 1950s. Whether the indications for an emptying procedure are similar after gastric mobilization and pull-up for esophageal reconstruction is a matter of debate. Concerns about the routine use of an emptying procedure after esophagectomy include the potential for surgical complications related to the emptying procedure itself, including leakage, shortening of the reconstructive organ, and the possibility that the blood supply to the stomach might be impaired. In addition, in the intermediate and long-term there is an increased risk of duodenogastric reflux and an appreciable incidence of dumping syndrome that can be quite bothersome to patients.

Anatomy and Physiology of the Pylorus

The stomach is composed of three muscle layers: outer longitudinal, middle circular, and inner oblique. At the distal extent of the gastric antrum, the middle circular gastric muscle thickens gradually to form the pyloric sphincter. This thickened region ends abruptly on the aboral, or duodenal, side. The pylorus is easily recognized by palpation of its muscular ring at the junction between the stomach and duodenum. When the sphincter is indistinct, however, it may also be located by its proximity to a vein which crosses anteriorly over the region of the pylorus known as the pyloric vein of Mayo. The arterial supply to the superior aspect of the pylorus is from branches of the right gastric and supraduodenal arteries

From Ferguson MK: *Reconstructive Surgery of the Esophagus* Armonk, NY: Futura Publishing Company, Inc., © 2002.

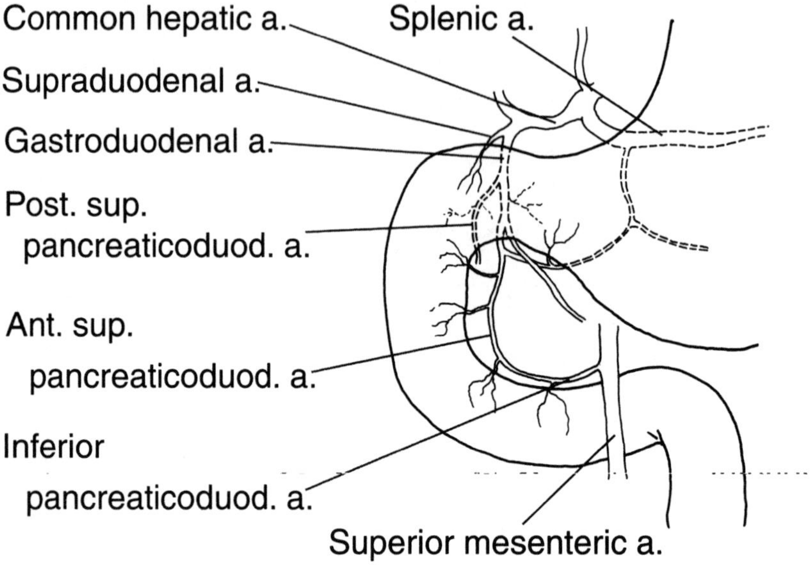

Figure 14-1. The arterial blood supply to the pyloric region.

(Figure 14-1). The inferior and medial aspects are supplied by the gastroduodenal artery via its pancreaticoduodenal or right gastroepiploic branches.

The pylorus acts as a true sphincter. It has a high pressure zone with a resting amplitude of about 5-mm Hg which relaxes in response to gastric antral peristalsis.[1] Infusion of substances into the duodenum or jejunum results in changes in pyloric tone. An increase in amplitude results from HCl, olive oil and other fats, amino acids, and glucose, whereas NaCl causes no apparent change in pyloric tone.[1] Pyloric closure is also prolonged after intestinal infusion of fats, while sugars, acids, and proteins do not appear to have a similar effect.[2]

Use of Emptying Procedures

There is a wealth of published reports regarding indications for pyloroplasty or other gastric drainage procedures as an adjunct to esophagectomy. Unfortunately, most contain observational or anecdotal information that is not amenable to critical analysis. Fortunately, a few formal trials regarding the utility of pyloroplasty have been performed. These randomized trials of a gastric drainage procedure compared to no gastric drainage at the time of gastric replacement of the esophagus have produced mixed results (Table 14-1).

Table 14-1.
Randomized Studies of the Efficacy of Gastric Emptying Procedures after Esophagectomy.

Author	Year	Patients in drainage/control groups	Type of reconstruction	Route of reconstruction	Short-term benefit	Long-term benefit
Mannell et al.[3]	1990	20/20	Whole stomach	Retrosternal	Yes	No
Fok et al.[4]	1991	100/100	Whole stomach	Posterior mediastinum	Yes	Yes
Chattopadhyay et al.[5]	1993	12/12	Whole stomach	Posterior mediastinum	Yes	No
Zieran et al.[6]	1995	52/55	Gastric tube	Variable	No	No
Fontes et al.[7]	1996	22/27	Gastric tube	Posterior mediastinum	—	No
Kobayashi et al.[8]	1996	34/33	Gastric tube	Variable	—	No

In a South African study, 40 patients who underwent substernal reconstruction with the whole stomach were randomized to pyloroplasty or no emptying procedure.[3] Patients without an emptying procedure were significantly more likely to suffer gastric stasis symptoms in the early postoperative period than were patients who had pyloroplasty, and three patients without pyloroplasty died of aspiration pneumonia. Evaluation of gastric emptying between 1 and 3 months after operation, however, showed that most symptoms had resolved and that the gastric emptying times were similar between the two groups.

In a study from Hong Kong involving 200 patients, the whole stomach was used for reconstruction and was passed through the bed of the resected esophagus.[4] No complications occurred due to the performance of the pyloroplasty. There were 13 patients in the control group who suffered delayed gastric emptying with regurgitation, two of whom died of aspiration pneumonia and one of whom required reoperation for drainage. The average gastric emptying time was much longer in the control group when measured at least 6 months postoperatively. There was no apparent difference between the groups after 6 months in the ability to ingest a solid diet or in the ability to eat normal amounts of food at a single sitting. More patients in the control group had symptoms during meals at long-term follow-up than did those who underwent pyloroplasty.

In a study from India, 24 patients who underwent subtotal esophagectomy and reconstruction with a gastric tube through the posterior mediastinum were randomized to pyloroplasty or control groups.[5] At 6 months after operation, bile acid concentrations within the stomach were similar between the two groups. Symptoms such as postprandial discomfort, bilious eructations, and vomiting occurred infrequently and did not appear to be related to whether or not an emptying procedure was performed.

A German study involved 107 patients who were reconstructed with a gastric tube placed in the posterior mediastinum and were randomized to pyloromyotomy or no emptying procedure.[6] One patient died as a result of a leak from the pyloromyotomy. Two additional patients suffered a fibrotic stricture at the site of pyloromyotomy resulting in severe vomiting. Between 2 weeks and 6 months postoperatively, there was no difference between the groups in symptoms of abdominal discomfort or in radiologic assessment of gastric emptying.

In a Brazilian study of 49 patients who underwent esophageal reconstruction with a gastric tube in the posterior mediastinum, the authors identified no important differences between the group undergoing pyloroplasty compared to the group that served as surgical controls.[7] Follow-up in the early period after discharge demonstrated similar symptoms, barium transit, and scintigraphic measurement of gastric emptying between the two groups.

In a Japanese study of 67 patients who had reconstruction performed with a gastric tube placed through any of three different mediastinal routes, the authors found mixed results at 1 and 6 months postoperatively.[8] The quantity of food ingested was similar between the pyloroplasty and control groups, but the control group had a higher incidence of regurgitation. There was no measurable difference in gastric emptying between the two groups at either time period. Nutritional indices were also similar.

Nonrandomized studies also fail to support the utility of routinely performing an emptying procedure after esophagectomy and gastric reconstruction. In particular, one Chinese report identified no advantage for pyloroplasty in normalizing gastric emptying.[9] In fact, patients who underwent pyloroplasty had a substantially higher incidence of bile regurgitation, dumping syndrome, aspiration pneumonia, and gastric ulceration.

The findings and the recommendation regarding routine use of an emptying procedure need to be viewed critically. It has been reported that gastric emptying is more rapid when a tubularized stomach rather than a whole stomach conduit is used for reconstruction.[10,11] However, recovery of gastric tone and motility has been reported after several years of follow-up, and the whole stomach appears to achieve better motility long-term than does the tubularized stomach.[12] Whether this influences gastric emptying or clinical function is a matter of conjecture. At least in the short term, the tubularized stomach appears to have advantages in terms of emptying compared to the whole stomach when used as an esophageal substitute. This fact may importantly impact on the need for a gastric drainage procedure accompanying esophageal reconstruction.

The technique of surgical decision analysis has been applied to determine the theoretic utility of an emptying procedure after esophagectomy with gastric reconstruction. As with the randomized studies, the results do not strongly indicate whether routine pyloroplasty or the use of no emptying procedure is optimal after esophagectomy.[13] Using the analysis, the authors concluded that routine performance of a gastric emptying procedure is appropriate if the risk of gastric outlet obstruction is greater than 10%, provided that the drainage procedure is 95% effective. The clinical results summarized above demonstrate neither that the efficacy of routine pyloroplasty approaches 95% nor that the incidence of outlet obstruction exceeds 10%. One approach is to use drainage procedures selectively based on a number of factors. Drainage procedures are strongly indicated in patients who have underlying problems that might affect gastric emptying, including preexisting pyloric pathology such as scarring or ulceration and gastroparesis. The fact that dumping symptoms are identified more often in younger patients and among women may mitigate against the routine use of emptying procedures in these patients.[14] In most other patients use of a gastric emptying procedure is based on the surgeon's training and preferences. There are currently no data to support the routine use of gastric emptying procedures based on long-term outcomes after esophagectomy. Whether there is a short-term advantage to its use with regards to acute postoperative complications depends in part on whether the whole stomach is used for reconstruction. In patients in whom a gastric tube is created for a reconstructive organ, routine use of a gastric emptying procedure is not necessary.

If an emptying procedure is to be used, there are a number of different procedures to choose from, including pyloromyotomy, different techniques for pyloroplasty, finger dilation, and finger fracture. A randomized comparison between pyloroplasty and pyloromyotomy demonstrated more rapid gastric emptying after pyloromyotomy when evaluated 6 months postoperatively.[15] However, longer term follow-up disclosed no differences between the groups in the type or quantity of food intake nor in the types of long-term complications such as regurgitation and dumping. Another randomized study of gastric emptying procedures after esophageal reconstruction using intrathoracic stomach demonstrated no difference between emptying of solids or liquids comparing pyloroplasty, pyloromyotomy, or pyloric dilation in the early postoperative period.[16] In another study, finger dilation was found to produce results that are similar to pyloroplasty while being simpler and safer.[17]

Options for managing patients who fail a trial of no emptying procedure include dietary modification, the use of prokinetic agents, pneumatic dilation, and reoperation. Dietary modifications include restricting intake to liquids and very soft solids, and eliminating foods with high fiber content that can create a gastric bezoar. Prokinetic agents include metaclopramide, bethanecol, domperidone, and the motilin agonist erythromycin.[18,19] In one report, erythromycin was superior to pyloroplasty in its salutary effects on gastric emptying after esophagectomy.[20] Pneumatic dilation is usually sufficient to provide adequate gastric emptying if these conservative measures fail.[21] As a last resort, the patient can undergo a reoperation with pyloromyotomy or pyloroplasty.

Techniques for Performing Emptying Procedures

Pyloromyotomy

Perhaps the most commonly used emptying procedure after esophagectomy and gastric reconstruction is pyloromyotomy. It is quick to perform and is as effective as pyloroplasty. Since it is designed to be accomplished without entry into the gastric or duodenal lumen, the risk of infection from a leak and of gastrointestinal bleeding is less than for

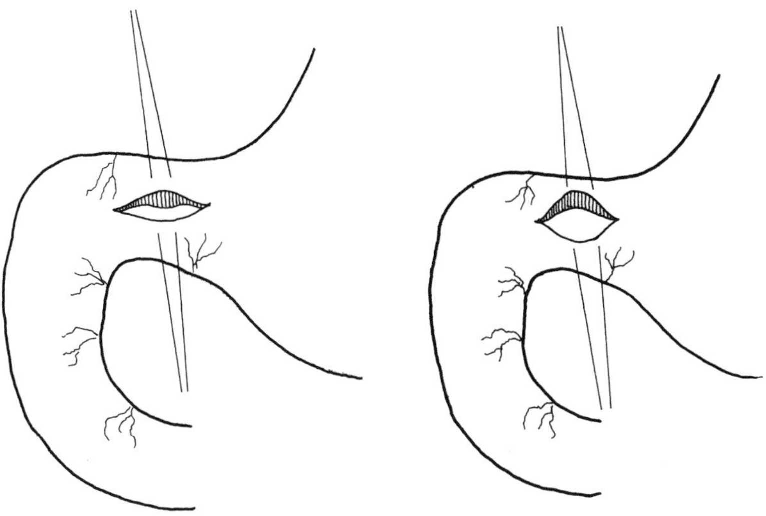

Figure 14-2. A pyloromyotomy is begun by placing stay sutures through the pyloric ring. While traction is placed on the sutures, the muscle of the ring is divided along the gastroduodenal axis (left). The muscle is then dissected from the mucosa to ensure that the cut edges do not heal back together (right).

pyloroplasty. Stay sutures are placed to incorporate the pyloric vein of Mayo, one on the antero-superior surface and the other on the antero-inferior surface of the pylorus. As traction is placed on these, the serosa is sharply incised along the gastroduodenal axis over a distance of 2 to 3 cm to encompass the width of the pyloric muscle (Figure 14-2). The fibers of the pylorus are elevated with a right-angle clamp and are divided until the bare gastroduodenal mucosa is completely exposed. The risk of mucosal injury increases as the duodenum is approached. The mucosa is gently separated bluntly from the overlying muscle to ensure that the edges of the muscle do not heal back together. Alternatively, a 1-cm wide section of pyloric muscle is removed. Inspection and palpation serve to demonstrate that the myotomy is complete. If inadvertent mucosal injury occurs, management options include repair with omental reinforcement or conversion to pyloroplasty.

Pyloroplasty

The most traditional method of providing gastric drainage after esophagectomy and gastric reconstruction is by performing a pyloroplasty. The standard form of pyloroplasty is the Heineke-Mikulicz version as modified by Weinberg.[22] Two stay sutures are placed superiorly and inferiorly into the pyloric ring as described for pyloromyotomy. A 6- to 7-cm

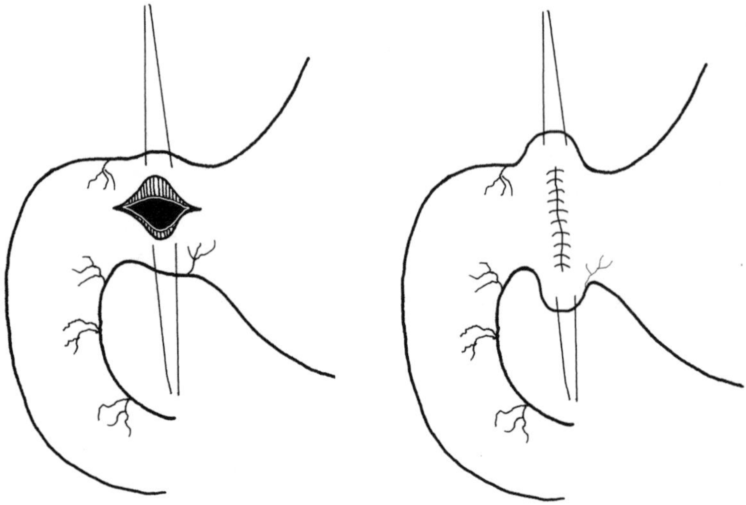

Figure 14-3. A pyloroplasty is begun by placing stay sutures through the pyloric ring. A full thickness incision is made through the ring along the gastroduodenal axis and traction is placed on the stay sutures to convert the longitudinal incision to a transverse one (left). The incision is closed with a running stitch (right).

full thickness incision is made across the pylorus along the gastroduodenal axis and is centered more on the gastric side of the pyloric ring (Figure 14-3). The gastric contents are aspirated. Tension is placed on the stay sutures to convert the longitudinal orientation of the incision to a transverse orientation. The incision is then closed with interrupted inverting sutures.

Pyloric Dilation

Pyloric dilation has been used as an alternative to more traditional emptying procedures for more than two decades. Some surgeons use a large clamp passed through a gastrotomy to stretch the pylorus.[23] A more elegant technique is to complete mobilization of the duodenum (Kocher maneuver) and then perform digital dilation of the pylorus. Using a single finger, the gastric antrum or duodenal bulb is invaginated into the pylorus, stretching or tearing the pyloric ring while leaving the mucosa and serosa intact.[17,24] The risk of leakage after this maneuver is considerably less than after pyloromyotomy or pyloroplasty.

References

1. Fisher R, Cohen S. Physiologic characteristics of the human pyloric sphincter. *Gastroenterology* 1973;64:67-75.

2. Kumar D, Ritman EL, Malagelada J-R. Three-dimensional imaging of the stomach: Role of pylorus in the emptying of liquids. *Am J Physiol* 1987;253:G79-G85.
3. Mannell A, McKnight A, Esser JD. Role of pyloroplasty in the retrosternal stomach: Results of a prospective, randomized, controlled trial. *Br J Surg* 1990;77:57-59.
4. Fok M, Cheng SWK, Wong J. Pyloroplasty versus no drainage in gastric replacement of the esophagus. *Am J Surg* 1991;162:447-452.
5. Chattopadhyay TK, Gupta S, Padhy AK, et al. Is pyloroplasty necessary following intrathoracic transposition of stomach? Results of a prospective clinical study. *Aust N Z J Surg* 1991;61:366-369.
6. Zieren HU, Muller JM, Jacobi CA, et al. Soll beim Magenhochzug nach subtotaler Oesophagektomie mit oesophago-gastraler Anastomose am Hals eine Pyloroplastik durchgefuhrt werden? Eine prospektiv randomisierte Studie. *Chirurg* 1995;66:319-325.
7. Fontes P, Nectoux M, Escobar A, et al. Esophagogastroplasty with and without pyloroplasty: A prospective study. In Peracchia A, Rosati R, Bonavina L, et al. (eds): **Recent Advances in Diseases of the Esophagus**. Bologna, Monduzzi Editore, 1996, pp 241-245.
8. Kobayashi A, Ide H, Eguchi R, et al. The efficacy of pyloroplasty in relation to food-taking quality of life in the reconstruction with gastric tube after esophagectomy. In Peracchia A, Rosati R, Bonavina L, et al. (eds): **Recent Advances in Diseases of the Esophagus**. Bologna, Monduzzi Editore, 1996, pp 247-254.
9. Wang L-S, Huang M-H, Huang B-S, et al. Gastric substitution for resectable carcinoma of the esophagus: An analysis of 368 cases. *Ann Thorac Surg* 1992;53:289-294.
10. Barbera L, Kemen M, Wegener M, et al. Effect of site and width of stomach tube after esophageal resection on gastric emptying. *Zentralb Chirurg* 1994;119:240-244.
11. Bemelman WA, Taat CW, Slors JF, et al. Delayed postoperative emptying after esophageal resection is dependent on the size of the gastric substitute. *J Am Coll Surg* 1995;180:461-464.
12. Collard J-M, Romagnoli R, Otte J-B, et al. The denervated stomach as an esophageal substitute is a contractile organ. *Ann Surg* 1998;227:33-39.
13. Olak J, Detsky A. Surgical decision analysis: Esophagectomy/esophagogastrectomy with or without drainage? *Ann Thorac Surg* 1992;53:493-497.
14. McLarty AJ, Deschamps C, Trastek VF, et al. Esophageal resection for cancer of the esophagus: Long-term function and quality of life. *Ann Thorac Surg* 1997;63:1568-1572.
15. Law S, Cheung M-C, Fok M, et al. Pyloroplasty and pyloromyotomy in gastric replacement of the esophagus after esophagectomy: A randomized controlled trial. *J Am Coll Surg* 1997;184:630-636.
16. Manjari R, Padhy AK, Chattopadhyay TK. Emptying of the intrathoracic stomach using three different pylorus drainage procedures - results of a comparative study. *Surgery Today* 1996;26:581-585.
17. Yamashita Y, Hirai T, Mukaida H, et al. Finger bougie method compared with pyloroplasty in the gastric replacement of the esophagus. *Surgery Today* 1999;29:107-110.

18. Burt M, Scott A, Williard WC, et al. Erythromycin stimulates gastric emptying after esophagectomy with gastric replacement: A randomized trial. *J Thorac Cardiovasc Surg* 1996;111:649-654.
19. Collard J-M, Romagnoli R, Otte J-B, et al. Erythromycin enhances early postoperative contractility of the denervated whole stomach as an esophageal substitute. *Ann Surg* 1999;229:337-343.
20. Hill ADK, Walsh TN, Hamilton D, et al. Erythromycin improves emptying of the denervated stomach after oesophagectomy. *Br J Surg* 1993;80:879-881.
21. Bemelman WA, Brummelkamp WH, Bartelsman JFWM. Endoscopic balloon dilation of the pylorus after esophagogastrostomy without a drainage procedure. *Surg Gynecol Obstet* 1990;170:424-426.
22. Weinberg JA, Stempein SJ, Movius HJ, et al. Vagotomy and pyloroplasty in the treatment of duodenal ulcer. *Am J Surg* 1956;92:202-207.
23. Siewert JR, Stein HJ, Liebermann-Meffert D, et al. The gastric tube as an esophageal substitute. *Dis Esoph* 1995;8:11-19.
24. Santi S, Ruol A, Baldan N, et al. Finger dilatation of the pylorus: Report on 1234 consecutive patients undergoing esophagectomy and esophagogastrostomy for cancer. In Peracchia A, Rosati R, Bonavina L, et al. (eds): **Recent Advances in Diseases of the Esophagus**. Bologna, Monduzzi Editore, 1996, p 254-259.

Chapter 15

The Esophageal Anastomosis

The anastomosis is often the "make or break" element of an esophageal reconstructive operation. As such, an esophageal anastomosis usually represents one of two extremes: a prideful, personal signature on a surgeon's work or a surgeon's Waterloo. Until only a few years ago, performing an esophageal anastomosis was said to be "suturing the unsuturable."[1] Advances in the past decade have substantially reduced the risk of morbidity associated with an esophageal anastomosis. In some centers with substantial experience in esophageal surgery, the risk of an anastomotic leak has become vanishingly small. However, collective reviews from unselected centers continue to illustrate the high risk of complications associated with an esophageal anastomosis.[2]

Most esophageal surgeons have a particular style used to perform their anastomoses that has been developed over years of training and experience. Once such a technique has been established it is often difficult to convince a surgeon to alter the "accepted" approach. Given the wide range of outcomes after performance of an esophageal anastomosis and the wide variety of techniques available, it is clear that understanding the secrets behind reducing the risks of anastomotic complications is challenging. Hopefully, this chapter will encourage some surgeons to reconsider the technique they are using and incorporate some of the recent elements that have been described which contribute to improved anastomotic techniques and outcomes.

Anastomotic Healing

Healing of the esophagus has been investigated since the 1920s, a time when esophageal surgery was beginning to become a practical possibility. Functionally, the esophagus has three layers, which may contribute to the strength of an anastomosis: mucosa, submucosa, and muscularis

---

From Ferguson MK: *Reconstructive Surgery of the Esophagus* Armonk, NY: Futura Publishing Company, Inc., © 2002.

propria. As early as 1923, the esophageal submucosa was identified as possessing the greatest suture holding power among these three layers, a finding that has analogy to most other parts of the gastrointestinal tract.[3] This fact has been confirmed by several other investigators.[4-6] The holding strength of the esophagus of a single through-and-through suture is the lowest of any portion of the alimentary tract.[5] The reasons for this are unclear, but may be due in part to the lack of an esophageal serosa.

Healing of an esophageal anastomosis progresses until the anastomotic tissues are as strong as the native tissues. The bursting strength of esophageal anastomoses initially decreases to a nadir 4 days postoperatively, corresponding to the inflammatory (or lag) phase of healing. During this time, the sutures or staples used to join the tissues together are the primary source of anastomotic integrity. Thus, it is primarily during the first week or two of anastomotic healing that surgical technique plays a significant role in anastomotic integrity.[7] During the ensuing days there is a gradual increase in the bursting strength, which does not plateau for at least 2 weeks postoperatively.[8-10] Similar findings have been reported in regards to the tensile strength of esophagogastric anastomoses and the suture holding capacity of the esophagus.[11,12] These findings can be explained by changes in hydroxyproline (a unique amino acid constituent of collagen) content in the anastomosis. Anastomotic tissue hydroxyproline content decreases during the first 4 days postoperatively and then increases during the subsequent 10 days, at the end of which time it is only two-thirds of normal tissue hydroxyproline content.[9,10]

The pathophysiology of wound healing has been studied extensively in the large intestine and to a lesser extent in the small intestine, and serves as a good model for understanding similar processes in the esophagus. Anastomotic healing is a complex process affected by a decrease in aerobic and anaerobic metabolism in the mucosa and muscularis propria, whereas metabolic activity in the submucosa is relatively preserved.[13] Aerobic metabolism does not return to normal until 3 weeks postoperatively, a condition that likely requires ingrowth of new blood vessels. Collagen content decreases for the first 2 days postoperatively and then increases to such an extent that it is equal to preoperative levels in the colon and exceeds that of the native ileal tissues by the end of the first postoperative week.[14] This reflects a complex process of collagen synthesis and breakdown that is regulated by a variety of cytokines and growth factors.[15] Collagenolytic activity is greater in the colon than in the small bowel, a fact that helps explain the differences in collagen content throughout the inflammatory and proliferative phases of healing.[16] Interestingly, the highest expression of the collagen genes is not evident until more than one week postoperatively.[13] Maturation of the newly formed collagen, with alterations in collagen types and amounts of cross-linking, continues for many weeks after anastomotic integrity is ensured, a process that has not been adequately studied.[17]

There is some evidence that the healing process of an esophageal anastomosis proceeds at a slower pace than does that of other gastrointestinal tissues. Large intestinal anastomoses reach a breaking strength or bursting strength equivalent to that of the native tissues by 7 days postoperatively.[18,19] In contrast, small intestinal anastomoses achieve anastomotic strength equivalent to that of normal tissue a few days later, while the healing rate of ileocolic anastomoses falls somewhere between the healing rates of the colon and the ileum.[20,21] These differences may reflect variations in collagen metabolism affected by intestinal contents (bacteria and intraluminal bulk). An esophageal anastomosis, in contrast, does not reach the strength of native tissues for at least 2 weeks postoperatively. Whether this is a reflection of differences in blood supply and the resulting metabolic rates, or reflects a higher collagenolytic activity, is not known. The finding does, however, suggest that surgical technique may be even more important in ensuring the integrity of an esophageal anastomosis than it is for intestinal anastomoses.

From a practical perspective, the mucosa/submucosa and muscularis propria comprise two layers that can be sutured separately or together. Most successful anastomotic techniques include the mucosa/submucosa because of its suture holding powers, although this appears, at least experimentally, to increase the risk of stricture formation.[22,23]

Types of Anastomoses

End-to-Side or End-to-End

The most common type of esophageal anastomosis performed is the end-to-side anastomosis (Figure 15-1). This is partly due to the fact that the most common organ used for esophageal replacement is the stomach. An esophagogastrostomy is usually constructed some distance from the tip of the gastric tube for a variety of reasons. Tissue viability increases as a function of the distance from the tip of the gastric tube. Performing the anastomosis more distally on the stomach often enables the creation of an anastomotic lumen with a cross sectional area that exceeds that of the native esophagus. Placing the anastomosis somewhat below the tip of the gastric tube provides some element of an antireflux valve. Leaving a portion of the stomach above the anastomosis also provides a protective effect, in essence partially or completely wrapping the anastomosis with gastric tissue which can prevent or localize an anastomotic leak (see below regarding invaginating anastomoses).

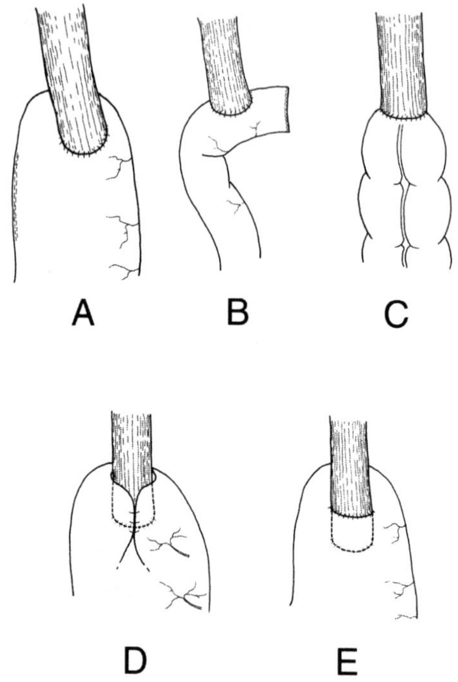

Figure 15-1. Types of anastomoses. A: end-to-side esophagogastrostomy; B: end-to-side esophagojejunostomy; C: end-to-end esophagocolostomy; D: invaginating esophagogastrostomy; E: tunneled esophagogastrostomy.

There are potential drawbacks to the performance of an end-to-side esophagogastrostomy. The blood supply to the tip of the gastric tube is entirely through an intramural network of vessels. Creation of an end-to-side anastomosis necessitates division of some of these vessels, which theoretically results in ischemia of the tip of the gastric tube. An end-to-side anastomosis also requires greater length of stomach tube and may result in greater tension on the anastomosis than would an end-to-end anastomosis.

End-to-side anastomoses are also often performed when constructing an esophagojejunostomy. The jejunum is often tethered on a somewhat short vascular pedicle that necessitates some curvature in the interposition if tension on the pedicle is to be avoided. Thus, even though the proximal end of the jejunum lies very close to the distal end of the esophagus, an end-to-side anastomosis is usually safer and presents little additional technical difficulty.

End-to-end anastomoses are most often performed when the colon is used as an esophageal replacement organ. Despite the slight size mismatch between the colon and the esophagus, such an anastomosis can be constructed with either suture or stapling techniques with good success. On occasion, tailoring of the proximal end of the colon interposition is necessary if there is too much size discrepancy.

There appears to be no *a priori* advantage to using an end-to-side instead of an end-to-end anastomosis with reference to the incidence of postoperative complications. A literature review from the 1970s concluded that outcomes favored end-to-side anastomoses.[24] However, a more recent retrospective study from a single institution identified similar complication rates after transhiatal esophagectomy and cervical esophagogastrostomy. The incidence of anastomotic leak (14% vs. 14%), anastomotic stricture (32% vs. 29%), and the number of dilations necessary to achieve freedom from dysphagia in patients who developed strictures (7 vs. 9) did not differ among patients who underwent end-to-end or end-to-side anastomoses.[25]

Invaginating

A number of options for embedding the esophagus within the stomach have been developed in an effort to decrease the rate of esophagogastric anastomotic leak. These include the inkwell anastomosis (wrapping the anastomosis with redundant gastric fundus) and the "tunnel" esophagogastrostomy, both of which provide circumferential reinforcement of an anastomosis.[26-31] Other options include partially circumferential reinforcement of the anastomosis such as is provided by the redundant gastric fundus that lies posterior to an end-to-side esophagogastrostomy.

Variables in Creating an Esophageal Anastomosis

Hand Sutured versus Mechanical

The most contentious variable encountered in the performance of an esophageal reconstructive operation is whether the anastomosis is sutured or stapled. However, given that many anastomoses are currently performed using a combination of suture and stapled techniques, the choice is not always dichotomous. The preeminence of the traditional hand sewn anastomosis that was developed during the early decades of esophageal surgery was challenged in the 1970s by the introduction of circular stapling techniques.[32] The latter techniques had the presumed advantage of reducing the incidence of postoperative anastomotic leak but quickly fell into some disrepute due to the higher incidence of anastomotic stricture associated with their use.[32-35] A decade of additional clinical experience was necessary to document safer techniques of stapler use for esophageal anastomoses.

There have been numerous randomized and nonrandomized comparisons between stapled (using circular stapling devices) and sutured anastomoses (Table 15-1).[32,36-47] Stapling techniques appear to reduce operative time somewhat and may reduce blood loss. Operative mortality is not affected by the anastomotic technique. Despite the initial promise of stapling techniques, the incidence of anastomotic leak does not seem to be affected by the method used to create an anastomosis. Of more importance is the fact that, even with decades of experience using stapling techniques, the incidence of anastomotic stricture is still significantly higher in patients who have a stapled anastomosis. To summarize, both suturing and stapling are acceptable anastomotic techniques, although stapled anastomoses have a higher rate of stricture. Because of the technical capabilities of stapling devices, there may be an advantage in creating stapled anastomoses in certain situations in which suturing may be difficult.[48-50]

Sutured Anastomoses

Types of Suture

Early debates regarding which type of suture is best for performing esophageal anastomoses centered around the utility of silk compared to linen, catgut, or chromic catgut.[51] Subsequent studies focused on the utility of monofilament sutures and suggested that wire or polypropylene were superior to the traditional suture materials.[52,53] Synthetic braided absorbable sutures (polyglycolic acid, polyglactin 910) were introduced in the 1970s in an effort to reduce local reaction to foreign material in the healing wound. Their overly rapid rates of hydrolysis, due in part to a large surface area of exposure, led to the development of monofilament absorbable sutures (polyglyconate, polydioxanone) in the 1980s.[54] The strength of the monofilament sutures far exceeds that of the synthetic braided sutures, polypropylene, silk, catgut, and chromic catgut.[55] Polyglyconate sutures have been shown to be less stiff than the initial formulation of polydioxanone sutures, although reformulation of the latter has largely compensated for this difference.[56,57]

There have been no controlled studies directly comparing the effectiveness of different synthetic suture materials for esophageal anastomoses. In randomized studies in which sutured esophageal anastomoses were studied, the suture material of choice varied considerably and in-

Table 15-5.
Characteristics of Linear and Linear Cutting Staplers.

Type	Name	Manufacturer[1]	Jaw length	Disposable (D) or Reusable (R)	Closed staple height	Staple material
Linear cutting	TLC	Ethicon	55, 75, 100 mm	D	1.5, 2 mm	Titanium
	GIA	USSC	60, 80 mm	D	1.5, 2 mm	Titanium
	GIA	USSC	50, 90 mm	R	1.5, 2 mm	Stainless steel
	ILA	3M	75 mm	D	1.5, 2 mm	Titanium
	ILA	3M	100 mm	R	1.5, 2 mm	Stainless steel
Linear	TX	Ethicon	30, 60, 90 mm	D	1.5, 2 mm	Titanium
	TL	Ethicon	30,60,90 mm	D	1.5, 2 mm	Titanium
	TLH[2]	Ethicon	30,60,90 mm	D	1.5, 2 mm	Titanium
	Access[3]	Ethicon	55	D	1.5, 2 mm	Titanium
	TA	USSC	30, 55 mm	D	1.5, 2 mm	Titanium
	Premium TA	USSC	30, 60, 90 mm	D	1.5, 2 mm	Titanium
	Premium TA	USSC	30, 55, 90 mm	R	1.5, 2 mm	Titanium
	PI	USSC	30, 55, 90 mm	D	1.5, 2 mm	Titanium
	PI	USSC	30, 55, 90 mm	R	1.5, 2 mm	Stainless steel
	Roticulator[3]	USSC	30, 55 mm	D	1.5, 2 mm	Titanium

1. Ethicon, Inc.; USSC - United States Surgical Corporation; 3M, Inc.
2. Heavy wire staples
3. These models have the capability of altering the angle of the head of the stapler up to 90°.

Table 15-1. (cont).
Randomized Evaluations

Author	Year	Anastomotic technique	Leaks	p value	Strictures	p value
Fujimoto et al.[40]	1991	Sutured	4/180	NS*	1/180	0.078
		Stapled	7/199		6/199	
West of Scotland[41]	1991	Sutured	0/25	NS	—	—
		Stapled	1/27		—	
Craig et al.[42]	1996	Sutured	3/50	NS	13/48	NS
		Stapled	4/50		13/46	
Valverde et al.[44]	1996	Sutured	12/74	NS	8/62	NS
		Stapled	12/78		7/53	
Law et al.[45]	1997	Sutured	1/61	NS	5/55	0.0003
		Stapled	3/61		20/50	
Laterza et al.[46]	1999	Sutured	1/21	NS	2/19	NS
		Stapled	4/20		3/19	
Totals	—	Sutured	21/411 (5.1%)	0.22	29/364 (8.0%)	0.018
		Stapled	31/435 (7.1%)		49/367 (13.3%)	

*NS: not significant

Table 15-2.
Anastomotic Complications after Single- and Double-layer Esophageal Anastomoses.

Author	Year	Single-layer	Leaks (%)	Double-layer	Leaks (%)
Giuli and Sancho-Garnier[36]	1986	225	9	321	19
Richelme and Baulieux[60]	1986	225	9	636	24.6
Muller et al.[58]	1990	3648	12	5078	12

cluded silk, synthetic absorbable braided sutures, and synthetic absorbable monofilament sutures. In one retrospective review, the incidence of anastomotic leak was higher (11% of 1222) in patients in whom a nonabsorbable suture was used than in those in whom an absorbable suture was used (7% of 1737 patients).[58] Although the mechanical and biological properties of synthetic monofilament absorbable sutures are superior to those of other suture types, successful esophageal anastomoses can be created with a variety of suture materials.

Number of Layers

The tradition technique of esophageal anastomosis in the middle of the 20th century employed multiple layers of silk, linen, or catgut, with the primary differences centered around whether the sutures were placed in a continuous or an interrupted fashion.[51] Current factors influencing the choice between single- and multiple-layer anastomoses have recently been summarized.[1,2] Proponents of multiple-layer suturing techniques claim that better tissue apposition is possible, whereas single-layer proponents believe that the technique is faster and results in a lower incidence of anastomotic stricture. Some surgeons report a low incidence of anastomotic leak using a two-layer technique.[59] In contrast, other summarized experiences suggest that a two-layer technique results in a higher incidence of anastomotic leak than does a single layer technique (Table 15-2).[36,58,60] One randomized study demonstrated that rates of anastomotic leak were similar for one- and two-layer anastomoses (19%), but that the incidence of anastomotic stricture was significantly higher in patients undergoing a two-layer anastomosis (48% compared to 22%).[61]

Interrupted versus Continuous Suturing

Personal preference and training have guided the use of either continuous or interrupted suture techniques for esophageal anastomoses. Only one prospective study has been performed comparing the two techniques in a singe-layer anastomosis.[62] This demonstrated one leak and two strictures in patients in whom an interrupted suture technique was used, whereas in the continuous suture group there was no leak or stricture development. In addition, operating time and costs were reduced in the continuous suture group. Good results have been reported by others using this technique.[63]

Stapled Anastomoses

The use of automatic stapling devices to create esophageal anastomoses has been widespread since their introduction during the 1970s. A variety of devices are manufactured and, as a result, there are numerous techniques available for performing anastomoses. Historically, the most common technique has been the use of a circular stapling device to create an end-to-end or end-to-side anastomosis. The 1980s witnessed the development of techniques for creating esophageal anastomoses using linear cutting staplers. These and hybrid techniques using partially stapled, partially sutured anastomoses are gaining increasing acceptance.

Circular Stapling Devices

End-to-side esophagogastric, end-to-side or end-to-end esophagojejunal, and end-to-end esophagocolic anastomoses are all routinely performed with circular staplers. A variety of circular stapling devices, all of which share similar design basics, are available.[64] The sizes and relative advantages of each are outlined in Table 15-3. The head of the circular staplers includes a staple cartridge and a detachable anvil. The cartridge contains two staggered, concentric rows of staples and a circular knife that lies inside the inner row of staples. Approximation of the cartridge against the anvil fires the staples and deploys the knife, which cuts tissue from within the rings of staples. The stapler must reside with the lumen of the esophagus or the reconstructive organ, and the anvil is positioned inside the lumen of the remaining organ. In order for the stapler to reside within the lumen, it may be passed orally, but more commonly it is placed through an incision in the wall of the stomach or an open end of the bowel.

There appear to be substantial differences in the proclivity of staplers to produce anastomotic strictures. The primary explanation for this appears to be the diameter of the stapler used (Table 15-4).[33,35,45,65-67] Small diameters (21 mm, 25 mm) produce strictures at unacceptable rates of 63% and 26%, respectively. Larger diameter staplers produce strictures at rates of about 15%, which are acceptable and compare favorably to stricture rates associated with manual suturing. There are mixed views

Table 15-3.
Characteristics of Circular Stapling Devices.

Name	Manufacturer[1]	Cartridge diameter (mm)	Stoma diameter (mm)	Straight or curved shaft	Disposable (D) or Reusable (R)	Closed staple height	Staple material
EEA	USSC	21, 25, 28, 31	11.4, 15, 18, 21.2	Both	R	2 mm	Stainless steel
Premium Plus CEEA	USSC	21, 25, 28, 31	11.4, 15, 18, 21.1	Both	D	2 mm	Titanium
Proximate ILS	Ethicon	21, 25, 29, 33	12.4, 16.4, 20.4, 24.4	Both	D	1 to 2.5 mm	Titanium

1. USSC - United States Surgical Corporation; Ethicon, Inc.

Table 15-4.
The Incidence of Anastomotic Stricture Associated with the Use of Circular Staplers for Esophageal Anastomoses.

Author	Year	Diameter	Diameter	Diameter	Diameter
		21 mm	25 mm	28 or 29 mm	31 or 33 mm
Wong et al.[33]	1987	—	7/27	7/65	2/18
Berrisford et al.[65]	1996	4/9	13/51	2/30	0/3
Law et al.[45]	1997	—	6/14	14/29	2/7
Dresner et al.[66]	2000	8/10	25/78	19/81	7/37
Petrin et al.[67]	2000	5/8	14/84	4/93	0/2
Totals		17/27 (63%)	65/254 (26%)	46/298 (15%)	11/67 (16%)

on whether staplers of similar diameter but produced by different manufacturers create anastomotic strictures at different rates.

Linear Stapling Devices

Linear staplers used in creating esophageal anastomoses come in two basic types. Linear cutting staplers consist of two assemblies (jaws, or forks) that are aligned in a "V" shape and are approximated, compressing between them the tissue that is to be stapled. A replaceable cartridge in one of the forks contains both staples and a knife blade, while the other fork serves as an anvil. After the assemblies are approximated, a slider is pushed that fires the staples and simultaneously drives a knife blade, which cuts the tissue between the staple lines. Different manufacturers provide variations in the length of the forks and the length of the staples (Table 15-5). Non-cutting linear staplers have two parallel jaws (one containing staplers and the other serving as an anvil) that are approximated, compressing the tissue between them. A handle is then squeezed which fires the staples, and a scalpel is used to trim away excess tissue if desired. Options for linear staplers are summarized in Table 15-5.

Most esophageal anastomoses created with linear stapling devices are anatomical side-to-side but functional end-to-side anastomoses and are variations of the classic anatomic side-to-side and functional end-to-end anastomosis developed for linear staplers in the late 1960s.[68] The typical esophageal anastomosis is created between the esophagus and stomach tube. One jaw of a linear-cutting stapler is placed through a small gastrotomy, and the other jaw is positioned in the open end of the remaining esophagus. Firing the stapler creates a V-shaped opening between the two organs, and serves as the back wall of the anastomosis. The remaining opening is sutured (hybrid anastomotic technique) or is closed with a linear stapler.

Techniques for Performing Anastomoses

Prerequisites for performing an anastomosis include optimal tissue viability, minimal contamination of the operative field, no tension on the tissues being anastomosed, adequate exposure, and the ability to examine the anastomosis for patency and completeness prior to moving to the next phase of the operation. Some authors recommend that tissues being anastomosed to the esophagus (most commonly the stomach) be fixed to the prevertebral fascia to eliminate tension.[69] Catastrophic complications associated with this technique have since resulted in recommendations against routine anchoring of the stomach.[70,71] Although some authors recommend techniques that incorporate a staple line within the anastomo-

Table 15-5.
Characteristics of Linear and Linear Cutting Staplers.

Type	Name	Manufacturer[1]	Jaw length	Disposable (D) or Reusable (R)	Closed staple height	Staple material
Linear cutting	TLC	Ethicon	55, 75, 100 mm	D	1.5, 2 mm	Titanium
	GIA	USSC	60, 80 mm	D	1.5, 2 mm	Titanium
	GIA	USSC	50, 90 mm	R	1.5, 2 mm	Stainless steel
	ILA	3M	75 mm	D	1.5, 2 mm	Titanium
	ILA	3M	100 mm	R	1.5, 2 mm	Stainless steel
Linear	TX	Ethicon	30, 60, 90 mm	D	1.5, 2 mm	Titanium
	TL	Ethicon	30,60,90 mm	D	1.5, 2 mm	Titanium
	TLH[2]	Ethicon	30,60,90 mm	D	1.5, 2 mm	Titanium
	Access[3]	Ethicon	55	D	1.5, 2 mm	Titanium
	TA	USSC	30, 55 mm	D	1.5, 2 mm	Titanium
	Premium TA	USSC	30, 60, 90 mm	D	1.5, 2 mm	Titanium
	Premium TA	USSC	30, 55, 90 mm	R	1.5, 2 mm	Titanium
	PI	USSC	30, 55, 90 mm	D	1.5, 2 mm	Titanium
	PI	USSC	30, 55, 90 mm	R	1.5, 2 mm	Stainless steel
	Roticulator[3]	USSC	30, 55 mm	D	1.5, 2 mm	Titanium

1. Ethicon, Inc.; USSC - United States Surgical Corporation; 3M, Inc.
2. Heavy wire staples
3. These models have the capability of altering the angle of the head of the stapler up to 90°.

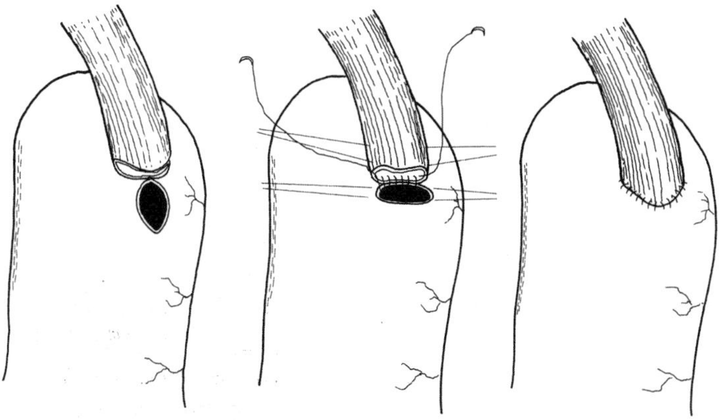

Figure 15-2. Technique for performing a sutured end-to-side esophagogastrostomy.

sis, particularly when performing end-to-end anastomoses between the esophagus and bowel, it is probably best to avoid this practice when possible because of the increased risk of suture line leak. Indeed, when performing esophagogastric anastomoses, the stapled or sutured gastric cardia or lesser curvature is positioned as far from the anastomosis as possible to prevent necrosis of the intervening tissues. In creating an anastomosis, care should be taken to maintain proper alignment of the tissues so that there is no kinking of the newly formed alimentary tract once the anastomosis has been completed. This minimizes the risk of postoperative dysphagia and makes dilation of anastomotic strictures, should they occur, straightforward.

Esophagogastrostomies

End-to-Side Hand Sewn Anastomoses

Two heavy silk stay sutures are placed on either side of the esophagus to help with positioning (Figure 15-2). A small gastrotomy is created near the greater curvature, opposite the closure of the cardia and lesser curvature. Alternatively, a small button of stomach is excised from a similar location. Two stay sutures are placed on either side of the gastrotomy. The back wall of the anastomosis is sutured first, either using a continuous technique or using interrupted sutures in one or two layers. It is sometimes useful to triangulate the anastomosis in order to straighten the tissue layers, thus avoiding narrowing of the anastomosis. Sutures are placed deep into the esophagus and care is taken to include the mucosa for the inner layer of a two-layer closure and for all bites of a single layer

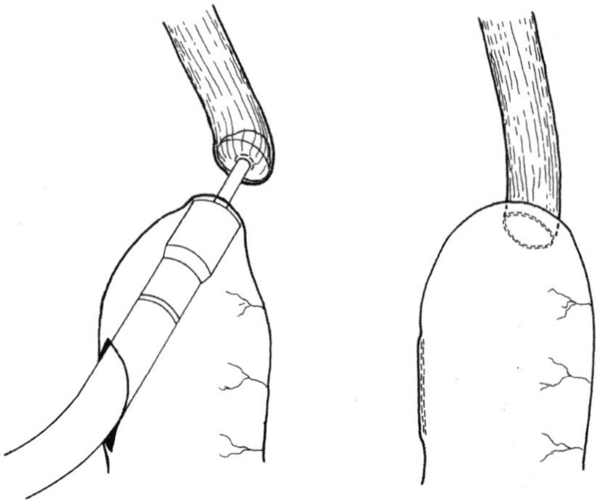

Figure 15-3. Technique for performing an end-to-side esophagagogastrostomy using a circular stapler.

closure to ensure that the submucosa is included. Knots for this portion of the anastomosis are tied on the inside of the lumen. A nasogastric tube is positioned across the anastomosis. The suture line is extended anteriorly, again tying the knots intraluminally. As the final portion of the anastomosis is approached, the inner layer of sutures of a two-layer closure are placed with the knots tied on the outside. The subsequent second layer stitches are placed in a Lembert fashion and are tied on the outside. For single layer closures, the final anterior sutures are placed in a Lembert fashion taking bites deep enough to encompass the submucosal layer.

End-to-Side Stapled Anastomoses

Several techniques are available for performing end-to-side stapled esophagogastrostomies.[72-74] The original technique involves use of the circular stapler for intrathoracic or high intra-abdominal anastomoses (Figure 15-3). A straight or curved circular stapler is introduced through one of several sites: an open pyloromyotomy before closure of a pyloroplasty, a small gastrotomy created for this purpose, or an opening in the lesser curvature of the stomach that exists prior to final closure of the lesser curvature resection.[75] The tapered rod to which the anvil connects is brought through the wall of the stomach at the site of the anastomosis. A purse-string suture is placed around the cut end of the esophagus, taking care to get full thickness bites so as to incorporate the submucosa. Devices for automatic placement of purse-string sutures fail to adequately incorporate the submucosa and result in a high leak rate.[76] The anvil is

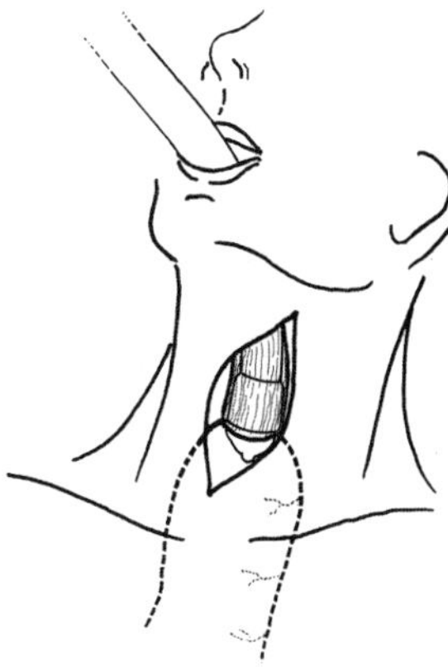

Figure 15-4. An alternative technique for performing a cervical end-to-side esophagogastrostomy using a circular stapler placed transorally.

placed within the esophageal lumen, taking care not to displace the mucosal layer cephalad. This is aided by placing stay sutures in each of four quadrants to permit countertraction on the esophagus. It is often somewhat difficult to get the appropriate sized anvil within the esophagus. In such instances the lumen may be gently dilated with Hegar dilators or a spreading instrument, or glucagon may be administered to cause smooth muscle relaxation.[77] The pursestring suture is tied down and the ends of the suture are cut. The surface of the cartridge is approximated against the anvil and the stapling device is fired. Upon removal of the device, it is important to ensure that a complete ring, or doughnut, of tissue has been excised. If the ring is not complete, the anastomosis should be reinforced with sutures circumferentially. The site used for introduction of the circular stapler is closed with sutures or with a linear stapling device. A nasogastric tube is positioned through the anastomosis and its position is confirmed by palpation. A similar technique has been described for creation of a cervical esophagogastrostomy, but requires amputation of a substantial portion of the gastric fundus after completion of the anastomosis.[78]

As an alternative to the technique described above for use of the circular stapler, the device can also be introduced through the mouth to perform a cervical esophagogastrostomy (Figure 15-4). In this situation, the gastric tube has been pulled into the neck and the esophagus has been transected. A small gastrotomy is created and a pursestring suture is placed around its edges. The stapler is introduced through the patient's mouth. The tapered rod is either brought through a staple line that has been used to close the distal end of the cervical esophagus, or is brought through the open end of the esophagus and a pursestring suture is used to approximate the tissues around the rod. The anvil is connected to the rod and is placed through the gastrotomy, after which the gastric pursestring suture is tied down. The cartridge is approximated against the anvil and the device is fired and then removed. A nasogastric tube is positioned across the anastomosis and its position is confirmed by palpation.

In addition to techniques for creating esophagogastric anastomoses using the circular stapler, there are a variety of techniques for creating end-to-side esophagogastrostomies using linear and linear cutting staplers. These were initially described in the late 1970s and have been popularized recently.[71,79-82] These methods can be used for creating intrathoracic esophagogastrostomies, but the size of the anastomotic lumen is generous, and reflux and regurgitation may occur more often than is the case with more traditional intrathoracic anastomotic techniques. The methods are quite useful for creating cervical esophagogastrostomies, but require a somewhat generous length of gastric tube. The esophagus is transected in the neck, sparing at least 6 to 8 cm below the cricopharyngeus (Figure 15-5). Stay sutures are placed to enable the application of traction. A site on the stomach 5 to 8 cm distal to the tip of the fundus is selected opposite the closure of the lesser curvature or cardia, and stay sutures are placed. A small gastrotomy is created, and the smaller of the two forks of a linear cutting stapler is inserted. After positioning the esophagus anterior to the gastric fundus, the other fork is inserted in the esophagus. The traction sutures are used to align the mucosal margins of the two organs, after which the linear cutting stapler is fired. This creates a "V"-shaped opening between the stomach and esophagus, which serves as the posterior wall of the anastomosis. A nasogastric tube is positioned across the partially completed anastomosis. The remaining edges of stomach and esophagus are closed either with interrupted sutures or with a linear stapler.

An alternative side-to-side technique has been described for creating a cervical esophagogastrostomy.[81] The stomach and cervical esophagus are each brought out of the cervical incision, and their back walls are brought into apposition. A gastrotomy is performed at the apex of the fundus, and the forks of the linear cutting stapler are inserted into the open esophagus and the gastrotomy. Firing the stapler creates a common opening between the two, and the open ends are then closed with a linear stapler. One potential disadvantage of this technique is that tension on the anastomosis will be transmitted to the tip of the staple line created by the linear cutting stapler rather than by having the tension distributed more evenly throughout the anastomosis. In addition, the geometry of the anastomosis does not permit it to lie flat within the neck.

Invaginating and Tunneled Anastomoses

Invaginating anastomoses are most commonly performed as part of an intrathoracic or high intra-abdominal anastomosis.[29] Redundant gastric

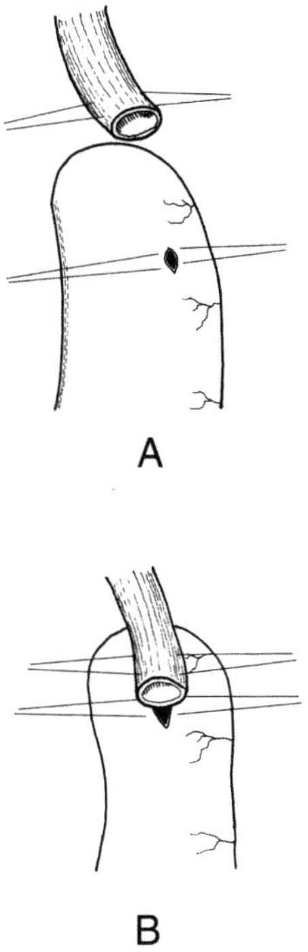

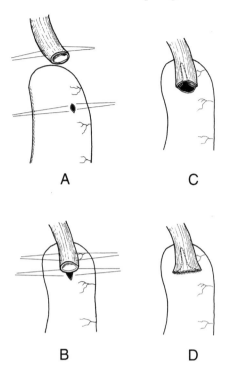

Figure 15-5. Technique for creating a cervical esophagogastrostomy using linear staplers. A: a small gastrotomy is made near the greater curvature of the stomach; B: the stomach is rotated to position the greater curvature more anteriorly, positioning the future anastomosis opposite the lesser curve resection line, and the open end of the esophagus is aligned with the gastrotomy; C: a linear cutting stapler has been fired across the back wall of the esophagus and the front wall of the stomach, creating a large V-shaped common opening which forms the majority of the anastomosis; D: a linear stapler has been fired across the open ends of the esophagus and stomach, closing the anterior portion of the anastomosis.

fundus is required, which is not usually available when performing a cervical esophagogastrostomy. A standard end-to-side esophagogastrostomy is performed using one of the techniques described above. The only difference is that the anastomosis is positioned somewhat more distal on the stomach than would normally be the case. After completing the anastomosis, the redundant gastric fundus proximal and posterior to the anastomosis is wrapped around the anastomosis and distal esophagus, completely enveloping the anastomosis in a type of fundoplication (Figure 15-6). Whether this technique carries with it any antireflux properties is unknown. It provides reinforcement of the anastomosis using well-vascularized tissue, and may reduce the incidence of anastomotic leak. Another similar technique involves separating the gastric mucosa and submucosa from the muscularis. The anastomosis is performed in a stan-

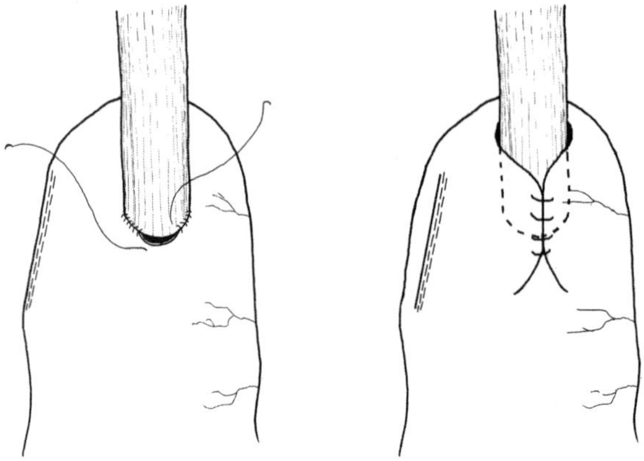

Figure 15-6. Technique for invaginating an anastomosis within a fundic wrap. An end-to-side esophagogastrostomy is performed (left), after which redundant gastric fundus is wrapped around the anastomotic site (right).

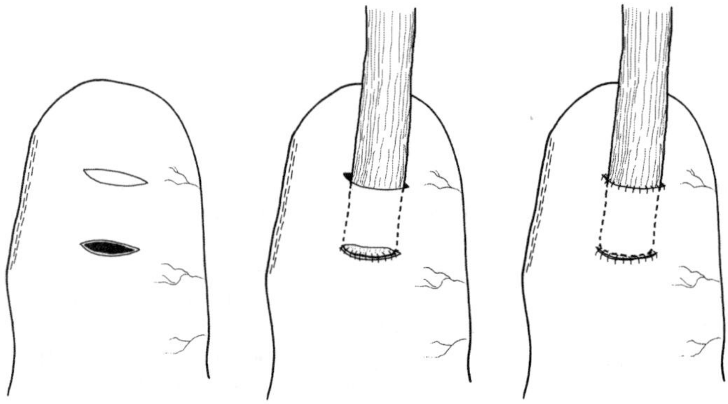

Figure 15-7. Technique for creating a tunneled anastomosis. A submuscular tunnel is created between a seromuscular opening proximally and a gastrotomy distally (left). The esophagus is brought through the tunnel and an end-to-side esophagogastrostomy is performed (right), after which the proximal edge of the tunnel is sutured to the esophagus and the distal edges are reapproximated.

dard fashion between the esophagus and the mucosa/submucosa. The muscularis flap is then sutured circumferentially around the esophagus 3 cm proximal to the anastomosis to reinforce it.[31]

Tunneled esophagogastric anastomoses are performed much less commonly than are other standard anastomoses, and are also relegated primarily to anastomoses performed within the thorax or upper abdomen.[26,30] A site for the anastomosis is selected that is more caudad from the fundic tip than usual (Figure 15-7). A counter incision is performed 3 to 5 cm proximal to this, extending through the muscularis propria but preserving the submucosa and mucosa. A submucosal plane is developed linking the two sites, through which the esophagus is tunneled. A standard end-to-side esophagogastrostomy is performed using a suture technique. The distal edge of the serosa and muscularis propria is then sutured to the gastric serosa, enveloping the anterior margin of the anastomosis. The proximal edges of the tunnel are sutured to the wall of the esophagus, closing the tunnel around it.

Esophageal Anastomoses to Small or Large Bowel

End-to-End Hand Sewn Anastomoses

Among the most easily performed anastomoses are those between the esophagus and the open end of a loop of intestine. The size match is the only potentially challenging factor, and judicious suture placement usually obviates any such concern. The ends of the esophagus and intestine are aligned with the help of stay sutures placed a centimeter or two from the open ends of the organs. Suturing is begun on the posterior wall, tying knots on the inside of the lumen. It sometimes helps to place triangulation stitches to ensure that the maximum anastomotic diameter is achieved. Either a single-layer or a two-layer anastomosis may be performed, although a single-layer anastomosis is preferred. Similarly, continuous or interrupted sutures may be used, depending on the personal preference of the surgeon. As the anastomotic line approaches the center of the anterior wall, a nasoenteral tube is positioned across the anastomosis. The anterior portion is completed with interrupted Lembert sutures.

End-to-End Stapled Anastomoses

It is somewhat unusual to perform end-to-end stapled anastomoses for esophagocolostomies or esophagojejunostomies. These procedures are performed less commonly than are esophagogastrostomies and the orientation of the tissues doesn't always lend itself to stapling. In general, end-to-end stapled anastomoses of esophagus to bowel are performed using circular staplers, although linear stapling techniques are also applicable. For circular stapled anastomoses, the primary issue is how to insert the shaft of the stapler through the bowel. For short segment interpositions, the stapler shaft is inserted through the distal end of the interposition segment (Figure 15-8). For longer interposition segments, which are almost always colonic in this case, the stapler can be inserted through a small colotomy performed through one of the taenia coli. A standard

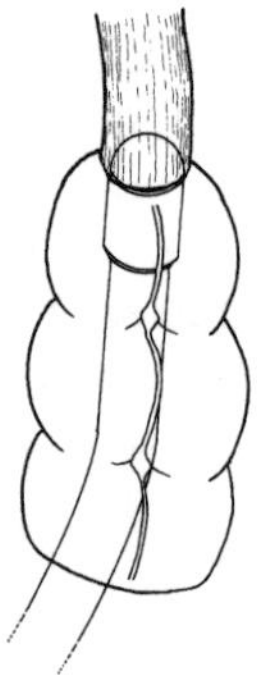

Figure 15-8. Technique for performing a stapled end-to-end esophagocolostomy for a short segment interposition.

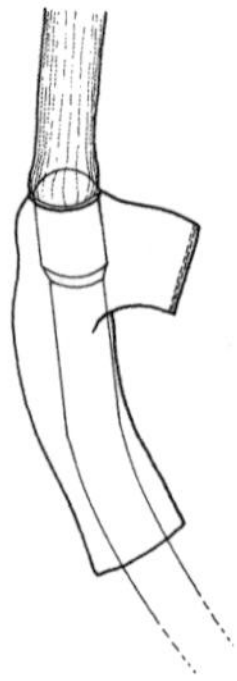

Figure 15-9. Technique for performing a stapled end-to-side esophagojejunostomy.

stapled anastomosis is performed with the aid of a purse-string suture around the open end of each organ.

End-to-Side Anastomoses

Most end-to-side esophago-intestinal anastomoses are performed between the esophagus and the jejunum either using stapling or suturing techniques. Stay sutures are placed through the esophagus and are positioned in the jejunum far enough apart to expose an appropriate length of jejunum to accommodate the anastomosis. For a sutured anastomosis, an appropriate length jejunotomy is performed and a standard anastomosis is accomplished as described above. For a stapled anastomosis, the instrument is introduced either through the distal end of a short segment interposition or through the proximal end of either a short or a long segment interposition (Figure 15-9).[83,84] The tapered rod is brought through the antimesenteric border of the jejunum, and the anvil is positioned within the esophagus after placement of a purse-string suture. The suture is tied down, the head of the stapler and the anvil are approximated, and the stapler is fired. A nasoenteral tube is positioned across the anastomosis either during (suture technique) or after (staple technique) its completion.

Complications

Anastomotic complications are common and are usually due to failures of technique or judgment. Complications that are specifically associated with an anastomosis, such as leak and stricture, will be discussed in this chapter. Complications that arise subsequently and which may be more generalized are discussed in Chapter 17.

Anastomotic Leak

Anastomotic leaks pose special challenges both in their diagnosis and their treatment. Leaks are classified according to site (cervical, thoracic, abdominal), clinical impact (symptomatic or asymptomatic [sometimes referred to as subclinical]), pathophysiology (minor suture line insufficiency, major suture line insufficiency, dehiscence, partial necrosis), and extent (contained or not contained). The overall incidence of leaks in randomized studies is summarized in Table 15-1, and ranges from 3% to 7%. A more realistic portrayal of the incidence of leaks in actual clinical practice can be gleaned from surveys of publications encompassing large numbers of patients. Such surveys suggest that the average anastomotic leak rate is between 7% and 12%, and that the incidence of leak is sometimes as high as 30%.[58,85] Anastomotic leaks are associated with an increase in operative mortality from a baseline rate of 7% to nearly 20%.

Pathophysiology

Factors leading to anastomotic leak are detailed earlier in this chapter and are discussed in prior chapters dealing with specific reconstructive organs and techniques. The primary factors leading to leakage are technical misadventures and the use of higher risk anastomotic techniques. Cervical anastomotic leaks are more common than are leaks from intrathoracic anastomoses due to increased anastomotic tension and poorer blood supply associated with cervical anastomoses. Multivariable analyses have demonstrated a number of other factors to be potentially related to an increased risk of anastomotic leak (Table 15-6). These include malnutrition, diabetes, operation for bypass rather than resection, excessive intraoperative blood loss, use of the colon as the reconstructive organ, delayed gastric emptying, and radical dissection.[37,86-91] Although one review suggests that tumor infiltration of the esophageal margin of resection is a risk factor for anastomotic leakage, others state that this is not an important factor increasing the risk of leakage.[88,92,93] An excellent overview of esophageal anastomotic leaks summarizes other factors commonly

Table 15-6.
Factors which may predispose to Anastomotic Leak.

Systemic factors:
Albumin concentration <3 gm/dL*
Diabetes mellitus
Hypotension
Hypoxia
Technical factors:
Retrosternal or subcutaneous rather than posterior mediastinal route for reconstruction
Use of colon rather than stomach for reconstruction
End-to-end rather than end-to-side stapled anastomosis
Cervical rather than intrathoracic anastomosis
Excess tension
Other factors:
Operation for bypass rather than resection
Esophageal margin involved by cancer*
Excess intraoperative blood loss
Delayed gastric emptying
Extended lymph node dissection
Extrinsic compression
Local contamination/infection

* Different studies report that these factors either are or are not associated with an increase in the incidence of anastomotic leak.

thought to be involved in the etiology of leaks which are listed in Table 15-6.[94]

Esophageal anastomotic leaks pose serious risks to patients. Cervical leaks, although they are usually contained and remain local problems, can dissect into the mediastinum, the retropharyngeal space, or into surrounding vital structures including the carotid artery or trachea. Mediastinal leaks have higher risks of dissection and erosion. The risks of intrathoracic leaks also are increased because of the exposure to negative intrathoracic pressure, which promotes rapid involvement of the mediastinum and the pleural spaces. Such widespread infection is accompanied by sepsis and multiple organ failure. Leaks from esophagogastrostomies are usually more serious than those from esophageal anastomoses to other organs. Gastric juices, which are acidic and contain powerful digestive enzymes, promote autodigestion of surrounding tissues and result in fulminant necrosis of surrounding tissues.

Prevention

It has been the goal of some investigators to prevent leaks. Use of a free peritoneal patch to wrap a cervical esophageal anastomosis does not influence the incidence of anastomotic leak but does increase the likelihood of an anastomotic stricture developing postoperatively.[95] The use of fibrin glue to reinforce an anastomosis has been shown experimentally to substantially reduce the incidence of anastomotic leak.[96] The clinical application of this technique results in a somewhat decreased rate of anastomotic leak, but not to a point that is statistically significant.[97] Use of topical antibacterials to effect local decontamination the at the time an anastomosis is performed results in a significant reduction in the incidence of both anastomotic leak and operative mortality after stapled esophagojejunostomy.[98]

Diagnosis

The diagnosis of anastomotic leak is sometimes not in doubt. In patients in whom a cervical anastomosis is performed, swelling of the cervical incision or leakage of saliva through the cervical incision or through a drain placed at the time of surgery makes the presence of an anastomotic leak obvious. Some patients with intrathoracic anastomoses will develop a septic picture and be found to have foul chest tube drainage containing a high level of amylase. In many other patients, however, a confusing postoperative clinical course may develop for which anastomotic leak is one of many potential explanations. In such situations, an aggressive evaluation of the patient is appropriate to rule out an anastomotic leak.

Clinical symptoms and signs of leak include acidosis, tachycardia, supraventricular arrhythmia (possibly due to inflammation of the pericardium), odynophagia, leukocytosis, confusion, hyperglycemia, and fever. When a suspicion of leak develops as a result of such clinical findings, further investigation is warranted. The manner in which the investigation proceeds is dependent on the condition of the patient and the site of the anastomosis. A plain chest film is routinely performed to look for subcutaneous or mediastinal air, pneumothorax, and pleural effusion. In patients suspected of having a cervical anastomotic leak who are not stable enough to undergo a contrast study, the most expedient step is to open the cervical incision and explore the depths of the wound at the bedside under local anesthesia possibly combined with mild sedation. The wound is drained and packed regardless of whether a leak is identified. This maneuver is often both diagnostic and therapeutic. Flexible endoscopy may also be of diagnostic benefit in such patients. This technique permits identification of partial necrosis of the reconstructive organ, and anastomotic dehiscence. Some small leaks may also be identified on the basis of air extravasation into the surrounding tissues during endoscopic air insufflation.

In patients who are otherwise stable and are able to tolerate transport to the radiology department, a contrast swallow is sometimes useful as an initial test. This is most often the case for patients who are at least several days out from surgery and are being cared for on a regular hospital ward. The choice of contrast material is important and is a matter of some controversy. Water-soluble agents (gastrografin) have a relatively low overall accuracy in the diagnosis of anastomotic leak.[99,100] In addition, aspiration of such material, which often occurs in patient who have recently undergone a cervical esophageal anastomosis and have impaired swallowing function, can cause a severe pneumonitis. Use of barium sulfate in patients in whom an initial swallow with water soluble contrast material is unrevealing, particularly when a leak is suspected, results in a substantially increased rate of detection of leaks.[101] Barium sulfate, either full-strength or diluted with water, also is appropriate for initial investigation of suspected leak unless there is a concern that leakage is extending into the peritoneal space. Barium sulfate is benign in the tracheobronchial tree and does not contribute to the severity of sepsis if it accumulates in the mediastinal or pleural spaces as a result of an anastomotic leak.

It is sometimes useful to perform a standard chest radiograph after a barium swallow has been completed. If no leak is identified on the swallow study, the follow-up chest radiograph may demonstrate retained barium at a previously unsuspected site, which is evidence for a leak. When a leak is identified on the barium contrast study, a follow-up chest radiograph provides information as to how completely the leak drains back into the esophagus, or, conversely, helps to indicate how poorly drained any resultant collection is.

In patients who have undergone routine placement of a neck drain after a cervical anastomosis, a swallow of methylene blue will sometimes be diagnostic of a leak if the dye comes out the drain shortly after a single swallow. With increasing time after the swallow, however, there is general staining of tissues due to absorption of the dye, which may lead to confusion about the outcome of the test.

Computed tomography (CT) is often useful to evaluate patients who are symptomatic and are suspected of having an anastomotic leak. Such a scan may reveal air in the surrounding tissues, air-fluid levels, or fluid collections that are not suspected on the basis of clinical examination or other radiographic studies (Figure 15-10). Administration of intraluminal and intravenous contrast optimizes the accuracy of such studies but may not be tolerated by all individuals. Use of a nasogastric tube to administer contrast to patients suspected of having an intrathoracic leak is necessary if they are unable to take anything by mouth. However, it is particularly difficult to effectively administer intraluminal contrast to an ill patient who is suspected of having a cervical anastomotic leak.

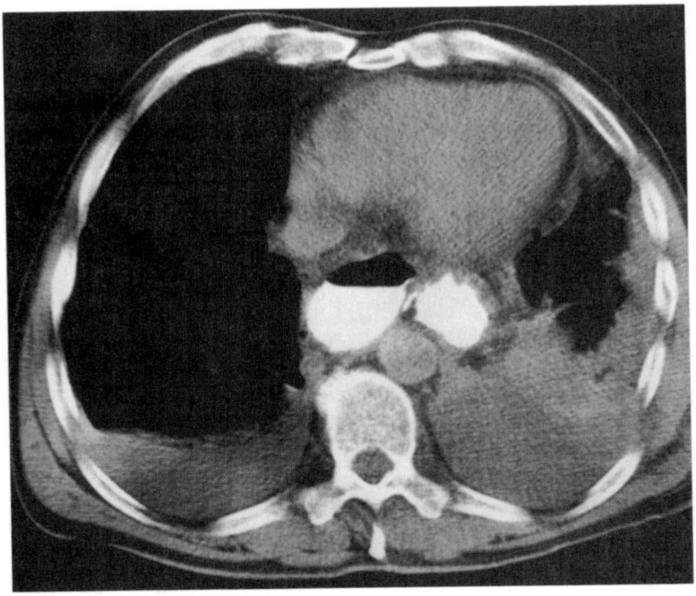

Figure 15-10. Computed tomographic scan demonstrating signs of an anastomotic leak.

Management

Patients who exhibit systemic signs of esophageal anastomotic leak require broad-spectrum antibiotic therapy and fluid resuscitation. It is difficult to predict the response of an individual patient to a leak. Fulminant changes in a patient's clinical course may occur. If there are signs suggestive of important systemic effects of leakage, such as respiratory insufficiency, low urine output, or hypotension, then management in a step-down or intensive care unit is appropriate. In patients in whom early institution of oral nutrition is unlikely, some method of providing nutrition must be identified early in their course. Most patients do best with enteral feedings through a jejunostomy tube since the stomach is usually not available or is inappropriate for feedings. In most instances, the stomach should be drained to minimize reflux of gastric contents through an anastomotic leak.

In patients in whom symptoms of sepsis are present, it is appropriate to administer systemic antibiotics to cover oral flora. In longstanding leaks the presence of candida species is often noted, and repeat culture of patients who do not appropriately respond to therapy should be directed towards fungi as well as a wide variety of bacteria.

Drainage is the mainstay of therapy for esophageal anastomotic leaks. Drains placed routinely at the time of esophageal reconstruction cannot

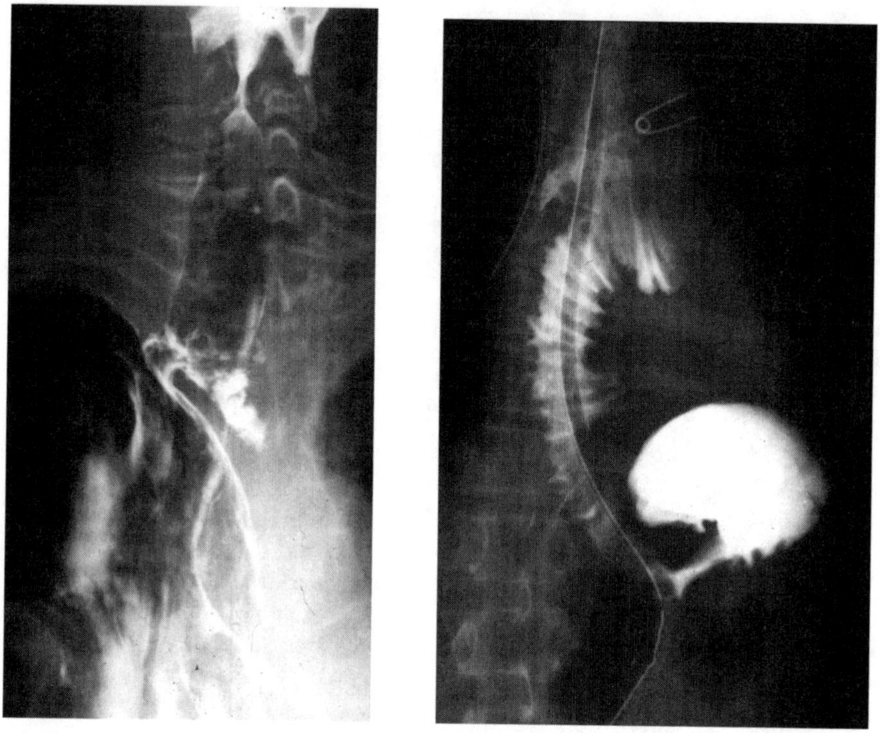

Figure 15-11. Contained anastomotic leaks from a cervical esophagogastrostomy (left) and an intrathoracic esophagojejunostomy (right).

be relied upon to provide adequate evacuation of a leak. Anastomotic leaks typically don't develop within the first 48 hours after surgery, during which time drainage tubes are often walled-off by inflammatory processes that are a natural response to surgery. Because of the proximity of cervical drains to a leak, there is a good likelihood that such a drain will facilitate evacuation of extravasated material. Thoracostomy tubes routinely placed after a thoracotomy with an intrathoracic anastomosis are usually not positioned near the anastomosis, and frequently do not evacuate extravasated material even when a large collection of such material develops postoperatively. Routine placement of additional drains adjacent to the anastomosis may reduce morbidity associated with a leak.[102]

Contained anastomotic leaks are defined as leaks in which contrast material extravasates outside of the alimentary tract lumen to a limited extent and gathers in a well-defined collection adjacent to the anastomosis (Figure 15-11). Patients with contained leaks are, by definition, relatively asymptomatic, a necessary condition for the conservative management that is usually recommended. Very small, contained cervical anastomotic leaks can be observed with the patient on a clear liquid diet for a few more days than is usually the case. Larger contained cervical anastomotic leaks are usually managed adequately with opening of the cervical incision, irrigation of the wound, possible placement of a drain, and wound packing. If small volumes of saliva drain through the wound, a clear liquid diet is begun. If larger volumes of drainage occur, a stoma bag is fitted over the neck wound for ease of wound care and alternative methods of providing nutrition are pursued. A repeat contrast swallow in 5 to 7 days will help define the progress of healing.

Some authors recommend early dilation for patients with contained cervical anastomotic leaks.[103-105] Theoretically, edema and the development of granulation tissue at the site of leakage contribute to maintenance of the fistula. Early dilation is believed to decrease the degree of obstruction and promote more rapid closure of the leak. Dilation may be performed with bougies passed over a guidewire or with fluoroscopically guided balloon dilators. Whether early dilation lessons the risk of anastomotic stricture is not known.

Contained leaks associated with intrathoracic anastomoses are more difficult to drain. If they are small and empty readily back into the alimentary tract, observation is all that is necessary. In other cases, internal drainage can be accomplished by endoscopic placement of a nasogastric tube (sump drain) through the anastomotic defect into the abscess cavity.[106-109] The drain is maintained on suction and may be irrigated intermittently. Contrast studies are performed at intervals to monitor the size of the abscess cavity, and the drain is gradually withdrawn as the size of the cavity decreases. This technique is relatively noninvasive and helps avoid the major pleural contamination that necessarily accompanies transthoracic drainage of infected mediastinal collections.

Leaks that are large, are not contained, or are associated with systemic changes suggestive of sepsis require more aggressive therapy (Figure 15-12). They pose a serious threat to patients due to the likelihood of developing multisystem organ failure and local problems such as erosion into vital structures. Noncontained cervical leaks are best explored with the patient under a general anesthetic. A thorough examination of the contaminated space is performed, and the region is copiously irrigated. A suction drain is placed. Use of a passive drain is usually not sufficient because the negative intramediastinal pressure will prevent evacuation through such a system. For leaks that are small or moderate in size, repair can be attempted, after which reinforcement with local tissues such as strap muscles is appropriate. Larger leaks occasionally may be patched with a local flap.[110] A leak of small or moderate size will evolve to a controlled fistula and spontaneously close within a few weeks if appropriately drained.[111]

Larger cervical anastomotic leaks that are due to substantial suture line disruption or gastric tip necrosis require more aggressive interven-

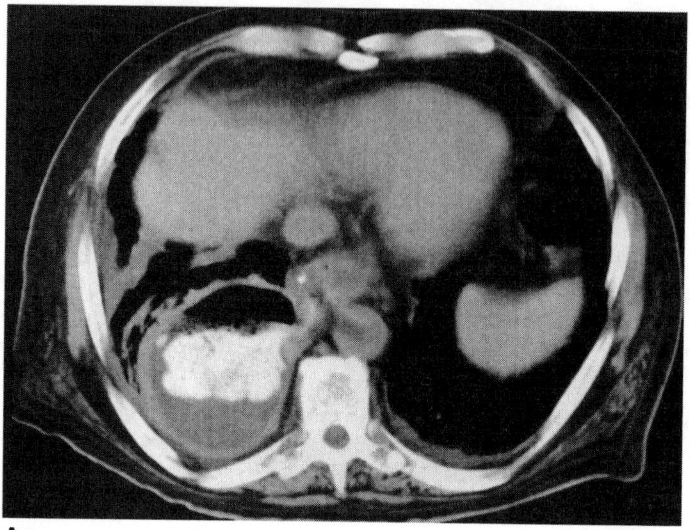

A

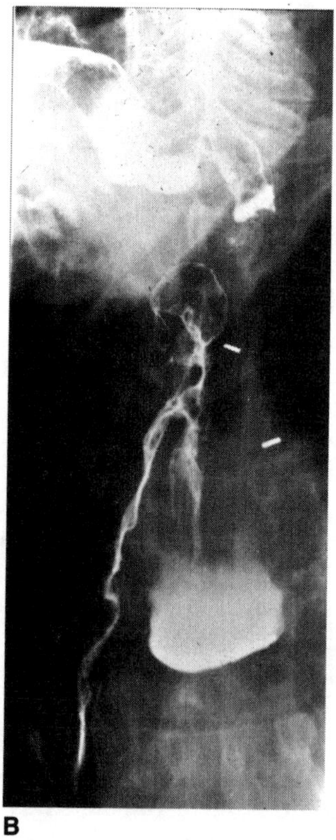

B

Figure 15-12. Large, noncontained anastomotic leaks from a cervical (**A**) and an intrathoracic (**B**) esophagogastrostomy.

tion. Simple repair and reinforcement is not sufficient. Instead, a salivary fistula is created by bringing the end of the esophagus to the cervical skin. The reconstructive organ, if viable and of sufficient length, can be closed and sutured to the muscular wall of the esophagus or to the sternocleidomastoid muscle to help maintain its position in the neck. After the patient has recovered and the region has healed, it is then a simple matter to free the end of the esophagus, locate the apex of the reconstructive organ, and create a new anastomosis. If the reconstructive organ is not viable or of sufficient length, it must be taken down and either returned to the abdomen or discarded, and a salivary fistula is established. A subsequent staged reconstruction is performed when all signs of sepsis have resolved and the patient is clinically well.

Noncontained intrathoracic leaks that contaminate the mediastinum or pleural spaces pose the biggest risk to patients and offer the greatest challenge to surgeons. Establishment of a controlled fistula may be possible with accurate placement of a thoracostomy tube or other percutaneous drain, but preferential drainage through the tube must be documented radiographically. When there is greater soilage of the mediastinum or pleural spaces, formal thoracotomy for evacuation of infected material, decortication, placement of drains, and reinforced closure of the anastomotic defect is necessary. Some surgeons prefer to place a "T"-tube to aid in establishing a controlled fistula. Bilateral pleural space involvement frequently occurs, and computed tomography is useful in defining the extent of the problem and in selecting appropriate drainage techniques for the contralateral pleural space.

Some intrathoracic leaks are the result of substantial disruption of a suture line due to necrosis of the reconstructive organ or major technical problems that occurred during the operation. In such instances spontaneous healing cannot be expected, and the reconstructive organ must be repaired for use at a subsequent time, returned to the abdomen, or discarded. It is appropriate in such cases to exteriorize the esophagus on the chest wall, preserving as much esophageal length as possible to help in future reconstruction.[112] This also makes it simpler to apply a stoma appliance than if the esophagus was brought out on the neck. Excluding the reconstructive organ may make it tempting to avoid thoracotomy altogether, but this puts the patient at risk for chronic empyema if the mediastinum and pleural spaces are not adequately decorticated. In addition, leaving a reconstructive organ midway in the posterior mediastinal space may not offer much advantage for subsequent reconstruction. It is difficult to bridge the gap between the exteriorized esophagus and the intrathoracic reconstructive organ because access to the reconstructive organ is difficult as a result of prior thoracotomies and inflammation resulting from the intrathoracic leak. Bridging the gap with a free segment of jejunum may be possible, but a subsequent reconstruction through another route is more expeditious.

Anastomotic stricture

Anastomotic strictures are classified as benign (due to scarring from leak or other inflammatory causes or due to surgical technique) or malignant (owing to local recurrence or persistence of tumor). Benign strictures typically become symptomatic early in the postoperative period, usually within 6 months and on average within 2 or 3 months of the operation.[66,113-115] Such strictures are usually a result of anastomotic leak with resultant scarring or a technical misadventure. Benign strictures may also occur late, many months or years after successful surgery. In such cases the cause is most likely chronic inflammation resulting from reflux across the anastomosis. Malignant strictures are usually identified many months or years after the operation. Distinguishing between the two etiologies is important in their management. Although a contrast esophagram may provide some useful information regarding this, endoscopy with brushings and biopsy is usually necessary to make a definitive distinction between the two causes. In this chapter only benign anastomotic strictures will be discussed.

Incidence and Etiology

The overall incidence of benign anastomotic stricture ranges from nearly 15% to 20% in randomized and nonrandomized studies which compare suture to staple techniques (Table 15-1).[32,36-47] The incidence among other publications is somewhat higher, ranging from 0% to more than 40% and averaging 25% among selected reports (Table 15-7).[38,66,67,90,113-115] As outlined previously, anastomotic strictures are often a consequence of an anastomotic leak. Up to 25% of strictures are preceded by a known leak, and it is possible that a substantial additional percentage of patients who develop strictures suffer a subclinical leak. The specific additional factors that contribute to the development of anastomotic stricture are not well understood, but likely include acid or alkaline reflux, technical errors in performing the anastomosis, use of small diameter circular staplers, a previous history of cardiac disease, the degree of intraoperative blood loss, and relative ischemia of the reconstructive organ as assessed intraoperatively.[87,113,114,116,117]

Table 15-7.
The Incidence of Benign Anastomotic Stricture after Esophagectomy and Reconstruction.

Author	Year	Patients	Anastomotic technique	Benign strictures
McManus et al.[38]	1990	221	Sutured or stapled	15
Dewar et al.[87]	1992	165	Sutured	50
Pierie et al.[113]	1993	81	Sutured	24
Siersma et al.[114]	1996	269	Sutured or stapled	114
Bruns et al.[90]	1997	173	Sutured	63
Heitmiller et al.[115]	1999	101	Sutured	26
Dresner et al.[66]	2000	222	Stapled	59
Petrin et al.[67]	2000	187	Stapled	23
Totals		1419		353 (24.9%)

Diagnosis

Clinical signs and symptoms of anastomotic stricture include dysphagia, regurgitation of undigested food, regurgitation of thick, tenacious mucus, and odynophagia. An anastomotic stricture may lead to proximal dilatation and a palpable, ballottable mass in the neck. The differential diagnosis of such symptoms includes slow emptying of a reconstructive organ and an anastomotic deformity affecting the anastomosis or the reconstructive organ. A contrast esophagram helps determine whether a stricture is present, delineates the anatomy of the reconstructive organ, and gives information about emptying of the reconstructive organ. Endoscopy is used to assess the etiology of a stricture and differentiates between a benign cause and recurrent cancer. It is rare that any other assessment of a stricture is necessary prior to embarking on therapy.

Management

Dilation is the only management necessary for most esophageal anastomotic strictures. Dilation may be performed blindly with Maloney-type bougies, but narrow, angulated, or very fresh strictures are more safely managed with wire-guided dilation using either Savary-type bougies or balloon dilators. Strictures that are complicated by residual sinus tracts or by severe angulation require fluoroscopic guidance of a guidewire, sometimes with endoscopic assistance, to ensure safe passage through the strictured region. Most patients are successfully managed with two to four episodes of dilation. When multiple dilations are necessary, the interval between episodes typically lengthens until no further intervention is necessary. The mean time to stricture resolution in patients who require more than a single episode of dilation is 2 to 3 months.[66] What constitutes successful dilation therapy is not well defined. In some reports, patients required dilation up to 17 times over periods ranging up to several years.[66,117,118] The overall success rate of dilation exceeds 80% in most series[43,113,117,119] but in some reports varies according to the etiology of the anastomotic stricture. Strictures which develop without an antecedent anastomotic leak resolve with dilation over 90% of the time, while dilation is successful for strictures associated with an anastomotic leak less than 60% of the time.[120]

Other Complications

A wide variety of other anastomotic complications have been described. They include vertebral body osteomyelitis, epidural abscess, internal jugular vein abscess with septic thromboemboli to the lungs resulting in pulmonary microabscesses, and fistulization between the anastomosis and the trachea.[70] Fortunately, these occur rarely. It is likely that expeditious intervention for suspected leak in such situations may minimize the risk of development of such catastrophic problems.

References

1. Bardini R, Asolati M, Ruol A, et al. Anastomosis. *World J Surg* 1994;18:373-378.
2. Pierie J-P EN, de Graaf PW, van Vroonhoven TJMV, et al. Healing of the cervical esophagogastrostomy. *J Am Coll Surg* 1999;188:448-454.
3. Miller RT Jr, WDW Andrus. Experimental surgery of the thoracic oesophagus. *Bull Johns Hopkins Hosp* 1923;34:109-114.
4. Gollighter JC. Visceral and parietal suture in abdominal surgery. *Am J Surg* 1976;131:130-140.
5. Tera H, Aberg C. Tissue holding power to a single suture in different parts of the alimentary tract. *Acta Chir Scand* 1976;142:343-348.
6. Dallman MJ. Functional suture-holding layer of the esophagus in the dog. *J Am Vet Med Assoc* 1988;192:638-640.
7. Ballantyne GH. Intestinal suturing. Review of the experimental foundations for traditional doctrines. *Dis Colon Rectum* 1983;26:836-843.
8. Postlethwait RW, Weinberg M, Jenkins LB, et al. Mechanical strength of esophageal anastomoses. *Ann Surg* 1951;133:472-476.
9. Levi A, Ramadan E, Gelber E, et al. Healing of the esophageal suture line: Does it differ from the rest of the alimentary tract? *Isr J Med Sci* 1996;32:1313-1316.
10. Cui Y, Urschel JD. Esophagogastric anastomotic wound healing in rats. *Dis Esoph* 1999;12:149-151.
11. Csikos M, Karacsony G, Petri I, et al. Mechanical capacity of esophagogastric anastomosis at early postoperative stage. *Acta Chir Hung* 1983;24:105-114.

12. Hogstrom H, Haglund U. Postoperative decrease in suture holding capacity in laparotomy wounds and anastomoses. *Acta Chir Scand* 1985;151:533-535.
13. Brasken P. Healing of experimental colon anastomosis. *Eur J Surg Suppl* 1991;566:1-51.
14. Hesp FL, Hendriks T, Lubbers EJ, et al. Wound healing in the intestinal wall. A comparison between experimental ileal and colonic anastomoses. *Dis Colon Rectum* 1984;27:99-104.
15. Thornton FJ, Barbul A. Healing in the gastrointestinal tract. *Surg Clin N Am* 1997;77:549-573.
16. van der Stappen JW, Hendriks T, de Boer HH, et al. Collagenolytic activity in experimental intestinal anastomoses. Differences between small and large bowel and evidence for the presence of collagenase. *Int J Colorectal Dis* 1992;7:95-101.
17. Hendriks T, Mastboom WJ. Healing of experimental intestinal anastomoses. Parameters for repair. *Dis Colon Rectum* 1990;33:891-901.
18. Blomquist P, Jiborn H, Zederfeldt B. The effect of relative bowel rest on healing of colonic anastomoses. Breaking strength and collagen content in the colonic wall following left colon resection and anastomosis in the rat. *Acta Chir Scand* 1984;150:671-675.
19. Christensen H, Langfelt S, Laurberg S. Bursting strength of experimental colonic anastomoses. A methodological study. *Eur Surg Res* 1993;25:38-45.
20. Jonsson K, Jiborn H, Zederfeldt B. Changes in collagen content of the small intestinal wall after anastomosis. *Am J Surg* 1985;150:315-317.
21. Jonsson K, Jiborn H, Zederfeldt B. Healing of ileocolic anastomoses. Breaking strength and collagen content in the intestinal wall after ileocolic resection and anastomosis in the rat. *Acta Chir Scand* 1985;151:629-633.
22. Livaditis A, Okmian L, Bjorck G, et al. Esophageal suture anastomosis. *Scand J Thorac Cardiovasc Surg* 1969;3:163-173.
23. Scheele J, Klupfel P, Pesch HJ, et al. Vergleichende morphologische Untersuchungen verschiedener Anastomosentechniken bei transthorakalen Oesophagogastrostomien am Hand. *Langenbecks Arch Chir* 1978;344:239-253.
24. Chassin JL. Esophagogastrectomy: Data favoring end-to-side anastomosis. *Ann Surg* 1978;188:22-27.
25. Pierie J-P EN, de Graaf PW, Poen H, et al. End-to-side and end-to-end anastomoses give similar results in cervical oesophagogastrostomy. *Eur J Surg* 1995;161:893-896.
26. Liu K, Zhang GC, Cai ZJ. Avoiding anastomotic leakage following esophagogastrostomy. *J Thorac Cardiovasc Surg* 1983;86:142-145.
27. Noirclerc M, Sastre B, Barthelemy A, et al. Anastomose oeso-gastrique continente intrathoracique. *Presse Med* 1983;12:2943-2945.
28. Maier WP, Lauby VW, Au FC, et al. Esophagogastric anastomosis. *Surg Gynecol Obstet* 1987;164:170-172.
29. Zhi H-X, Ma J-S, Wang S-Y, et al. Intussusception anastomosis of the esophagus: A new method of anastomosis after resection of esophageal or cardiac carcinoma. *J Surg Oncol* 1989;42:161-164.
30. Liu K, Zhang KC, Fan D, et al. Assessment of "Tunnel" esophagogastrostomy based on laboratory findings, clinical analysis and 24-hours esophageal pH monitoring. *Dis Esoph* 1991;4:111-117.

31. Cheng CS, Zhang MK, Zhang JL, et al. Oesophagogastric intramural implantation anastomosis after oesophagectomy. *Br J Surg* 1992;79:1325-1326.

32. Hopkins RA, Alexander JC, Postlethwait RW. Stapled esophagogastric anastomosis. *Am J Surg* 1984;147:283-287.

33. Wong J, Cheung H, Lui R, et al. Esophagogastric anastomosis performed with a stapler: The occurrence of leakage and stricture. *Surgery* 1987;101:408-415.

34. Peracchia A, Bardini R, Asolati M, et al. Mechanical sutures in esophageal surgery. In Siewert JR, Holscher AH (eds): **Diseases of the Esophagus**. Berlin, Springer-Verlag, 1988, pp 474-476.

35. Muehrcke DD, Kaplan DK, Donnelly RJ. Anastomotic narrowing after esophagogastrectomy with the EEA stapling device. *J Thorac Cardiovasc Surg* 1989;97:434-438.

36. Giuli R, Sancho-Garnier H. Diagnostic, therapeutic, and prognostic factors of cancers of the esophagus: Results of the international prospective study conducted by the OESO group (790 patients). *Surgery* 1986;99:614-622.

37. Peracchia A, Bardini R, Ruol A, et al. Esophagovisceral anastomotic leak. A prospective statistical study of predisposing factors. *J Thorac Cardiovasc Surg* 1988;95:685-691.

38. McManus KG, Ritchie AJ, McGuigan J, et al. Sutures, staplers, leaks and strictures. A review of anastomoses in oesophageal resection at Royal Victoria Hospital, Belfast 1977-1986. *Eur J Cardio-Thorac Surg* 1990;4:97-100.

39. Fok M, Ah-Chong AK, Cheng SWK, et al. Comparison of a single layer continuous hand-sewn method and circular stapling in 580 oesophageal anastomoses. *Br J Surg* 1991;78:342-345.

40. Fujimoto S, Takahashi M, Endoh F, et al. Stapled or manual suturing in esophagojejunostomy after total gastrectomy: A comparison of outcome in 379 patients. *Am J Surg* 1991;162:256-259.

41. West of Scotland and Highland Anastomosis Study Group. Suturing or stapling in gastrointestinal surgery: A prospective randomized study. *Br J Surg* 1991;78:337-341.

42. Craig SR, Walker WS, Cameron EW, et al. A prospective randomized study comparing stapled with handsewn oesophagogastric anastomoses. *J R Coll Surg Edinb* 1996;41:17-19.

43. Honkoop P, Siersema PD, Tilanus HW, et al. Benign anastomotic strictures after transhiatal esophagectomy and cervical esophagogastrostomy: Risk factors and management. *J Thorac Cardiovasc Surg* 1996;111:1141-1148.

44. Valverde A, Hay JM, Fingerhut A, et al. Manual versus mechanical esophagogastric anastomosis after resection for carcinoma: A controlled trial. French Associations for Surgical Research. *Surgery* 1996;120:476-483.

45. Law S, Fok M, Chu K-M, et al. Comparison of hand-sewn and stapled esophagogastric anastomosis after esophageal resection for cancer. *Ann Surg* 1997;226:169-173.

46. Laterza E, de' Manzoni G, Veraldi GF, et al. Manual compared with mechanical cervical oesophagogastric anastomosis: A randomized trial. *Eur J Surg* 1999;165:1051-1054.

47. Takeyoshi I, Ohwada S, Ogawa T, et al. Esophageal anastomosis following gastrectomy for gastric cancer: Comparison of hand-sewn and stapling techniques. *Hepatogastroenterology* 2000;47:1026-1029.

48. Walther BS, Oscarson JE, Graffner HO, et al. Esophagojejunostomy with the EEA stapler. *Surgery* 1986;99:598-603.
49. Smirniotis V, Morritt GG. EEA stapler in oesophagogastrectomies. *Int Surg* 1990;75:36-38.
50. Adams RD, Allen KB, Millikan K, et al. Transhiatal stapled esophagojejunostomy without a pursestring suture in patients with previous gastric resection. *Ann Thorac Surg* 1994;58:254-256.
51. Postlethwait RW, Deaton WR Jr, Bradshaw HH, et al. Esophageal anastomosis: Types and methods of suture. *Surgery* 1950;28:537-542.
52. Orringer MB, Appleman HD, Argenta L, et al. Polypropylene suture in esophageal and gastrointestinal operations. *Surg Gynecol Obstet* 1977;144:67-70.
53. Senyk J, Rank F. Oesophageal tissue reaction to different suture materials. An experimental study in the cat. *Scand J Thorac Cardiovasc Surg* 1978;12:265-273.
54. Bourne RB, Bitar H, Andreae PR, et al. In-vivo comparison of four absorbable sutures: Vicryl, Dexon Plus, Maxon and PDS. *Can J Surg* 1988;31:43-45.
55. Greenwald D, Shumway S, Albear P, et al. Mechanical comparison of 10 suture materials before and after *in vivo* incubation. *J Surg Res* 1994;56:372-377.
56. Rodeheaver GT, Powell TA, Thacker JG, et al. Mechanical performance of monofilament synthetic absorbable sutures. *Am J Surg* 1987;154:544-547.
57. Knoop M, Lunstedt B, Thiede A. Maxon und PDS - Bewertung physikalischer und biologischer Eigenschaften monofiler, absorbierbarer Nahtmaterialien. *Langenbecks Arch Chir* 1987;371:13-28.
58. Muller JM, Erasmi H, Stelzner M, et al. Surgical therapy of oesophageal carcinoma. *Br J Surg* 1990;77:845-857.
59. Mathisen DJ, Grillo HC, Wilkins EW, et al. Transthoracic esophagctomy: A safe approach to carcinoma of the esophagus. *Ann Thorac Surg* 1988;45:137-143.
60. Richelme H, Baulieux J. **Le Traitement des Cancers de l'Oesophage**. Paris, Masson, 1986.
61. Zieren HU, Muller JM, Pichlmaier H. Prospective randomized study of one- or two-layer anastomosis following oesophageal resection and cervical oesophagogastrostomy. *Br J Surg* 1993;80:608-611.
62. Bardini R, Bonavina L, Asolati M, et al. Single-layered cervical esophageal anastomoses: A prospective study of two suturing techniques. *Ann Thorac Surg* 1994;58:1087-1090.
63. Fok M, Wong J. Cancer of the oesophagus and gastric cardia. Standard oesophagectomy and anastomotic technique. *Ann Chir Gynaecol* 1995;84:179-183.
64. McGuire J, Wright IC, Leverment JN. Surgical staplers: A review. *J R Coll Surg Edinb* 1997;42:1-9.
65. Berrisford RG, Page RD, Donnelly RJ. Stapler design and strictures at the esophagastric anastomosis. *J Thorac Cardiovasc Surg* 1996;111:142-146.
66. Dresner SM, Lamb PJ, Wayman J, et al. Benign anastomotic stricture following transthoracic oesophagectomy and stapled oesophago-gastrostomy: Risk factors and management. *Br J Surg* 2000;87:370-371.

67. Petrin G, Ruol A, Battaglia G, et al. Anastomotic stenoses occurring after circular stapling in esophageal cancer surgery. *Surg Endosc* 2000;14:670-674.

68. Steichen FM. The use of staplers in anatomical side-to-side and functional end-to-end enteroanastomoses. *Surgery* 1968;64:948-953.

69. Orringer MB, Stirling MC. Cervical esophagogastric anastomosis for benign disease. *J Thorac Cardiovasc Surg* 1988;96:887-893.

70. Iannettoni MD, Whyte RI, Orringer MB. Catastrophic complications of the cervical esophagogastric anastomosis. *J Thorac Cardiovasc Surg* 1995;110:1493-1501.

71. Orringer MB, Marshall B, Iannettoni MD. Eliminating the cervical esophagogastric anastomotic leak with a side-to-side stapled anastomosis. *J Thorac Cardiovasc Surg* 2000;119:277-288.

72. Chassin JL, Rifkind KM, Turner JW. Errors and pitfalls in stapling gastrointestinal tract anastomoses. *Surg Clin N Am* 1984;64:441-459.

73. Humphrey EW. Stapling techniques in esophageal replacement. *Surg Clin N Am* 1984;64:499-510.

74. Steichen FM. Varieties of stapled anastomoses of the esophagus. *Surg Clin N Am* 1984;64:481-498.

75. Kawano T, Yoshino K, Endo M. Cervical esophagogastric anastomosis by the cuff technique using a stapler. *J Am Coll Surg* 1996;183:157-159.

76. O'Riordain DS, Buckley DJ, Waldron DJ, et al. Purse-string suture for stapled oesophagogastric anastomosis: Hand-sewn versus automatic. *Br J Surg* 1993;80:734-736.

77. Robinson LA, Moulton AL, Fleming WH. Techniques to simplify esophagogastric circular stapled anastomoses. *J Surg Oncol* 1994;57:266-269.

78. Mafune K-I, Tanaka Y. Stapled anastomotic technique for cervical esophagogastrostomy. *J Am Coll Surg* 1995;181:85-87.

79. Chassin JL. Stapling techniques for esophagogastrostomy after esophagogastric resection. *Am J Surg* 1978;136:399-404.

80. Bird P, Daniel F, MacLellan D. Oesophagogastrectomy with an anastomosis using linear staplers. *Aust N Z J Surg* 1996;66:757-763.

81. Collard J-M, Romagnoli R, Goncette L, et al. Terminalized semimechanical side-to-side suture technique for cervical esophagogastrostomy. *Ann Thorac Surg* 1998;65:814-817.

82. Singh D, Maley RH, Santucci T, et al. Experience and technique of stapled mechanical cervical esophagogastric anastomosis. *Ann Thorac Surg* 2001;71:419-424.

83. Walther BS, Oscarson JEA, Graffner HOL, et al. Esophagojejunostomy with the EEA stapler. *Surgery* 1986;99:598-603.

84. Pol B, LeTreut YP, Hardwigsen J, et al. Mechanically stapled esophagojejunostomy. Results of a prospective series of 176 cases. *Hepatogastroenterology* 1997;44:458-466.

85. Ferguson MK. Management of esophageal anastomotic leaks. In Franco KL, Putnam JB Jr: **Advanced Therapy in Thoracic Surgery**. Hamilton, B.C. Decker Inc., 1998, pp 464-471.

86. Lorentz T, Fok M, Wong J. Anastomotic leakage after resection and bypass for esophageal cancer: lessons learned from the past. *World J Surg* 1989;13:472-477.

87. Dewar L, Gelfand G, Finley RJ, et al. Factors affecting cervical anastomotic leak and stricture formation following esophagogastrectomy and gastric tube interposition. *Am J Surg* 1992;163:484-489.
88. Patil PK, Patel SG, Mistry RC, et al. Cancer of the esophagus: Esophagogastric anastomotic leak - a retrospective study of predisposing factors. *J Surg Oncol* 1992;49:163-167.
89. Lee Y, Fujita H, Yamana H, et al. Factors affecting leakage following esophageal anastomosis. *Surg Today* 1994;24:24-29.
90. Bruns CJ, Gawenda M, Wolfgarten B, et al. Collare Anastomosenstenosen nach Magenhochzug beim Osophaguskarzinom. Auswertung des eigenen Patienkenguts von 1989-1995. *Langenbecks Arch Chir* 1997;382:145-148.
91. Isozaki H, Okajima K, Ichinona T, et al. Risk factors of esophagojejunal anastomotic leakage after total gastrectomy for gastric cancer. *Hepatogastroenterology* 1997;44:1509-1512.
92. Lin XS, Wu X, Chen BT, et al. Significance of residual tumor at the esophageal stump after resection for carcinoma. *Semin Surg Oncol* 1986;2:257-262.
93. Law S, Arcilla C, Chu KM, et al. The significance of histologically infiltrated resection margin after esophagectomy for esophageal cancer. *Am J Surg* 1998;176:286-290.
94. Urschel JD. Esophagogastrostomy anastomotic leaks complicating esophagectomy: A review. *Am J Surg* 1995;169:634-640.
95. van Oosterom FJ, van Lanschot JJ, Oosting J, et al. A free peritoneal patch does not affect the leakage rate but increases stricture formation of a cervical esophagogastrostomy. *Dig Surg* 1999;16:379-384.
96. McCarthy PM, Trastek VF, Schaff HV, et al. Esophagogastric anastomoses: The value of fibrin glue in preventing leakage. *J Thorac Cardiovasc Surg* 1987;93:234-239.
97. Fernandez Fernandez L, Tejero E, Tieso A. Randomized trial of fibrin glue to seal mechanical oesophagojejunal anastomosis. *Br J Surg* 1996;83:40-41.
98. Schardey HM, Joosten U, Finke U, et al. The prevention of anastomotic leakage after total gastrectomy with local decontamination. *Ann Surg* 1997;225:172-180.
99. Fan ST, Lau WY, Yip WC, et al. Limitations and dangers of gastrografin swallow after esophageal and upper gastric operations. *Am J Surg* 1988;155:495-497.
100. Goel AK, Sinha S, Chattopadhyay TK. Role of gastrografin study in the assessment of anastomotic leaks from cervical oesophagogastric anastomosis. *Aust NZ J Surg* 1995;65:8-10.
101. Tanomkiat W, Galassi W. Barium sulfate as contrast medium for evaluation of postoperative anastomotic leaks. *Acta Radiol* 2000;41:482-485.
102. Kuwano H, Matsushima T, Ikebe M, et al. Mediastinal drainage prevents fatal pyothorax from anastomotic leakage after intrathoracic anastomosis in reconstruction for carcinoma of the esophagus. *Surg Gynecol Obstet* 1993;177:131-134.
103. Orringer MB, Lemmer JH. Early dilation in the treatment of esophageal disruption. *Ann Thorac Surg* 1986;42:536-539.
104. de Lange EE, Shaffer HA Jr, Holt PD. Esophagoenteric anastomotic leaks: Treatment with fluoroscopically guided balloon dilatation. *AJR* 1994;162:51-54.

105. Bhasin DK, Sharma BC, Gupta NM, et al. Endoscopic dilation for treatment of anastomotic leaks following transhiatal esophagectomy. *Endoscopy* 2000;32:469-471.
106. Damm P, Hoffman J. An alternative treatment for anastomotic leakage after oesophageal resection. *Ann Chir Gynaecol* 1988;77:164-165.
107. McNamee CJ, Meyns B, Pagliero KM. New method for dealing with late-presenting spontaneous esophageal perforations. *Ann Thorac Surg* 1991;52:151-153.
108. Jorgensen JO, Hunt DR. Endoscopic drainage of esophageal suture line leaks. *Am J Surg* 1993;165:362-364.
109. Infante M, Valente M, Andreani S, et al. Conservative management of esophageal leaks by transluminal endoscopic drainage of the mediastinum or pleural space. *Surgery* 1996;119:46-50.
110. Heitmiller RF, McQuone SJ, Eisele DW. The utility of the pectoralis myocutaneous flap in the management of select cervical esophageal anastomotic complications. *J Thorac Cardiovasc Surg* 1998;115:1250-1254.
111. Fan ST, Lau WY, Yip WC, et al. Healing of esophageal fistulas after surgical treatment for carcinoma of the esophagus and the upper part of the stomach. *Surg Gynecol Obstet* 1988;166:307-310.
112. Orringer MB, Stirling MC. Esophagectomy for esophageal disruption. *Ann Thorac Surg* 1990;49:35-43.
113. Pierie JPEN, de Graaf PW, Poen H, et al. Incidence and management of benign anastomotic stricture after cervical oesophagogastrectomy. *Br J Surg* 1993;80:471-474.
114. Siersma PD, Honkoop P, Tilanus HW. Risk factors for benign strictures after oesophagectomy and gastric tube reconstruction with cervical anastomosis. In Peracchia A, Rosati R, Bonavina L, et al (eds): **Recent Advances in Diseases of the Esophagus**. Bologna, Monduzzi Editore, 1996, pp 261-266.
115. Heitmiller RF, Fischer A, Liddicoat JR. Cervical esophagogastric anastomosis: Results following esophagectomy for carcinoma. *Dis Esoph* 1999;12:264-269.
116. Wang LS, Huang MH, Huang BS, Chien KY. Gastric substitution for resectable carcinoma of the esophagus: An analysis of 368 cases. *Ann Thorac Surg* 1992;53:289-294.
117. Trentino P, Pompeo E, Nofroni I, et al. Predictive value of early postoperative esophagoscopy for occurrence of benign stenosis after cervical esophagogastrostomy. *Endoscopy* 1997;29:840-844.
118. Johansson J, Zilling T, von Holstein CS, et al. Anastomotic diameters and strictures following esophagectomy and total gastrectomy in 256 patients. *World J Surg* 2000;24:78-85.
119. Inagake M, Yamane T, Kitao Y, et al. Balloon dilatation for anastomotic stricture after upper gastro-intestinal surgery. *World J Surg* 1992;16:541-544.
120. Ikeya T, Ohwada S, Ogawa T, et al. Endoscopic balloon dilation for benign esophageal anastomotic stricture: Factors influencing its effectiveness. *Hepatogastroenterology* 1999;46:959-966.

Chapter 16

Postoperative Management

Most of the information and guidelines in this chapter pertain to the management of patients who have undergone combined esophagectomy and esophageal reconstruction. It is uncommon for a reconstruction to be performed apart from esophagectomy except during staged reconstruction or esophageal bypass operations, and little information specific to the postoperative management of such patients exists. As a result, it is often difficult to sort out which perturbations are a result of esophagectomy and which are due primarily to the effects of reconstruction. For purposes of this chapter, a general overview will be provided for postoperative management of patients who undergo combined esophagectomy and esophageal reconstruction. However, the commentary will focus on the specific effects and management of postoperative issues related to reconstruction when feasible. Although general management issues will be addressed in detail, true critical care management of desperately ill patients is beyond the scope of this textbook and more authoritative sources should be sought out regarding patient management in such situations.

Maintaining Oxygenation and Perfusion

Supplemental Oxygen

The need for supplemental oxygen in patients who have undergone major surgery such as esophageal reconstruction is determined by a variety of factors, including the degree of alveolar hypoventilation, problems with oxygen diffusion into the blood, difficulties with oxygen transport, and increased oxygen extraction, to name a few. Decreased oxygen delivery correlates with postoperative complications and may be a determinant of hospital mortality after esophagectomy.[1] Measurement of arterial oxygen saturation is routine in the early postoperative period following esophageal reconstruction and supplemental oxygen is provided by face mask or nasal cannula to maintain arterial saturations above 90%.[2] In addition to maintaining adequate blood oxygen concentrations for cardiac and central nervous system function, supplemental oxygen has other less obvious benefits. These include more rapid postoperative rewarming, a reduction in the usual degree of postoperative tachycardia, a decrease in the incidence of nausea and vomiting, and lower wound infection rates.[3-8]

Intravenous Fluids

Opinions diverge widely as to the optimal rate to administer intravenous fluids during the immediate postoperative period after esophageal reconstruction. Some surgeons caution that patients should not be given fluid at rates that exceed their normal requirements because of the risk of promoting pulmonary edema with resultant respiratory insufficiency. On the other hand, esophagectomy and reconstruction usually requires extensive dissection in at least one and frequently in two or three body cavities, which results in capillary leakage and so-called "third spacing" of fluids during the first few postoperative days. This pathophysiology requires that fluid in addition to usual intravenous requirements be given so that intravascular volumes are sufficient to enable adequate perfusion of vital organs. A delicate balance must be achieved, since excess fluid leads not only to pulmonary insufficiency but also to edema of the reconstructive organ, which may influence its oxygen partial pressures and thus its viability.

Once the period of capillary leakage has passed, patients will mobilize the excess fluid and intravenous requirements will be equal to or less than their normal maintenance levels. The process of mobilization sometimes is aided by judicious use of intravenous diuretics. The administration of tube feedings in an effort to provide early postoperative nutrition may complicate the estimate of how much fluid is being absorbed in an individual patient.

Monitoring

During the initial postoperative period careful monitoring of renal, cardiac, pulmonary, and central nervous system function is essential for minimizing postoperative complications and optimizing short-term outcomes. Blood pressure, heart rate, respiratory rate, body temperature, and percutaneous oxygen saturation are all measured frequently. Measurement of central venous pressure and use of a pulmonary artery cathe-

Table 16-1.
Pain Management after Esophageal Reconstruction.

Pain management options
Epidural catheter
Patient controlled analgesia (PCA) pump for intravenous infusion
Local anesthetics injected into the incisions
Intercostal nerve block
Continuous extrapleural analgesia
Intravenous or oral nonsteroidal analgesics
Advantages of reduced postoperative pain
Improved quality of life
Shortened ICU stay
Shortened hospital stay
Decreased cost of hospitalization
Reduced respiratory morbidity
Reduced operative mortality
Decreased incidence of chronic postthoracotomy pain

ter to monitor cardiac filling pressures or cardiac output is not often necessary. The measurement or calculation of the serum base deficit is a useful clue to the adequacy of fluid resuscitation during the first postoperative days. Daily estimates of total net fluid loss or gain, aided by measurement of body weight, provide guidance as to the overall fluid status of a patient and helps in deciding if and when judicious diuresis is appropriate.

Pain Management

Possibly the most important and welcomed improvement in surgical care in the 1990s was the widespread acceptance of the need for adequate postoperative pain relief. This is true at no time more than after major esophageal surgery. Preemptive pain management is provided by preoperative insertion of an epidural catheter for continuous administration of local anesthetics and/or narcotics intraoperatively and postoperatively (Table 16-1).[9] In patients in whom epidural analgesia is contraindicated, continuous extrapleural analgesia in the postoperative period is a useful alternative that provides excellent results, especially when long-acting analgesics are used.[10-12] Local anesthetics may be applied intraoperatively to incisions and as intercostal nerve blocks to limit immediate postoperative pain. Nonsteroidal analgesics, especially when administered preemptively, dramatically reduce the severity of postoperative pain.[13-15] Frequent monitoring of pain levels and multidisciplinary management of postoperative pain are important elements in assuring optimal pain relief after major surgery.[16]

There is growing evidence for the advantages of adequate pain management. Quality of life as measured by relief of pain in the early postoperative period after major esophageal surgery is reduced with the use of epidural analgesia.[17] The use of epidural rather than intravenous narcotics for pain relief after esophagectomy and reconstruction shortens ICU and overall hospital length of stay and results in substantial cost savings.[18,19] There is also evidence that pain management with an epidural catheter reduces respiratory morbidity and mortality after esophagectomy.[19,20] Better pain management results in higher postoperative subcutaneous oxygen partial pressures which may translate into reduced rates of wound infection.[21] Providing adequate perioperative pain relief may reduce the incidence of chronic postoperative pain that occurs after thoracotomy.[22]

Antibiotics

The use of prophylactic perioperative antibiotics is discussed in some detail in Chapter 6. Most esophageal reconstructive operations are classified as clean contaminated procedures. On occasion, particularly if emergency reconstruction is necessary, the procedure is classified as contaminated. Patients who undergo major surgery that is classified in either category have been shown to benefit from perioperative systemic antibiotics.[23,24] Use of an antibiotic dose just prior to beginning the operation, maintenance of adequate antibiotic levels throughout the operation, and possible administration of an additional dose after completion of the operation reduces wound infection rates and may lessen the incidence of other infectious complications.[25,26] Single dose therapy directed at potentially contaminating organisms is the theoretical ideal for prophylactic antibiotic treatment.[27,28] The choice of antibiotic for most procedures is a second generation cephalosporin, but third generation cephalosporins which cover gram negative organisms should be considered for colon interpositions or if a high degree of contamination from oral flora has occurred.

Nutrition

The immediate postoperative systemic effects of major surgery are beginning to be elucidated and are profound. They include neuroendocrine stimulation which occurs in proportion to the magnitude of the operation, immunosuppression (especially in patients with cancer, who form the vast majority of those undergoing esophageal reconstructive surgery), and net-negative nitrogen balance. Preexisting malnutrition, which is also common among patients undergoing esophageal reconstruction, and the presence of cancer also adversely affect nitrogen balance and have immunosup-

Table 16-2.
Systemic Effects of Major Surgery, Malnutrition, and Cancer.

Macrophage dysfunction due to injury:
- Diminished effector functions
  - antibacterial
  - antitumoral
  - tissue modeling associated with wound healing and repair
- Diminished immunoregulatory functions
  - antigen presentation to T cells
  - T-helper-1 response
  - production of interferon-gamma
  - contributions to natural killer cell functions
- Increased immunoregulatory functions
  - T-helper-2 response
  - interleukin-4 (IL-4), interleukin-10 (IL-10) production

Effects of malnutrition:
- Decreased immune function
  - T-cell mitogenesis
  - cytotoxic T-cell activity
  - natural killer activity
  - lysozyme production
- Increased catecholamine and cortisol release
- Increased postoperative polymorphonuclear (PMN) elastase, C-reactive protein (CRP), interleukin-6 (IL-6)

Effects of cancer:
- Release of circulating factors (tumor necrosis factor-alpha [TNF-alpha], interleukin-1 [IL-1], IL-6, interferon gamma, leukocyte inhibitory factor)
  - increased whole body and liver protein synthesis, decreased skeletal muscle synthesis and nitrogen balance
  - increase in glucose production and consumption
  - increased Cori cycle activity
  - decreased glycogen synthesis and storage, decreased peripheral insulin effect
  - increased lipid and triglyceride levels, increased fat breakdown and decreased total body fat stores
- Monocyte and macrophage dysfunction (due to release of prostanoids, IL-10, and transforming growth factor-beta [TGF-beta])
  - impaired intracellular killing
  - decreased migration and chemotaxis

pressive effects (Table 16-2).[29,30] Beginning as early as the 1940s, techniques for parenteral and enteral nutrition were devised that helped reverse negative nitrogen balance after major surgery.[31] More recently, nutritional therapies, especially total parenteral nutrition, have been demonstrated to have positive effects on body composition, nitrogen balance, and body fat in cancer patients. However, this evident biologic value has not clearly translated into improved immune function, and there is little demonstrable effect of such therapy on the underlying malignancies.

Patients who suffer malnutrition experience a decrease in lean body mass, a relative decrease in extracellular water, impaired grip strength, a decrement in respiratory function, and an inability to cough and clear secretions. These findings translate to an increased incidence of postoperative complications including pneumonia and a prolongation of hospital stay after major gastrointestinal surgery.[32,33] Nutritional repletion prior to major surgery has been shown to reduce postoperative complications and mortality, but these benefits are only evident for the most seriously malnourished patients.[34,35] Therefore, postoperative nutritional therapy is recommended for select groups of patients: those who are severely malnourished (defined as > 15% weight loss accompanied by major organ dysfunction) prior to surgery, those who have severe complications, and those who are not expected to be able to eat adequately within 7 to 10 days of their operation.[36] Whether the administration of postoperative enteral or parenteral nutrition is of benefit in other surgical patients, especially those who are expected to resume normal alimentation within a week of operation, has not been conclusively demonstrated. In fact, there is some evidence to suggest that such therapy may be harmful.

Postoperative Parenteral Nutrition

The routine use of postoperative total parenteral nutrition (TPN) after gastrointestinal surgery has been controversial since the concept was introduced in the 1970s. Early retrospective reports suggested that TPN was beneficial in shortening hospital stay and in reducing the incidence of postoperative complications. More recent evidence indicates that the incidence of infectious complications is increased with routine use of postoperative TPN. These infections often are related to the presence of a central venous catheter but may also be associated with more ominous changes such as increased bacterial translocation and systemic infections. It has even been suggested that routine use of TPN exposes some patients to an increased risk of postoperative mortality.[37-39] Some of these complications may be due to inappropriate nutritional supplementation, both underfeeding and overfeeding. In fact, overfeeding may be a more common source of morbidity than underfeeding.

The advent of techniques for simplified administration of enteral feedings and the development of appropriate enteral formulas have helped to highlight the relative advantages of enteral feeding compared to parenteral feeding. These include cost savings, ease of administration, and possibly immunologic and nutritional benefits that may improve overall postoperative outcomes.[40-42] The net result has been a strong preference for enteral rather than parenteral nutritional support for selected patients postoperatively. Current recommendations suggest that the use of postoperative TPN should be restricted to specific situations: when enteral or oral feeding is not anticipated within 7 to 10 days postoperatively; in patients in whom major complications develop and in whom enteral or oral feedings are not possible; and in patients in whom preoperative TPN was utilized.[43,44]

Postoperative Enteral Nutrition

The clinical evidence for an increased risk of infectious and other complications related to the routine use of postoperative TPN led to the investigation of enteral feedings as an alternative means of protein repletion after trauma or sepsis. Experimental studies using a sepsis model demonstrated that a substantial decrease in mortality was provided by enteral feedings regardless of the initial nutritional state.[45-47] Subsequent clinical studies demonstrated the advantage of early enteral feeding compared to delayed enteral or parenteral feeding in reducing infectious complications after major abdominal trauma.[48] They also demonstrated an advantage of early enteral compared to early parenteral feeding in abdominal trauma patients in reducing septic complications, especially in the most severely injured patients.[49-51]

Why enteral feeding reduces septic complications compared to parenteral feeding is a matter of debate. Possible explanations include immunosuppressive effects of TPN and maintenance of gut-barrier function provided by enteral feedings.[52,53] The intestinal tract is thought to be the driving force behind progressive multiple organ dysfunction after exposure to any of a variety of insults such as shock, sepsis, and starvation. Proinflammatory cytokines are released from the mucosa and other immunologic cells, neutrophils are activated in the gut and relocate to other organs including the lungs, bacteria and endotoxin may translocate into the bloodstream, and gut immunoglobulin production is reduced. In normal volunteers following endotoxin infusion, TPN administration results in increased levels of serum tumor necrosis factor (TNF) and interleukin-6 (IL-6) compared to those maintained on an enteral diet.[54] Beneficial effects of enteral feedings have been demonstrated clinically in patients undergoing esophagectomy. Perioperative administration of enteral feedings led to reduced serum levels of IL-6 and interleukin-10 (IL-10) and lower endotoxin concentrations compared to patients receiving perioperative TPN.[55]

Despite the demonstrated advantages of enteral feeding compared to parenteral feeding after trauma and major surgery, whether routine immediate enteral feeding is beneficial compared to advancing an oral diet postoperatively as tolerated remains controversial.[35] An early randomized study demonstrated that no benefit was provided by early enteral feedings after major surgery, and the early feeding group also had an excessively high complication rate associated with the feeding tube.[56] Mixed results have accumulated from subsequent randomized trials. Early enteral nutrition has been shown to prevent an increase in gut mucosal permeability, produce a positive nitrogen balance, and reduce infectious complications.[57-60] However, other studies suggest that routine use of protein-sparing therapy after major surgery provides no clinical benefit and may not alter intestinal permeability.[61-63] In addition, one report has suggested that immediate postoperative jejunal feeding is associated with impaired respiratory mechanics and overall mobility without influencing loss of muscle strength or the development of fatigue.[64]

Use of either a needle catheter jejunostomy or a standard Witzel-type tube jejunostomy after major surgery is associated with a small incidence of complications. The risk of major catheter-related complications is less than 2%, and formula-related complications such as diarrhea occur with an incidence of less than 10%.[65-72] There is also a cost savings realized as a result of routine use of early postoperative enteral nutrition.[73] Given this low incidence of complications, the likelihood that esophageal reconstruction patients may encounter complications that will delay the onset of adequate oral intake, potential cost savings, and the ease of use of jejunostomy feeding tubes, it is logical that use of such catheters should be routine after esophageal reconstructive surgery. Because insertion of needle catheter jejunostomies is technically easier than placement of a Witzel-type catheter, it is recommended as the first choice for postoperative enteral nutrition after esophageal reconstructive surgery.

Immunonutrition

The persistent incidence of postoperative infectious complications, which is presumably related in part to perioperative immunosuppression, has led to the investigation of immune-modulating additives to enteral formulas. The typical supplements include arginine, ribonucleic acid (RNA), and omega-3 fatty acids. Such formulas have been shown to enhance host immunologic responses, induce a switch from acute-phase to constitutive proteins, and improve gut function.[74-79] Clinically, this translates to a decrease in postoperative infectious complications, shortened length of stay in some instances, and reduced costs of care.[80-84] Further investigation of the potential advantages of these supplements is warranted.

Oral Intake

Some surgeons prefer not to feed patients for a period of up to 2 weeks after surgery, while others begin oral intake as soon as there is evidence of gut motility. Since patients swallow up to 2 liters of saliva per day, the anastomosis is being tested clinically as soon as the patient emerges from the anesthetic. Rather than set some arbitrary time for beginning oral intake, decisions should be individualized based on a patient's clinical condition. The use of feeding jejunostomy tube feedings permits the slow introduction of oral nutrition without the need for concern about rapid progression to full oral nutrition and helps prevent postoperative malnutrition. As soon as airway protection is adequate, bowel activity has begun, and there is no evidence for anastomotic leak, it is appropriate to begin a clear liquid diet. Early institution of swallowing restores strength and coordination to the muscles of deglutition, hastens the return of full bowel function, and boosts the patient's morale. There is evidence that protein depletion continues for many weeks after major surgery, and that oral supplements or jejunostomy tube feedings during this period of time can reverse such tendencies, limit complications, and improve quality of life.[85]

Drainage Tubes

Nasoenteral Tubes

The use of nasoenteral tubes for draining reconstructive organs after esophageal reconstruction is standard. Such tubes have a number of benefits. They permit an assessment of the degree of emptying of the reconstructive organ, help prevent accumulation of saliva and food in the reconstructive organ which can predispose to aspiration, and, in some cases, stent narrowed, inflamed, or partially necrotic anastomoses. However, there are a number of potential drawbacks to the use of such tubes. They are uncomfortable and substantially interfere with a patient's quality of life in the immediate postoperative period. The presence of such a tube in a patient who also has an indwelling endotracheal tube can predispose to the development of erosion between the endotracheal tube and the reconstructive organ or esophagus, leading to the creation of an airway-enteric fistula. Nasoenteral tubes adversely affect pulmonary toilet exercises, leading to an increased risk of pneumonia. It is often argued the placement of such a tube across an intact esophagogastric junction eliminates the antireflux barrier provided by that structure and promotes reflux, increasing the risk of aspiration. Whether such a concern applies to patients having undergone esophageal reconstruction is unclear, since, under most circumstances, they have already lost their normal antireflux mechanisms.

In a patient in whom a nasoenteral tube is placed for initial postoperative management, the timing of tube removal is a matter of the surgeon's personal preference. Some surgeons prefer to leave the tube in until a contrast radiograph is performed that demonstrates no anastomotic leak and adequate emptying of the reconstructive organ. Many surgeons, however, remove the tube when feasible based on the absence of abdominal distension, the presence of bowel sounds, evidence for bowel activity such as passage of flatus, and low outputs from the tube. It is useful to remember that bowel gas is necessary to produce bowel sounds, and that most bowel gas originates as swallowed air. Removal of a segment of the esophagus interferes with passage of swallowed air into the bowel, and may substantially reduce the presence of bowel sounds postoperatively. Early removal of nasoenteric drainage tubes, when physiologically appropriate, promotes the return of normal bowel activity and facilitates early restoration of oral intake.

Local Drains

The use of local drains after esophageal reconstruction is primarily limited to drainage of the cervical wound after creation of a cervical anastomosis.

Placement of local drains adjacent to intrathoracic or intra-abdominal anastomoses is unusual and is unlikely to be effective except in unusual clinical circumstances. Whether or not cervical drains are used is more a matter of dogma than established surgical principle. Scant information exists in the literature which addresses this issue, and the available data support diametrically opposed viewpoints. One report suggests that the use of rubber drains locally promotes the development of anastomotic leaks in an experimental model.[86] Clinical experience with the use of drains after cervical esophagogastrostomy is mixed. One report suggests that the risk of anastomotic leak and other local complications is actually reduced if a drain is placed,[87] whereas another demonsrates no benefit to routine placement of a drain after cervical esophagogastrostomy.[88] Rational explanations for either of these contentions are lacking. If an anastomotic leak develops, whether placement of a drain decreases the likelihood of catastrophic complications is not known. The use of drains, therefore, is a matter that is best left to the judgment of surgeons based on their experience and the individual needs of their patients.

Chest Tubes

Thoracostomy tubes are routinely placed when a thoracotomy or sternotomy is used as part of esophageal reconstructive surgery. Such tubes are sometimes used when the pleura has been violated during other procedures, such as during a transhiatal esophagectomy and reconstruction or after development of a substernal tunnel as a route for esophageal replacement (if it is anticipated that fluid will accumulate in the pleural space), or if there has been parenchymal lung injury leading to an air leak. The routine use of chest tubes in other situations is best avoided, because of the risk of complications such as injury of the intercostal neurovascular bundle and because the presence of such tubes interferes with adequate pulmonary toilet postoperatively due to increased levels of pain. Removal of thoracostomy tubes is accomplished when certain standard criteria have been met: the patient is not on positive pressure ventilation, there has been no air leak through the tube for 12 to 24 hours, and drainage volume is at an acceptable level, usually less than 300 mL/24 hours. Leaving a thoracostomy tube in place routinely until a contrast radiograph is performed to rule out anastomotic leakage is of no advantage. It is uncommon for an intrathoracic or cervical anastomotic leak to be effectively drained by a standard thoracostomy tube placed at the time of esophageal reconstruction, since adhesions form quickly postoperatively that seal the tube tract from the region of the anastomosis. Placing the tube in close proximity to the anastomosis risks erosion by the typically stiff thoracostomy tube into the reconstructive organ. However, if there is clinical evidence for a leak and there appears to be effective drainage of that leak by an indwelling thoracostomy tube, confirmation of adequate drainage with a contrast study permits confident use of such a tube as a primary means of drainage of the region of the leak.

Evaluation of the Anastomosis

A substantial amount of information regarding evaluation of the esophageal anastomosis for patency and competency is provided in Chapter 15. This section will briefly summarize recommendations for appropriate evaluation of the anastomosis after surgery. There is considerable disagreement as to the need for and utility of routine tests of an anastomosis after esophageal reconstructive surgery. In the absence of clinical signs of an anastomotic leak, whether intervention is necessary for a small and asymptomatic (subclinical) leak/sinus tract is controversial. Surgeons who feel that no change in management is necessitated by the discovery of subclinical leaks also believe that there is little advantage in documenting such abnormalities.

Postoperative contrast radiographs assess anatomic and functional components after esophageal reconstruction. These studies provide potentially useful information regarding the anatomy of the reconstruction, possibly showing stricturing of the anastomosis, redundancy of the reconstruction, and any narrowing where the reconstruction crosses the level of the diaphragm. Some information regarding the completeness of emptying is also available, which helps determine whether the addition of prokinetic agents might be useful in the management of an individual patient.

The accuracy and utility of swallowing studies in determining the presence of an anastomotic leak is a matter of some debate. As discussed in Chapter 15, the use of water soluble contrast agents such as meglumine deatrizoate (gastrografin) has a false negative incidence of up to 40%, and such agents produce important pneumonitis if they are accidentally aspirated during the swallow, a common occurrence in the early postoperative period.[89,90] Water soluble agents, if used as the initial medium during a postoperative swallow assessing for a leak, are more likely to demonstrate clinically important leaks than subclinical leaks. The use of barium sulfate, either full strength or diluted, improves the accuracy of leak detection and produces a much lower risk of pulmonary complications if accidentally ingested during the swallow study.[91] However, more of the demonstrated leaks are clinically unimportant. Some surgeons have concerns that, if a leak is discovered, barium will be retained in the neck or mediastinum that may interfere with healing or with subsequent radiographic evaluation of healing, but neither of these concerns has proven to be clinically important.[92] In fact, some authors suggest that the presence of barium in a fistula tract encourages the development of granulation tissue and hastens closure of the fistula.[93]

Radiographic contrast swallows may also provide information about the risk of aspiration in patients who have recently undergone esophageal reconstruction. Reconstructive surgery in the neck often results in neuropraxia or permanent injury of the ipsilateral recurrent or superior laryngeal nerve, resulting in discoordinated swallowing and, in the case of injury to a recurrent laryngeal nerve, failure of adequate protection of the airway during swallowing. Most swallowing studies directed towards identifying the status of an anastomosis are not performed to provide an assessment of the swallowing mechanism, and the reasons for the development of aspiration, should it occur, are often not obvious. A more formal cineradiographic swallowing study is usually necessary to make such distinct delineations.[94-96]

Although interpretation of contrast studies after use of the stomach for reconstruction may be relatively straightforward, the reading of such studies after more complex esophageal reconstruction can be challenging.[97] The presence of jejunum, colon, or composite reconstructive tissues naturally creates impediments to rapid emptying, including retention of contrast material in haustra or other natural tissue folds. The presence or absence of contractile activity during the short period of the contrast study also affects interpretation of the anatomy and estimation of emptying. Care should be taken so that interpretation of such studies does not lead to erroneous conclusions about the relative success of esophageal reconstruction.

The overall accuracy of contrast radiographic studies in assessing an esophageal anastomosis, particularly with regards to the presence of an anastomotic leak, is difficult to estimate. The definition of a leak varies with the author or institution. Moreover, the frequency with which clinically important leaks occur and the number of routine studies that is performed are important determinants of accuracy. Accuracy is calculated by dividing the sum of true positive and true negative studies by the total number of studies performed. In institutions where swallow studies are not performed routinely, but are ordered so as to confirm the clinical suspicion of a leak, the percentage of true positive studies is likely to be high, and the total number of studies will be relatively low, leading to a high degree of accuracy. A better estimate of accuracy may be gleaned from institutions in which studies are performed routinely and in which the incidence of leaks is not low but approaches the average rate of around 10% quoted in Chapter 15. Such data suggest that the true positive rate approaches 100% but that the false negative rate is about 30%, leading to an overall accuracy of 60% to 70%.[98] More important, perhaps, is the likelihood of identifying a leak that is important but is not clinically evident. Some authors suggest that up to 50% of leaks that are detected radiographically may not be clinically evident.[99] Whether leaks that are not initially clinically evident eventually cause clinical problems is a matter of some debate. Most authors suggest that there is no important morbidity associated with such findings, although substantial morbidity was reported by at least one group.[99-101]

Some authors routinely provide methylene blue for oral ingestion by their patients to test the integrity of esophageal anastomoses prior to instituting oral feedings. This technique is best applied to patients who have indwelling cervical drains after a cervical esophageal anastomosis has been performed, but is also of potential benefit in patients who have a thoracostomy tube in place after either a cervical or intrathoracic anastomosis.[102] In patients who have already had their cervical wound opened because of a clinically diagnosed infection, administration of methylene blue may also serve to document the etiology of the infection. Immediate extravasation of methylene blue through a drain or through an open cervical wound is diagnostic of an anastomotic leak, although the exact site and size of the leak cannot be determined with this technique. Delayed appearance of blue-stained material through drains or in an open wound leaves the existence of an anastomotic leak in some doubt because the dye is rapidly absorbed and tends to cause a blue discoloration in bodily fluids.

Many surgeons do not routinely perform any type of study to assess the anastomosis postoperatively, but begin their patients on oral intake when appropriate. The decision to begin water ingestion or a liquid diet is made when a patient is able to control oral secretions, is able to protect the airway, has no evidence of delayed emptying of the reconstructive organ, and has no clinical signs of an anastomotic leak. If the water or liquid diet is well tolerated, the diet is advanced to soft solids over a period of a few days. Under these circumstances, studies are performed to assess the anastomosis only when there is clinical evidence for problems such as leak, aspiration, partial obstruction, or delayed emptying of the reconstructive organ.

Respiratory Therapy

Pulmonary complications are among the most common problems affecting patients after esophageal reconstruction (see Chapter 17). The key to their management is prevention, which encompasses a wide spectrum of efforts. Preoperative assessment of respiratory status is important in estimating the risk of postoperative complications. Smoking cessation, ambulation, and pulmonary toilet exercises can be instituted preoperatively which can decrease the risk of postoperative pulmonary complications after major surgery.[103] In the immediate postoperative period, the risks of pneumonia and respiratory insufficiency can be minimized by providing adequate pain relief, early ambulation, and pulmonary toilet exercises such as coughing and deep breathing.[104,105] Incentive spirometry devices may help in the effective performance of the latter exercises.[106-108] In patients with a history of chronic bronchitis, percussion and postural drainage can help clear secretions and may reduce the incidence of pulmonary infection.[109]

Some surgeons and anesthesiologists customarily maintain their patients on positive pressure ventilation until at least the first postoperative day after esophagectomy and reconstruction. The rationale for this includes the need for a prolonged anesthetic, substantial pain that may interfere with postoperative respiratory effort, the need for large amounts of intravenous fluid during and after the operation to maintain intravascular volume, division of innervation to the pulmonary hila which could impair ventilatory function, large volumes of blood transfusion, the presence of an upper abdominal incision that interferes with diaphragmatic function, and the use of prolonged single lung anesthesia during transthoracic operations which may lead to unilateral pulmonary edema. It is believed by some physicians that elective ventilatory support under these circumstances is best for preventing pulmonary complications after esophageal reconstruction.

In contrast, most surgeons prefer to extubate their patients as soon after esophageal reconstruction as possible. A variety of improvements in postoperative management permit this to be done with no risk to the patient, and there are some documented advantages to this approach. Such changes include better postoperative pain management (see above), improved algorithms for fluid management, reduced operating times, and limited blood transfusions. In fact, some centers don't make use of intensive care units for their typical reconstruction patient, but send the patients to the regular hospital ward after a few hours in the postanesthesia care unit. When patients have adequate pain control and breathe spontaneously, pulmonary toilet is more efficient when executed through coughing and deep breathing maneuvers than if endotracheal suctioning is performed, the risk of atelectasis is reduced, and bronchoalveolar barotrauma is avoided. Early extubation after esophagectomy and reconstruction reduces intensive care unit days and postoperative respiratory complications, and does not lead to an increased risk of reintubation, especially in patients who undergo reconstruction not requiring a thoracotomy.[110,111]

Patients who are not artificially ventilated may at times develop retained secretions leading to hypoxia. There is growing experience in such a setting with the use of a minitracheostomy tube placed through the cricothyroid membrane, which provides a means to effectively suction tracheobronchial secretions and permits administration of supplemental oxygen. The location of the minitracheostomy does not usually interfere with reconstructive surgery that has been performed, insertion is straightforward, and the risk of complications associated with the use of such a device is low. Therapeutic use of the device has been very satisfactory after a variety of major operations, but results of prophylactic use of the device after esophageal reconstruction has not been reported.[112,113]

References

1. Kusano C, Baba M, Takao S, et al. Oxygen delivery as a factor in the development of fatal postoperative complications after oesophagectomy. *Br J Surg* 1997;84:252-257.
2. Powell JF, Menon DK, Jones JG. The effects of hypoxaemia and recommendations for postoperative oxygen therapy. *Anaesthesia* 1996;51:769-772.
3. Knighton DR, Halliday B, Hunt TK. Oxygen as an antibiotic. The effect of inspired oxygen on infection. *Arch Surg* 1984;119:199-204.
4. Stausholm K, Kehlet H, Rosenberg J. Oxygen therapy reduces postoperative tachycardia. *Anaesthesia* 1995;50:737-739.
5. Greif R, Laciny S, Rapf B, et al. Supplemental oxygen reduces the incidence of postoperative nausea and vomiting. *Anesthesiology* 1999;91:1246-1252.
6. Rosenberg-Adamsen S, Lie C, Bernhard A, et al. Effect of oxygen treatment on heart rate after abdominal surgery. *Anesthesiology* 1999;90:380-384.
7. Frank SM, Hesel TW, El-Rahmany HK, et al. Warmed humidified inspired oxygen accelerates postoperative rewarming. *J Clin Anesth* 2000;12:283-287.

8. Greif R, Akca O, Horn EP, et al. Supplemental perioperative oxygen to reduce the incidence of surgical wound infection. Outcomes Research Group. *N Engl J Med* 2000;342:161-167.
9. Brodner G, Pogatzki E, Van Aken H, et al. A multimodal approach to control postoperative pathophysiology and rehabilitation in patients undergoing abdominothoracic esophagectomy. *Anesth Analg* 1998;86:228-234.
10. Francois T, Blanloeil Y, Pillet F, et al. Effect of intrapleural administration of bupivacaine or lidocaine on pain and morphine requirement after esophagectomy with thoracotomy: A randomized, double-blind and controlled study. *Anesth Analg* 1995;80:718-723.
11. Kaiser AM, Zollinger A, De Lorenzi D, et al. Prospective, randomized comparison of extrapleural versus epidural analgesia for postthoracotomy pain. *Ann Thorac Surg* 1998;66:367-372.
12. Bimston DN, McGee JP, Liptay MJ, Fry WA. Continuous paravertebral extrapleural infusion for post-thoracotomy pain management. *Surgery* 1999;126:650-657.
13. Power I, Bowler GM, Pugh GC, et al. Ketorolac as a component of balanced analgesia after thoracotomy. *Br J Anaesth* 1994;72:224-226.
14. Joris J. Efficacy of nonsteroidal antiinflammatory drugs in postoperative pain. *Acta Anaesthesiol Belg* 1996;47:115-123.
15. Sabanathan S, Shah R, Tsiamis A, et al. Oesophagogastrectomy in the elderly high risk patients: role of effective regional analgesia and early mobilisation. *J Cardiovasc Surg* 1999;40:153-156.
16. Stevens DS, Edwards WT. Management of pain in intensive care settings. *Surg Clin N Am* 1999;79:371-386.
17. Tsui SL, Chan CS, Chan AS, et al. Postoperative analgesia for oesophageal surgery: A comparison of three analgesic regimens. *Anaesth Intensive Care* 1991;19:329-337.
18. Smedstad KG, Beattie WS, Blair WS, Buckley DN. Postoperative pain relief and hospital stay after total esophagectomy. *Clin J Pain* 1992;8:149-153.
19. Tsui SL, Law S, Fok M, et al. Postoperative analgesia reduces mortality and morbidity after esophagectomy. *Am J Surg* 1997;173:472-478.
20. Watson A, Allen PR. Influence of thoracic epidural analgesia on outcome after resection for esophageal cancer. *Surgery* 1994;115:429-432.
21. Akca O, Melischek M, Scheck T, et al. Postoperative pain and subcutaneous oxygen tension. *Lancet* 1999;354:41-42.
22. d'Amours RH, Riegler FX, Little AG. Pathogenesis and management of persistent postthoracotomy pain. *Chest Surg Clin N Am* 1998;8:703-722.
23. Ludwig KA, Carlson MA, Condon RE. Prophylactic antibiotics in surgery. *Annu Rev Med* 1993;44:385-393.
24. Page CP, Bohnen JM, Fletcher JR, et al. Antimicrobial prophylaxis for surgical wounds. Guidelines for clinical care. *Arch Surg* 1993;128:79-88.
25. Classen DC, Evans RS, Pestotnik SL, et al. The timing of prophylactic administration of antibiotics and the risk of surgical wound infection. *N Engl J Med* 1992;30:281-286.
26. Bricard H, Deshayes JP, Sillard B, et al. Antibiotic prophylaxis in surgery of the esophagus. *Ann Fr Anesth Reanim* 1994;13:S161-S168.
27. DiPiro JT. Short-term prophylaxis in clean-contaminated surgery. *J Chemother* 1999;11:551-555.

28. Polk HC, Christmas AB. Prophylactic antibiotics in surgery and surgical wound infections. *Am Surg* 2000;66:105-111.
29. Nakamura K, Moriyama Y, Kariyazono H, et al. Influence of preoperative nutritional state on inflammatory response after surgery. *Nutrition* 1999;15:834-841.
30. Daly JM. In defense of the surgical cancer patient: Nutrition may be key. *Bull Am Coll Surg* 2001;86:18-23.
31. Wilmore DW. Postoperative protein sparing. *World J Surg* 1999;23:545-552.
32. Windsor JA, Hill GL. Weight loss with physiologic impairment. A basic indicator of surgical risk. *Ann Surg* 1988;207:290-296.
33. Windsor JA, Hill GL. Risk factors for postoperative pneumonia. The importance of protein depletion. *Ann Surg* 1988;208:209-214.
34. Veterans Affairs Total Parenteral Nutrition Cooperative Study Group. Perioperative total parenteral nutrition in surgical patients. *N Engl J Med* 1991;22:525-532.
35. Torosian MH. Perioperative nutrition support for patients undergoing gastrointestinal surgery: critical analysis and recommendations. *World J Surg* 1999;23:565-569.
36. Waitzberg DL, Plopper C, Terra RM. Postoperative total parenteral nutrition. *World J Surg* 1999;23:560-564.
37. Sandstrom R, Drott C, Hyltander A, et al. The effect of postoperative intravenous feeding (TPN) on outcome following major surgery evaluated in a randomized study. *Ann Surg* 1993;217:185-195.
38. Brennan M, Pisters PW, Posner M, et al. A prospective randomized trial of total parenteral nutrition after major pancreatic resection for malignancy. *Ann Surg* 1994;220:436-444.
39. Baigrie RJ, Devitt PG, Watkin DS. Enteral versus parenteral nutrition after oesophagogastric surgery: A prospective randomized comparison. *Aust N Z J Surg* 1996;66:668-670.
40. Eeftinck Schattenkerk M, Obertop H, Bruining HA, et al. Needle catheter jejunostomy (NCJ) for early postoperative feeding: Experience in 210 patients. *Neth J Surg* 1983;35:163-166.
41. Sand J, Luostarinen M, Matikainen M. Enteral of parenteral feeding after total gastrectomy: Prospective randomized pilot study. *Eur J Surg* 1997;163:761-766.
42. Lipman TO. Grains or veins: Is enteral nutrition really better than parenteral nutrition? A look at the evidence. *J Parenter Enteral Nutr* 1998;22:167-182.
43. Buzby GP. Overview of randomized clinical trials of total parenteral nutrition for malnourished surgical patients. *World J Surg* 1993;17:173-177.
44. Bozzetti F, Gavazzi C, Miceli R, et al. Perioperative total parenteral nutrition in malnourished, gastrointestinal cancer patients: A randomized clinical trial. *J Parenter Enteral Nutr* 2000;24:7-14.
45. Petersen SR, Kudsk KA, Carpenter G, et al. Malnutrition and immunocompetence: Increased mortality following an infectious challenge during hyperalimentation. *J Trauma* 1981;21:528-533.
46. Kudsk KA, Carpenter G, Petersen S, et al. Effect of enteral and parenteral feeling in malnourished rats with *E. coli*-hemoglobin adjuvant peritonitis. *J Surg Res* 1981;31:105-110.

47. Kudsk KA, Stone JM, Carpenter G, et al. Enteral and parenteral feeding influences mortality after hemoglobin-*E. coli* peritonitis in normal rats. *J Trauma* 1983;23:605-609.
48. Moore EE, Jones TN. Benefits of immediate jejunostomy feeding after major abdominal trauma—a prospective, randomized study. *J Trauma* 1986;26:874-881.
49. Moore FA, Moore EE, Jones TN, et al. TEN versus TPN following major abdominal trauma - reduced septic morbidity. *J Trauma* 1989;29:916-922.
50. Kudsk KA, Croce MA, Fabian TC, et al. Enteral versus parenteral feeding. Effects on septic morbidity after blunt and penetrating abdominal trauma. *Ann Surg* 1992;215:503-513.
51. Moore FA, Feliciano DV, Andrassy RJ, et al. Early enteral feeding, compared with parenteral, reduces postoperative septic complications. The results of a meta-analysis. *Ann Surg* 1992;216:172-183.
52. Minard G, Kudsk KA. Nutritional support and infection: Does the route matter? *World J Surg* 1998;22:213-219.
53. MacFie J. Enteral versus parenteral nutrition: The significance of bacterial translocation and gut-barrier function. *Nutrition* 2000;16:606-611.
54. Braxton CC, Coyle SM, Montegut WJ, et al. Parenteral nutrition alters monocyte TNF receptor activity. *J Surg Res* 1995;59:23-28.
55. Takagi K, Yamamori H, Toyoda Y, et al. Modulating effects of the feeding route on stress response and endotoxin translocation in severely stressed patients receiving thoracic esophagectomy. *Nutrition* 2000;16:366-360.
56. Smith RC, Hartemink RJ, Hollinshead JW, et al. Fine bore jejunostomy feeding following major abdominal surgery: A controlled randomized clinical trial. *Br J Surg* 1985;72:458-461.
57. Beier-Holgersen R, Boesby S. Influence of postoperative enteral nutrition on postsurgical infections. *Gut* 1996;39:833-835.
58. Carr CS, Ling KD, Boulos P, et al. Randomised trial of safety and efficacy of immediate postoperative enteral feeding in patients undergoing gastrointestinal resection. *Br Med J* 1996;312:869-871.
59. Harrison LE, Hochwald SN, Heslin MJ, et al. Early postoperative enteral nutrition improves peripheral protein kinetics in upper gastrointestinal cancer patients undergoing complete resection: A randomized trial. *J Parenter Enteral Nutr* 1997;21:202-207.
60. Hochwald SN, Harrison LE, Heslin MJ, et al. Early postoperative enteral feeding improves whole body protein kinetics in upper gastrointestinal cancer patients. *Am J Surg* 1997;174:325-330.
61. Doglietto GB, Gallitelli L, Pacelli F, et al. Protein-sparing therapy after major abdominal surgery: Lack of clinical effects. Protein-Sparing Therapy Study Group. *Ann Surg* 1996;223:357-362.
62. Heslin MJ, Latkany L, Leung D, et al. A prospective, randomized trial of early enteral feeding after resection of upper gastrointestinal malignancy. *Ann Surg* 1997;226:567-580.
63. Brooks AD, Hochwald SN, Heslin MJ, et al. Intestinal permeability after early postoperative nutrition in patients with upper gastrointestinal malignancy. *J Parenter Enteral Nutr* 1999;23:75-79.

64. Watters JM, Kirkpatrick SM, Norris SB, et al. Immediate postoperative enteral feeding results in impaired respiratory mechanics and decreased mobility. *Ann Surg* 1997;226:369-380.
65. Haun JL, Thompson JS. Comparison of needle catheter versus standard tube jejunostomy. *Am Surg* 1985;51:466-469.
66. Gerndt SJ, Orringer MB. Tube jejunostomy as an adjunct to esophagectomy. *Surgery* 1994;115:164-169.
67. Myers JG, Page CP, Stewart RM, et al. Complications of needle catheter jejunostomy in 2,022 consecutive applications. *Am J Surg* 1995;170:547-551.
68. Swails WS, Babineau TJ, Ellis FH, et al. The role of enteral jejunostomy feeding after esophagogastrectomy: A prospective, randomized study. *Dis Esoph* 1995;8:193-199.
69. Wakefield SE, Mansell NJ, Baigrie RJ, et al. Use of a feeding jejunostomy after oesophagogastric surgery. *Br J Surg* 1995;82:811-813.
70. McCarter MD, Gomez ME, Daly JM. Early postoperative enteral feeding following major upper abdominal surgery. *J Gastrointest Surg* 1997;1:278-285.
71. De Gottardi A, Krahenbuhl L, Farhadi J, et al. Clinical experience of feeding through a needle catheter jejunostomy after major abdominal operations. *Eur J Surg* 1999;165:1055-1060.
72. Yagi M, Hashimoto T, Nezuka H, et al. Complications associated with enteral nutrition using catheter jejunostomy after esophagectomy. *Surg Today* 1999;29:214-218.
73. Hedberg AM, Lairson DR, Aday LA, et al. Economic implications of an early postoperative enteral feeding protocol. *J Am Diet Assoc* 1999;99:802-807.
74. Kemen M, Senkal M, Homann HH, et al. Early postoperative enteral nutrition with arginine-omega-3 fatty acids and ribonucleic acid-supplemented diet versus placebo in cancer patients: An immunologic evaluation of Impact. *Crit Care Med* 1995;23:652-659.
75. Senkal M, Kemen M, Homann HH, et al. Modulation of postoperative immune response by enteral nutrition with a diet enriched with arginine, RNA, and omega-3 fatty acids in patients with upper gastrointestinal cancer. *Eur J Surg* 1995;161:115-122.
76. Braga M, Gianotti L, Cestari A, et al. Gut function and immune and inflammatory responses in patients perioperatively fed with supplemented enteral formulas. *Arch Surg* 1996;131:1257-1265.
77. Braga M, Vignali A, Gianotti L, et al. Immune and nutritional effects of early enteral nutrition after major abdominal operations. *Eur J Surg* 1996;162:105-112.
78. Gianotti L, Braga M, Vignali A, et al. Effect of route of delivery and formulation of postoperative nutritional support in patients undergoing major operations for malignant neoplasms. *Arch Surg* 1997;1332:1222-1230.
79. Gianotti L, Braga M, Fortis C, et al. A prospective, randomized clinical trial on perioperative feeding with an arginine-, omega-3 fatty acid-, and RNA-enriched enteral diet: Effect on host response and nutritional status. *J Parenter Enteral Nutr* 1999;23:314-320.
80. Daly JM, Lieberman MD, Goldfine J, et al. Enteral nutrition with supplemental arginine, RNA, and omega-3 fatty acids in patients after operation: Immunologic, metabolic, and clinical outcome. *Surgery* 1992;112:56-67.

81. Hill ADK, Shou J, Weintraub FN, et al. Enteral nutrition with supplemental arginine in patients following esophageal resection. In Peracchia A, Rosati R, Bonavina L, et al. (eds): **Recent Advances in Diseases of the Esophagus**. Bologna, Monduzzi Editore, 1996, pp 1067-1071.
82. Senkal M, Mumme A, Eickoff U, et al. Early postoperative enteral immunonutrition: Clinical outcome and cost-comparison analysis in surgical patients. *Crit Care Med* 1997;25:1489-1496.
83. Braga M, Gianotti L, Radaelli G, et al. Perioperative immunonutrition in patients undergoing cancer surgery: Results of a randomized double-blind phase 3 trial. *Arch Surg* 1999;134:428-433.
84. Senkal M, Zumtobel V, Bauer KH, et al. Outcome and cost-effectiveness of perioperative enteral immunonutrition in patients undergoing elective upper gastrointestinal tract surgery: A prospective randomized study. *Arch Surg* 1999;134:1309-1316.
85. Beattie AH, Prach AT, Baxter JP, et al. A randomized controlled trial evaluating the use of enteral nutritional supplements postoperatively in malnourished surgical patients. *Gut* 2000;46:813-818.
86. Cui Y, Urschel JD. Latex rubber (Penrose drain) is detrimental to esophagogastric anastomotic healing in rats. *J Cardiovasc Surg* (Torino) 2000;41:479-481.
87. Horstmann O, Becker H, Verreet PR, et al. Insufficiency of cervical esophagogastrostomy: Results of a prospective randomized trial. In Peracchia A, Rosati R, Bonavina L, et al. (eds): **Recent Advances in Diseases of the Esophagus**. Bologna, Monduzzi Editore, 1996, pp 1023-1027.
88. Choi HK, Law S, Chu KM, e al. The value of neck drain in esophageal surgery: A randomized trial. *Dis Esoph* 1998;11:40-42.
89. Fan ST, Lau WY, Yip WC, et al. Limitations and dangers of gastrografin swallow after esophageal and upper gastric operations. *Am J Surg* 1988;155:495-497.
90. Goel AK, Sinha S, Chattopadhyay TK. Role of gastrografin study in the assessment of anastomotic leaks from cervical oesophagogastric anastomosis. *Aust NZ J Surg* 1995;65:8-10.
91. Tanomkiat W, Galassi W. Barium sulfate as contrast medium for evaluation of postoperative anastomotic leaks. *Acta Radiol* 2000;41:482-485.
92. Gollub MJ, Bains MS. Barium sulfate: A new (old) contrast agent for diagnosis of postoperative esophageal leaks. *Radiology* 1997;202:360-362.
93. Reichelt S, Eising EG, Pelster FW. Radiologische Kontrolle von Anastomoseninsuffizienzen nach Osophagusteilresektionen oder Gastrektomien. Effekte bariumhaltiger Kontrastmittel. *Rofo Fortschr Geb Rontgenstr Neuen Bildgeb Verfahr* 1991;154:388-392.
94. Hambraeus GM, Ekberg O, Fletcher R. Pharyngeal dysfunction after total and subtotal oesophagectomy. *Acta Radiol* 1987;28:409-413.
95. Heitmiller RF, Jones B. Transient diminished airway protection after transhiatal esophagectomy. *Am J Surg* 1991;162:442-446.
96. Easterling CS, Bousamra M II, Lang IM, et al. Pharyngeal dysphagia in postesophagectomy patients: Correlation with deglutitive biomechanics. *Ann Thorac Surg* 2000;69:989-992.
97. Cordeiro PG, Shah K, Santamaria E, et al. Barium swallows after free jejunal transfer: Should they be performed routinely? *Plast Reconstr Surg* 1999;103:1167-1175.

98. Ferguson MK. Management of esophageal anastomotic leaks. In Franco KL, Putnam JB Jr: **Advanced Therapy in Thoracic Surgery**. Hamilton, B.C. Decker Inc., 1998, pp 464-471.
99. Valverde A, Hay J-M, Fingerhut A, et al. for the French Association for Surgical Research. Manual versus mechanical esophagogastric anastomosis after resection for carcinoma: A controlled trial. *Surgery* 1996;120:476-483.
100. Fekete F, Breil P, Ronsse H, et al. EEA stapler and omental graft in esophagogastrectomy: Experience with 30 intrathoracic anastomoses for cancer. *Ann Surg* 1981;192:825-830.
101. Zieren HU, Muller JM, Pichlmaier H. Prospective randomized study of one- or two-layer anastomosis following oesophageal resection and cervical oesophagogastrostomy. *Br J Surg* 1993;80:608-611.
102. Ancona E, Bardini R, Nosadini A, et al. Esophagogastric anastomotic leakage. *Int Surg* 1982;67:143-145.
103. Moores LK. Smoking and postoperative pulmonary complications. An evidence-based review of the recent literature. *Clin Chest Med* 2000;21:139-146.
104. Hall JC, Tarala RA, Tapper J, et al. Prevention of respiratory complications after abdominal surgery: A randomised clinical trial. *Br Med J* 1996;312:148-153.
105. Chumillas S, Ponce JL, Delgado F, et al. Prevention of postoperative pulmonary complications through respiratory rehabilitation: A controlled clinical study. *Arch Phys Med Rehabil* 1998;79:5-9.
106. Celli BR, Rodriguez KS, Snider GL. A controlled trial of intermittent positive pressure breathing, incentive spirometry, and deep breathing exercises in preventing pulmonary complications after abdominal surgery. *Am Rev Respir Dis* 1984;130:12-15.
107. Hall JC, Tarala R, Harris J, et al. Incentive spirometry versus routine chest physiotherapy for prevention of pulmonary complications after abdominal surgery. *Lancet* 1991;337:953-956.
108. Gosselink R, Schrever K, Cops P, et al. Incentive spirometry does not enhance recovery- after thoracic surgery. *Crit Care Med* 2000;28:679-683.
109. Stiller KR, Munday RM. Chest physiotherapy for the surgical patient. *Br J Surg* 1992;79:745-749.
110. Caldwell MT, Murphy PG, Page R, et al. Timing of extubation after oesophagectomy. *Br J Surg* 1993;80:1537-1539.
111. Bartels H, Stein HJ, Siewert JR. Early extubation vs. late extubation after esophagus resection: A randomized, prospective study. *Langenbecks Arch Chir Suppl Kongressbd* 1998;115:1074-1076.
112. Wain JC, Wilson DJ, Mathisen DJ. Clinical experience with minitracheostomy. *Ann Thorac Surg* 1990;881-886.
113. Balkan ME, Ozdulger A, Tastepe I, et al. Clinical experience with minitracheotomy. *Scand J Thorac Cardiovasc Surg* 1996;30:93-96.

Chapter 17

Complications and Their Management

Complications occur frequently after esophageal reconstructive surgery. The ability to predict which patients are more likely to develop complications, an awareness of which complications are most common, knowledge of methods for prevention of complications, and the ability to manage complications when they occur ensure optimal outcomes for patients undergoing esophageal reconstruction. Complications that are related to specific types of reconstruction, such as anastomotic leak, anastomotic stricture, delayed gastric emptying, and necrosis of the reconstructive organ, are discussed in detail in previous chapters. Many complications associated with esophageal reconstruction are more likely due to the resection portion of the procedure than to the reconstructive portion. This chapter will focus on general short-term and long-term complications associated with esophageal reconstruction and will highlight aspects of those complications that are particularly related to reconstruction rather than resection. As a result, general complications that occur, such as bleeding, infection (apart from those due to anastomotic leak or dehiscence), stroke, renal insufficiency, and mortality are not discussed in this text. A good summary of such problems is available in a number of general surgical or thoracic surgical texts. Table 17-1 summarizes the overall risk of complications which were retrospectively assessed after esophagectomy and reconstruction for both benign and malignant causes.[1-11] More accurate estimates are generated by prospective assessments of specific complications, which are detailed below.

Pulmonary Complications

The incidence of pulmonary complications after esophagectomy and reconstruction in series analyzed specifically for these types of adverse

From Ferguson MK: *Reconstructive Surgery of the Esophagus* Armonk, NY: Futura Publishing Company, Inc., © 2002.

Table 17-1.
Complications after Esophageal Reconstruction.

Author	Year	Patients	Pulmonary	Cardiac	RLN[1] injury	CVA[2]	Renal insufficiency	Hemorrhage	Chylothorax	PE[3]
Pac et al.[1]	1993	238	22	2[4]	16	5	1	—	—	—
Putnam et al.[2]	1994	221	20	41	4	—	—	5	9	—
O'Rourke et al.[3]	1995	116	27	7	1	—	—	3	—	5
Svanes et al.[4]	1995	83	25	—	7	—	—	—	4	3
Anikin et al.[5]	1997	113	5	—	3	—	1	—	2	1
Ferguson et al.[6]	1997	269	86	98	—	—	1	—	10	2
Orringer et al.[7]	1999	1076	—	—	74	—	—	8	18	—
Johansson et al.[8]	2000	120	7	17	3	—	—	2	1	—
Karl et al.[9]	2000	143	20	19	—	—	—	—	—	1
Kolh et al.[10]	2000	130	25	5	4	1	3	3	—	—
Young et al.[11]	2000	142	59	45	15	—	—	2	—	—
Totals		2651	296/1575 (18.8%)	232/1141 (20.3%)	127/2239 (5.7%)	6/368 (1.6%)	6/750 (0.8%)	23/1805 (1.3%)	44/1882 (2.3%)	12/724 (1.7%)

1. Recurrent laryngeal nerve injury
2. Cerebrovascular accident
3. Pulmonary embolism
4. Arrhythmias not included in the analysis; this value is excluded from the calculation of the overall total incidence for the table.

events is about 40%, including pneumonia in almost 30%, respiratory failure in 15%, and atelectasis in nearly 5% of patients. There is also an assortment of other less common pulmonary complications, which include pleural effusion, pneumothorax, hypoxemia, adult respiratory distress syndrome, prolonged initial ventilation, bronchopleural fistula, and airway-enteric fistula.[12-14] The development of pulmonary complications is associated with a five- to ten-fold increase in the risk of operative mortality, and pulmonary complications are responsible for up to 60% of operative deaths after esophagectomy and reconstruction.[13-15]

There is a growing understanding of the etiology of some of these complications.[16] Dysfunction of respiratory muscles and changes in chest wall mechanics lead to a 30% decrease in functional residual capacity (FRC) during the first postoperative week after thoracotomy or upper abdominal surgery. FRC also decreases in patients who are supine or obese and as a result of general anesthesia. Another element that is important in the development of respiratory complications after esophageal reconstruction is the closing volume (CV), which is the lung volume at which the flow from dependent parts of the lungs stops during expiration due to airway closure. Closing volume increases in patients with advanced age and due to tobacco use, fluid overload, bronchospasm, and the presence of airway secretions. As FRC decreases and CV increases, portions of the lung undergo premature airway closure and develop atelectasis. This causes ventilation-perfusion mismatch resulting in hypoxemia and trapping of secretions leading to pneumonia. Most patients who are candidates for esophageal reconstruction have some of the risk factors leading to a decrease in FRC and an increase in CV, which helps explain the high rate of pulmonary complications in this group of individuals.

In addition to general factors that promote changes in FRC and CV, other clinical factors have been identified which predispose patients undergoing esophagectomy and reconstruction to the development of pulmonary complications. Preoperative factors include such things as decreased spirometric values, the presence of hepatic cirrhosis, advanced stage of cancer (for patients undergoing reconstruction after resection for malignancy), advanced age, reduced diffusing capacity, poor performance capacity, evidence for chronic obstructive pulmonary disease (COPD), poor nutritional status, and abnormalities on the chest radiograph.[12,13,15,16] Intraoperative factors that predispose patients to respiratory complications include excessive blood loss, use of the substernal rather than the posterior mediastinal route for reconstruction, routine use of ventilatory support rather than early extubation postoperatively, inclusion of laparotomy as part of the surgical approach, and palliation as an indication for surgery.[13,15,17-19] The creation of a cervical esophageal anastomosis predisposes patients to aspiration, and the risk of aspiration is greatly magnified in patients in whom a recurrent laryngeal nerve injury occurs.[20-22]

Management of pulmonary complications must be individualized. Patients are evaluated for a possible pneumothorax, and a thoracostomy tube is placed if one is identified. Most patients will have some element of hypoxemia, and administration of supplemental oxygen sufficient to maintain arterial oxygen saturation above 90% is appropriate. In some patients, there may be an element of bronchospasm due either to underlying COPD or to microaspiration, and administration of bronchodilators is effective in reversing this problem. Minimizing postoperative pain aids in the performance of pulmonary toilet exercises, which include coughing, deep breathing, and the use of an incentive spirometer. Broad spectrum antibiotics are administered to patients in whom pneumonia is suspected, and if aspiration pneumonia is suspected, antibiotics effective against gram positive oral anaerobes are provided. If the patient is having difficulty clearing secretions, nasotracheal suctioning is performed by a skilled practitioner; excessive trauma to a newly created anastomosis should be avoided. The use of a minitracheostomy may be considered to help in the clearance of retained secretions.[23-25] In more tenuous situations treatment of hypoxemia and respiratory impairment is provided noninvasively by use of biphasic positive airway pressure (BiPAP) delivered through a mask.[26] This is particularly effective in patients with underlying COPD and may help avoid reintubation. Reintubation and positive pressure ventilation are necessary when true respiratory failure develops.

The need for prolonged intubation raises the issue of the timing and appropriateness of temporary tracheostomy. There is no general agreement as to whether a tracheostomy should be created relatively early (within 7 to 10 days of intubation) or delayed until efforts at ventilatory weaning have failed.[27] Most clinicians agree that patients who require ventilatory support for less than 10 days do not require a tracheostomy, and that patients who require support for more than 2 or 3 weeks should have a tracheostomy.[28] The problem arises in predicting which patient is going to require prolonged intubation. Although airway trauma resulting from long-term use of either translaryngeal intubation or tracheostomy is common, earlier conversion to a tracheostomy may decrease the risk of trauma to the posterior commissure of the larynx and may shorten the duration of mechanical ventilation, ICU stay, and hospital stay.[29-31] Even though evidence generally supports the early use of a tracheostomy in critically ill patients who require ventilatory support for more than 10 days, caution must be exercised in patients who have undergone recent esophageal reconstruction, particularly those who have a cervical anastomosis. The creation of a tracheostomy in a patient who is already prone to problems of aspiration due to deglutitive dysfunction may make satisfactory swallowing very difficult for an extended period of time after

Table 17-2.
Clinical Predictors of Increased Perioperative Cardiac Events.*

Major:
Unstable coronary syndromes
Recent myocardial infarction with evidence of important ischemic risk by clinical symptoms or noninvasive study
Unstable or severe angina (Canadian Class III or IV)
Decompensated congestive heart failure
Significant arrhythmias
High-grade atrioventricular block
Symptomatic ventricular arrhythmias in the presence of underlying heart disease
Sever valvular disease
Intermediate:
Mild angina pectoris (Canadian Class I or II)
Prior myocardial infarction by history or pathological Q waves
Compensated or prior congestive heart failure
Diabetes mellitus
Minor:
Advanced age
Abnormal ECG (left ventricular hypertrophy, left bundle branch block, ST-T abnormalities)
Rhythm other than sinus (e.g., atrial fibrillation)
Low functional capacity (e.g., inability to climb one flight of stairs with a bag of groceries)
History of stroke
Uncontrolled systemic hypertension

*Modified from: ACC/AHA Task Force Report: Guideline for perioperative cardiovascular evaluation for non-cardiac surgery. J Am Coll Cardiol 27:910-948, 1996.

successful wean from the ventilator. In addition, local wound problems related to a cervical anastomotic leak may be difficult to manage if a tracheostomy is created.

Cardiovascular Complications

Cardiovascular complications occur with alarming frequency in patients after esophageal reconstruction despite the careful preoperative screening that most patients receive. The overall incidence of such complications of about 15% quoted in Table 17-1 is likely an underestimate of the real rate of their occurrence. General risk factors for perioperative cardiovascular complications have been stratified and are listed in Table 17-2.[32] It is unlikely that many patients who have major clinical predictors of perioperative cardiac events will undergo esophageal reconstruction, but the presence of intermediate predictors is likely to be quite high in this patient population.

Arrhythmias

The most common cardiovascular complications that occur after esophagectomy and reconstruction are tachydysrhythmias. These are usually supraventricular and include atrial fibrillation in two-thirds of affected patients as well as atrial flutter and supraventricular tachycardia. About one-third of patients who undergo esophagectomy and reconstruction suffer such arrhythmias, which tend to develop during the first three postoperative days.[33] Some rhythm disturbances do not produce clinical symptoms, but two-thirds are associated with hypotension.[34,35] The etiology of such arrhythmias is thought to be injury to and subsequent inflammation in sympathetic and parasympathetic fibers supplying the heart (cardiac plexus) which modulate the response of atrial myocardial cells to circulating catecholamines.[36] The fact that arrhythmias occur more frequently in patients with advanced age may be related to the fact that only 10% of normal sinus node pacemaker cells remain in patients over 75 years of age.[37]

The development of supraventricular arrhythmias is associated with an increased duration of hospital stay, indicating that prevention and effective treatment of these abnormalities are important goals.[35,38] Efforts at reducing the incidence of tachydysrhythmias have focused on chemical prophylaxis. Studies investigating the utility of perioperative digoxin for this purpose have shown no benefit to its use.[34,39] Beta blockade with propranolol has demonstrated potential benefit in reducing the incidence of supraventricular arrhythmias after general thoracic surgical procedures, although the incidence of associated side effects is high.[40] Whether this approach is appropriate for patients undergoing esophageal reconstruction is not known.

Initial management of supraventricular arrhythmias is focused on rate control and possible chemical conversion to sinus rhythm. For patients with atrial fibrillation, an appropriate ventricular response rate is best established with digoxin, a calcium channel blocker, or beta blockade. Conversion to sinus rhythm is most effectively achieved with amiodarone, although digoxin and procainamide are sometimes successful. If chemical conversion fails, electrical conversion may be considered.[41] The likelihood of achieving a sustained conversion to sinus rhythm with any of these treatments is lessened by underlying risk factors such as a history of prior arrhythmias, left ventricular dysfunction, and atrial dilatation. If fibrillation persists, then consideration should be given to anticoagulation to prevent thromboembolic complications.

Atrial flutter does not occur commonly as a complication of esophagectomy and reconstruction. Its etiology is much different than that of atrial fibrillation, having been traced to the existence of a flutter circuit within the atrium which permits slow conduction that facilitates the development of atrial flutter.[42] Chemical conversion with ibutilide is successful in three-quarters of patients whereas procainamide is effective in fewer than 20% of affected patients.[43] Because of the existence of a single reentrant circuit, radiofrequency catheter ablation is now favored as an initial therapy for atrial flutter, with success rates of about 90% in patients with normal ventricular function and no history of prior atrial arrhythmias.[44]

Supraventricular tachycardia is often a physiologic response to stress or an early sign of sepsis or pericardial irritation. Efforts at evaluating these types of underlying causes are appropriate before investigation of other etiologies is undertaken. On occasion it is important to slow the heart rate with judicious use of beta blockade if no specific source of tachycardia is discovered. In some patients, supraventricular tachycardia is caused by an accessory pathway, reentry within the atrioventricular node, or atrial tachycardia. In such instances, radiofrequency ablation has a high likelihood of eliminating the tachycardia.[45]

Ventricular arrhythmias occur relatively infrequently after esophageal resection and reconstruction in the absence of preoperative evidence for such abnormalities.[33] Ventricular premature contractions (VPCs) are the most common types of ventricular arrhythmias that occur postoperatively and are usually evident within the first 24 hours after surgery. Ventricular tachyarrhythmias such as flutter and fibrillation are uncommon and will not be discussed further. Management of VPCs must be individualized because their etiology is usually multifactorial and they rarely cause symptoms or hemodynamic compromise. Most often they are related to relative hypoxia or potassium imbalance, and simple correction of these problems is all that is required.

Myocardial Infarction

Esophageal reconstruction poses stresses to cardiac performance that patients do not often experience during their normal daily activities. If an assessment of an individual patient's risk for cardiac events as outlined in Table 17-2 is performed routinely, patients at higher than average risk will be referred for appropriate preoperative evaluation, permitting underlying problems to be corrected preoperatively. Avoidance of prolonged elevations or decreases in mean arterial blood pressure also reduces the incidence of myocardial ischemia or infarct in patients undergoing noncardiac major surgery.[46] Use of these algorithms results in an incidence of myocardial infarction in esophageal reconstruction patients of less than 2%.[1,6,8,10,18] Ischemic events generally occur during the first or second postoperative day, which is the period of maximum cardiac stress. Such events can be classified according clinical, electrocardiographic, and laboratory abnormalities as follows: grade 1) asymptomatic ischemic ECG changes without evidence of myocardial necrosis; grade 2) symptomatic ischemic ECG changes without evidence of myocardial necrosis; grade 3) acute myocardial infarction (documented myocardial necrosis); grade 4) acute myocardial infarction requiring intervention (inotrope support, intra-aortic balloon pump, coronary artery bypass grafting). Recommendations for clinical management of myocardial ischemia or necrosis are beyond the scope if this text.

Pulmonary Embolism

Pulmonary embolism is an infrequent complication of esophageal reconstructive surgery, occurring in about 2% of patients postoperatively.[3,5,9,47] Risk factors for postoperative pulmonary embolism in patients undergoing major surgery include age greater than 40 years, prolonged immobility, prior venous thromboembolism, malignancy, obesity, varicose veins, congestive heart failure, myocardial infarction, stroke, any hypercoagulable state, and possibly the use of high dose estrogens.[36] Prevention of thromboembolic problems is the key to success. The use of perioperative low dose heparin may decrease the incidence of such complications, as may the use of intermittent pneumatic compression devices for the lower extremities.[47]

The diagnosis of pulmonary embolism is not always straightforward in patients who have undergone thoracic surgery. Clinical signs and symptoms include tachycardia, respiratory distress, an altered mental state, and possibly chest pain. In more serious instances patients exhibit cyanosis, shock, and loss of consciousness. A common method of diagnosing pulmonary embolism is with a lung scintigram. There is frequently evidence for segmental hypoperfusion in individuals after thoracic surgery, and correlating areas of hypoperfusion with those of underventilation on a lung scintigram is not always accurate.[48] Other diagnostic techniques include spiral computed tomography, D-dimer assay, or pulmonary arteriogram. Some patients who are critically ill as a result of a pulmonary embolism are not candidates for computed tomography or arteriography because of their unstable clinical condition, and arteriography has its own inherent risks despite its high degree of accuracy.[49,50] Initial management of pulmonary embolism includes heparinization and consideration may be given to the use of thrombolytic agents in some patients. A more detailed discussion of the management of pulmonary embolism is beyond the scope of this text.

Recurrent Laryngeal Nerve Injury

Injury to one or both recurrent laryngeal nerves is most often a consequence of esophageal resection but may also be due to the technique used for esophageal reconstruction. Nerve injuries occur on the side on which the reconstruction is performed in 85% of patients, about 10% of patients have contralateral nerve palsy, and fewer than 5% have bilateral injuries.[51,52] Recurrent nerve injury is more common as a result of a reconstruction using a cervical anastomosis as compared to an intrathoracic anastomosis.[1,18,53,54] The course of the recurrent laryngeal nerves dictates the relative risk of injury, which is higher if the anastomosis is created through a right neck incision than if a left neck incision is used.[55,56] Nerve injury may be more common following a transhiatal resection than after a transthoracic resection in which the anastomosis is created in the neck, suggesting that blunt dissection of the upper thoracic esophagus rather than the site of the anastomosis may put patients at excess risk for recurrent nerve injury.[1,2,5,18,51-54] However, some surgeons who use the transhiatal approach for esophagectomy report very low rates of recurrent laryngeal nerve injury, suggesting that experience in performing the operation is more important than the technique used.[7]

The presence of a recurrent nerve injury is suspected on the basis of postoperative hoarseness, although up to 25% of patients with hoarseness after esophageal reconstruction do not have a nerve injury and nearly 20% of patients with a nerve injury do not exhibit signs of hoarseness of ineffective cough.[51] In some reports, recurrent nerve injury is associated with an increase in pulmonary complications and a prolonged ICU stay.[52] These injuries are associated with postoperative dysphagia which is usually self-limiting.[57]

In the majority of patients, hoarseness and ineffective cough due to recurrent nerve injury resolve with time. This does not necessarily indicate that the nerve injury and vocal cord dysfunction are transient, because in many instances glottic function normalizes due to compensation by the unaffected vocal cord. When resolution of symptoms does not occur within 3 to 6 months, medialization of the affected vocal cord may be considered by any of a variety of techniques, including injection of foreign material, neuromuscular transfer, or implant via thyroplasty.[58-60] Under unusual circumstances, urgent medialization during the initial hospitalization may be necessary if a patient's pulmonary function is significantly impaired due to ineffective cough or a substantially increased risk of aspiration. Over 90% of patients will have resolution of their symptoms after such procedures.

Chylothorax

The development of a chylothorax after esophagectomy and reconstruction is almost exclusively a function of the resection rather than of reconstruction portion of the operation. However, a brief discussion of this complication is useful because there is a lack of an appropriate sense of urgency in its management on the part of many surgeons and because new techniques have recently been introduced for its correction. Chylothorax develops in fewer than 5% of patients after esophagectomy and reconstruction and is usually a result of injury to the thoracic duct.[2,5-7,61-64] The variable anatomy of the thoracic duct puts it at risk for injury as a result of almost any surgical approach to esophagectomy and reconstruction.[65] The diagnosis of chylothorax is usually straightforward. A pleural fluid collection develops, or there is excessive thoracostomy tube drainage, either of which is milky white and contains trigylcerides at a concentration greater than 110 mg/100 mL.[66] Caution must be exercised in situations in which there is a suspicion of a chyle leak but the triglyceride level is low. Lack of oral or enteral intake of fatty foods may lead to a falsely low triglyceride level. If this is suspected to be the case, test feeding and repeat measurement of the fluid triglyceride level is appropriate.

A persistent chyle leak can lead to immune suppression, malnutrition, and fluid and electrolyte imbalances. Immediate intervention is appropriate, which includes fluid repletion, allowing the patient nothing by mouth, and drainage of the pleural space. In two-thirds of patients, such conservative management will lead to spontaneous closure of the injury. A relatively low output of chyle through the thoracostomy tube during the initial period of observation may indicate the likelihood of success with this therapy.[63] In patients who do not experience spontaneous closure of the chyle leak within 7 days it is appropriate to consider surgical intervention to prevent ongoing debilitation and associated complications. Intervention consists of ligation of the site of leak if it can be identified, or mass ligation of tissues which encompass the thoracic duct as it emerges into the chest through the aortic hiatus, a procedure that is usually performed through the right chest. Thoracoscopic ligation of the thoracic duct has proven successful in selected patients with postoperative chylothorax.[67,68]

Herniation of Abdominal Contents

Herniation of abdominal contents through the esophageal hiatus fortunately is a rare complication of esophageal reconstructive surgery which occurs in fewer than 5% of patients. About half of the instances are identified acutely and the remainder become evident during long-term postoperative follow-up of patients. Herniated contents usually include small bowel or colon, and herniation of other structures such as liver or spleen is unusual (Figure 17-1). Most hernias produce symptoms such as epigastric or postprandial pain, nausea, vomiting, chest pressure, and dyspnea.

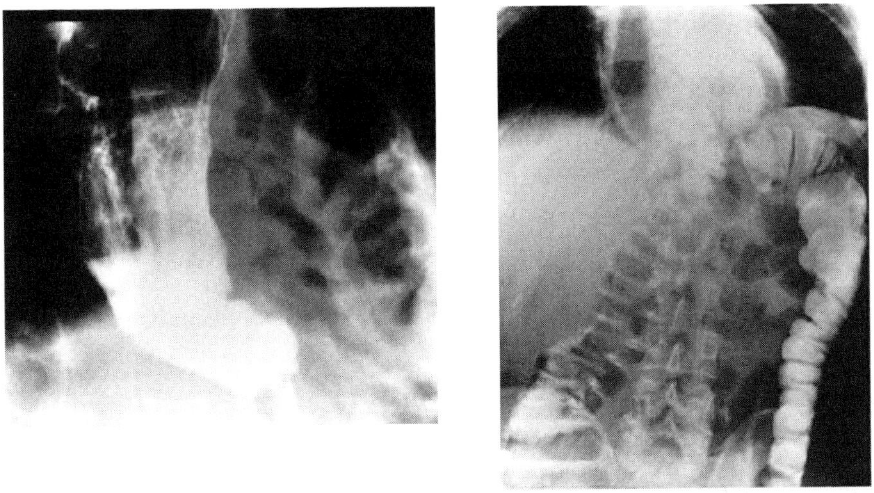

Figure 17-1. Herniation of colon through the esophageal hiatus after esophageal surgery. Reprinted by permission of the Society of Thoracic Surgeons, *Annals of Thoracic Surgery* 1997;63:554-556.

Risk factors for the development of herniation are use of an incision to enlarge the esophageal hiatus or partial diaphragmatic resection as part of an en bloc esophagectomy.[69] Intraoperative techniques to help prevent this complication include suturing the reconstructive organ to the crura at multiple sites and narrowing of the hiatus with crural stitches while maintaining a sufficient opening so that the reconstructive organ will not be obstructed. When herniation of abdominal contents through the esophageal hiatus is diagnosed, it is usually necessary to perform a repair to prevent obstruction and strangulation.

Late Complications

Dumping Syndrome

Dumping syndrome is a constellation of postprandial symptoms including abdominal distension, cramping abdominal pain, diaphoresis, tachycardia, palpitations, and urgent diarrhea. The etiology of the syndrome has been variously ascribed to rapid hyperglycemia followed by hypoglycemia, jejunal distension, or intraluminal sequestration of fluid caused by hyperosmolar jejunal content.[70] More recently, activation of the renin-aldosterone axis accompanied by a decrease in plasma atrial natriuretic peptide, reflecting a hypovolemic state, have been identified as causative factors.[71] These symptoms occur in up to 20% of patients after esophageal reconstruction and are more common among patients who have undergone a gastric emptying procedure.[72] Fortunately, severe symptoms occur in fewer than 5% of patients, symptoms are usually self-limiting after 6 months, and relief is provided by simple dietary modifications in most patients. Effective dietary modifications include eating slowly, avoiding drinking fluids during meals, ingesting small, frequent meals, and avoiding high carbohydrate meals and milk products. The use of antidiarrheal agents may also be of benefit. In patients with refractory symptoms, administration of the somatostatin analogue octreotide slows gastric emptying, reduces monosaccharide absorption, and prevents hemodynamic changes.[73,74]

Delayed Gastric Emptying

Delayed gastric emptying affects about 10% of patients in the early postoperative period, and symptoms persist in a substantial portion of these patients even 6 months postoperatively. Symptoms of gastric stasis are more common among patients who have not undergone an emptying procedure, and include early satiety, regurgitation, and epigastric discomfort.[75] Initial management is outlined in Chapter 14. Patients who have persistent symptoms despite the use of dietary modifications may respond to prokinetic agents such as metoclopramide or erythromycin. When these measures are ineffective, consideration should be given to performance of a gastric emptying procedure. This can be accomplished with balloon dilation or surgical pyloromyotomy or pyloroplasty.[76]

Unusual complications

Esophageal Mucocele

The esophagus is not resected in some reconstructive operations necessitated by esophageal injury and in all esophageal bypass operations for obstructive malignancy. The excluded esophagus develops into a cystic structure, and there is some evidence that the growth of this cyst is regulated by the pressure that develops within it, resulting in destruction of mucus glands by higher pressures. In other patients, chronic inflammation or caustic injury destroy the esophageal mucosa, resulting in obliteration of the lumen after exclusion has been accomplished. In some individuals, however, low intraluminal pressures and retained normal mucosa may lead to the continued generation of mucus and the development

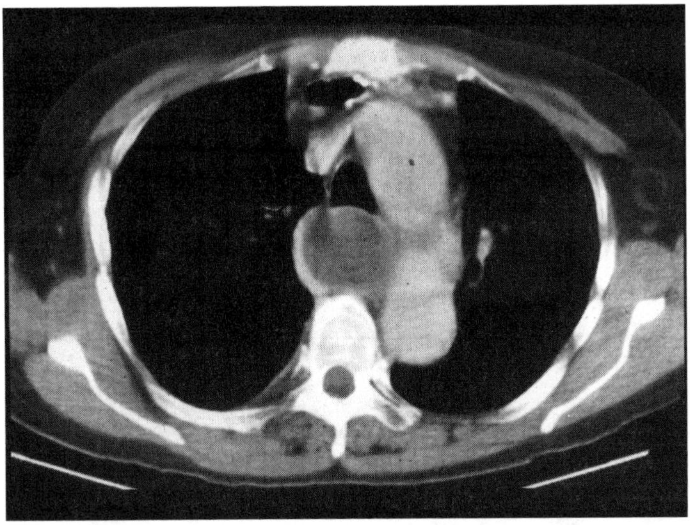

Figure 17-2. Esophageal mucocele after exclusion and reconstruction following spontaneous perforation.

of a mucocele (Figure 17-2). In two series, the incidence of mucocele development in the excluded esophagus was 40% to 50%.[77,78] Mucoceles typically develop within the first couple of months after esophageal exclusion, and are recognized as a posterior mediastinal fluid-filled mass on computed tomography. Mucoceles may cause pain, respiratory distress, or nausea, and there are reports of their becoming infected.[79,80] Most mucoceles remain small and asymptomatic, and require no specific therapy.[77,78] Resection is recommended if symptoms develop. In patients in whom resection is not possible, internal drainage or percutaneous drainage may be appropriate.

Recanalization of the Excluded Esophagus

Esophageal peristalsis is preserved after reconstructive operations for patients in whom the native esophagus is retained and excluded.[81] This condition predisposes such patients to spontaneously recanalize the distal esophagus, resulting in the development of an esophageal fistula.[82] The problem is best avoided by decompressing the excluded esophagus. Decompression is intrinsically provided when an esophageal-airway fistula exists as the indication for esophageal bypass surgery. Placement of a drainage catheter into the proximal thoracic esophagus as a means to decompress the distal esophagus does not always prevent recanalization and fistula formation. Some surgeons have suggested that a distal esopha-

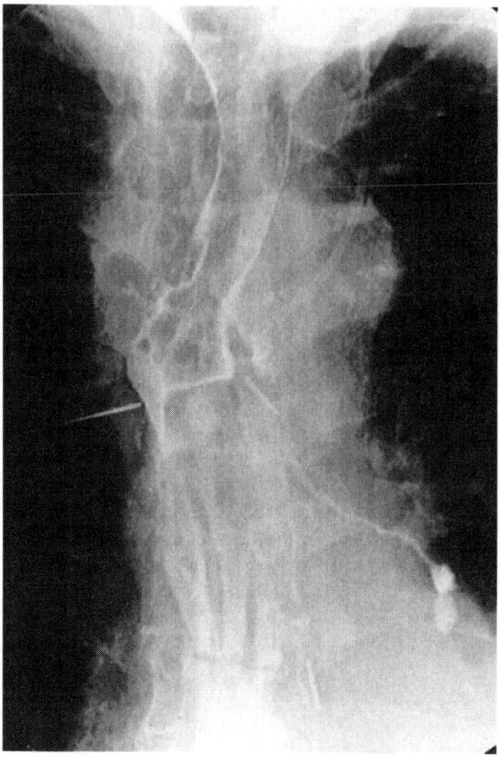

Figure 17-3. Gastro-bronchial fistula which occurred 2 years after esophagectomy and stomach pull-up for esophageal cancer. Reprinted by permission of the Society of Thoracic Surgeons, *Annals of Thoracic Surgery*, 2001;72:221-224.

gostomy should be created posteriorly at the level of the eighth rib in patients in whom decompression is otherwise not possible.[83]

Enteric-Airway Fistula

Placement of an esophageal reconstructive organ in the posterior mediastinum, adjacent to the major airways, invites the development of a fistula between the reconstructive organ and the airway. Fortunately, this is a rare complication of esophageal reconstructive surgery. Acute fistula formation may result from intraoperative trauma to the airway or dissection of an anastomotic leak into the airway. The mechanisms for development of a fistula many months or years after esophageal reconstructive surgery are not well understood. Most such fistulas occur after gastric pull-up, which is the most common means for esophageal reconstruction (Figure 17-3). Certain characteristics of the gastric conduit may help explain why fistulas develop almost exclusively in these organs. It is hypothesized that the long staple line used to close the lesser curvature may erode into the airway over time.[84,85] Alternatively, supradiaphragmatic gastric stasis may predispose patients to the development of benign gastric ulcers, which in some instances burrow into the airway. Most of the reported fistulas are benign and are not associated with recurrence of an esophageal cancer.

Enteric-airway fistulas seldom close spontaneously and eventually lead to fatal aspiration pneumonia if they are not closed. In patients who cannot tolerate open repair through a thoracotomy, placement of a coated stent in the airway may provide temporary relief. Long-term success with this technique is unlikely because of erosion of the stent into surrounding soft tissues. Most patients with a benign airway-enteric fistula after esophageal reconstructive surgery should undergo repair through a right thoracotomy or a cervical incision, depending on the level of the fistula. The fistula is divided and the reconstructive organ is repaired primarily. When possible the airway defect is closed primarily, and in all patients a muscle flap is placed over the airway defect to secure its closure.

References

1. Pac M, Basoglu A, Kocak H, et al. Transhiatal versus transthoracic esophagectomy for esophageal cancer. *J Thorac Cardiovasc Surg* 1993;106:205-209.
2. Putnam JB Jr, Suell DM, McMurtrey MJ, et al. Camparison of three techniques of esophagectomy within a residency training program. *Ann Thorac Surg* 1994;57:319-325.
3. O'Rourke I, Tait N, Bull C, et al. Oesophageal cancer: Outcome of modern surgical management. *Aust NZ J Surg* 1995;65:11-16.
4. Svanes K, Stangeland L, Viste A, et al. Morbidity, ability to swallow, and survival, after oesophagectomy for cancer of the oesophagus and cardia. *Eur J Surg* 1995;161:669-675.
5. Anikin VA, McManus KG, Graham AN, et al. Total thoracic esophagectomy for esophageal cancer. *J Am Coll Surg* 1997;185:525-529.
6. Ferguson MK, Martin TR, Reeder LB, Olak J. Mortality after esphagectomy: Risk factor analysis. *World J Surg* 1997;21:599-604.
7. Orringer MB, Marshall B, Iannettoni MD. Transhiatal esophagectomy: Clinical experience and refinements. *Ann Surg* 1999;230:392-403.
8. Johansson J, Walther B. Clinical outcome and long-term survival rates after esophagectomy are not determined by age over 70 years. *J Gastrointest Surg* 2000;4:55-62.
9. Karl RC, Schreiber R, Boulware D, et al. Factors affecting morbidity, mortality, and survival in patients undergoing Ivor Lewis esophagogastrectomy. *Ann Surg* 2000;231:635-643.
10. Kolh P, Honore P, Degauque C, et al. Early stage results after oesophageal resection for malignancy - colon interposition vs. gastric pull-up. *Eur J Cardio-Thorac Surg* 2000;18:293-300.

11. Young MM, Deschamps C, Trastek VF, et al. Esophageal reconstruction for benign disease: Early morbidity, mortality, and functional results. *Ann Thorac Surg* 2000;70:1651-1655.
12. Nagawa H, Kobori O, Muto T. Prediction of pulmonary complications after transthoracic oesophagectomy. *Br J Surg* 1994;81:860-862.
13. Ferguson MK, Martin TR, Reeder LB, et al. Determinants of pulmonary complications following esophagectomy. In Peracchia A, Rosati R, Bonavina L, et al. (eds): **Recent Advances in Diseases of the Esophagus**. Bologna, Monduzzi Editore, 1996, pp 527-532.
14. Hennessy TPJ. Respiratory complications in oesophageal surgery. In Peracchia A, Rosati R, Bonavina L, et al. (eds): **Recent Advances in Diseases of the Esophagus**. Bologna, Monduzzi Editore, 1996, pp 533-535.
15. Law SY, Fok M, Wong J. Risk analysis in resection of squamous cell carcinoma of the esophagus. *World J Surg* 1994;18:339-346.
16. Ferguson MK. Preoperative assessment of pulmonary risk. *Chest* 1999;115:58S-63S.
17. Bartels H, Thorban S, Siewert JR. Anterior versus posterior reconstruction after transhiatal oesophagectomy: A randomized controlled trial. *Br J Surg* 1993;80:1141-1144.
18. Stark SP, Romberg MS, Pierce GE, et al. Transhiatal versus transthoracic esophagectomy for adenocarcinoma of the distal esophagus and cardia. *Am J Surg* 1996;172:478-482.
19. Bartels H, Stein HJ, Siewert JR. Early extubation vs. late extubation after esophagus resection: A randomized, prospective study. *Langenbecks Arch Chir Suppl Kongressbd* 1998;115:1074-1076.
20. Hambraeus GM, Ekberg O, Fletcher R. Pharyngeal dysfunction after total and subtotal oesophagectomy. *Acta Radiol* 1987;28:409-413.
21. Heitmiller RF, Jones B. Transient diminished airway protection after transhiatal esophagectomy. *Am J Surg* 1991;162:442-446.
22. Easterling CS, Bousamra M II, Lang IM, et al. Pharyngeal dysphagia in postesophagectomy patients: Correlation with deglutitive biomechanics. *Ann Thorac Surg* 2000;69:989-992.
23. Wain JC, Wilson DJ, Mathisen DJ. Clinical experience with minitracheostomy. *Ann Thorac Surg* 1990;881-886.
24. Balkan ME, Ozdulger A, Tastepe I, et al. Clinical experience with minitracheotomy. *Scand J Thorac Cardiovasc Surg* 1996;30:93-96.
25. Van Raemdonck D, Cooseman W, De Leyn P, et al. Experience with minitracheostomy following oesophageal resection. In Peracchia A, Rosati R, Bonavina L, et al (eds): **Recent Advances in Diseases of the Esophagus**. Bologna, Monduzzi Editore, 1996, pp 541-545. 26. Kramer N, Meyer TJ, Meharg J, et al. Randomized, prospective trial of noninvasive positive pressure ventilation in acute respiratory failure. *Am J Respir Crit Care Med* 1995;151:1799-1806.
27. Blosser SA, Stauffer JL. Intubation of critically ill patients. *Clin Chest Med* 1996;17:355-378.
28. Gibbons KJ. Tracheostomy: Timing is everything. *Crit Care Med* 2000;28:1663-1664.
29. Stauffer JL, Olson DE, Petty TL. Complications and consequences of endotracheal intubation and tracheotomy. A prospective study of 150 critically ill adult patients. *Am J Med* 1981;70:65-76.

30. Whited RE. A prospective study of laryngotracheal sequelae in long-term intubation. *Laryngosope* 1984;94:367-377.
31. Rodriguez JL, Steinberg SM, Luchetti FA, et al. Early tracheostomy for primary management in the surgical critical care setting. *Surgery* 1990;108:655-659.
32. ACC/AHA Task Force Report: Guideline for perioperative cardiovascular evaluation for non-cardiac surgery. *J Am Coll Cardiol* 1996;27:910-948.
33. Konno O, Haga Y, Ogawa T, et al. Study of postoperative arrhythmias after operation for esophageal cancer. In Nabeya K, Hanaoka T, Nogami H (eds): **Recent Advances in Diseases of the Esophagus**. Tokyo, Springer-Verlag, 1993, pp 1072-1078.
34. Ritchie AJ, Whiteside M, Tolan M, et al. Cardiac dysrhythmia in total thoracic oesophagectomy. *Eur J Cardio-Thorac Surg* 1993;7:420-422.
35. Amar D, Burt ME, Bains MS, et al. Symptomatic tachydysrhythmias after esophagectomy: Incidence and outcome. *Ann Thorac Surg* 1996;61:1506-1509.
36. Amar D. Cardiopulmonary complications of esophageal surgery. *Chest Surg Clin N Am* 1997;7:449-456.
37. Wei JY. Age and the cardiovascular system. *N Engl J Med* 1992;327:1735-1739.
38. Polanczyk CA, Goldman L, Marcantonio ER, et al. Supraventricular arrhythmia in patients having noncardiac surgery: Clinical correlates and effect on length of stay. *Ann Intern Med* 1998;129:279-285.
39. Ritchie AJ, Tolan M, Whiteside M, et al. Prophylactic digitalization fails to control dysrhythmia in thoracic esophageal operations. *Ann Thorac Surg* 1993;55:86-88.
40. Bayliff CD, Massel DR, Inculet RI, et al. Propranolol for the prevention of postoperative arrhythmias in general thoracic surgery. *Ann Thorac Surg* 1999;67:182-186.
41. Hammill SC, Hubmayr RD. The rapidly changing management of cardiac arrhythmias. *Am J Respir Crit Care Med* 2000;161:1070-1073.
42. Daoud EG, Morady F. Pathophysiology of atrial flutter. *Ann Rev Med* 1998;49:77-83.
43. Volgman AS, Carberry PA, Stambler B, et al. Conversion efficacy and safety of intravenous ibutilide compared with intravenous procainamide in patients with atrial flutter or fibrillation. *J Am Coll Cardiol* 1998;31:1414-1419.
44. Paydak H, Kall JG, Burke MC, et al. Atrial fibrillation after radiofrequency ablation of type I atrial flutter: Time to onset, determinants, and clinical course. *Circulation* 1998;28:315-322.
45. Morady F. Radio-frequency ablation as treatment for cardiac arrhythmias. *N Engl J Med* 1999;340:534-544.
46. Charlson ME, MacKenzie CR, Gold JP, et al. The preoperative and intraoperative hemodynamic predictors of postoperative myocardial infarction or ischemia in patients undergoing noncardiac surgery. *Ann Surg* 1989;210:637-648.
47. Tsutsumi K, Udagawa H, Kajiyama Y, et al. Pulmonary thromboembolism after surgery for esophageal cancer: Its features and prophylaxis. *Surg Today* 2000;30:416-420.
48. Worsley DF, Alavi A. Comprehensive analysis of the results of the PIOPED study. Prospective Investigation of Pulmonary Embolism Diagnosis Study. *J Nucl Med* 1995;36:2380-2387.

49. Gotway MB, Edinburgh KJ, Feldstein VA, et al. Imaging evaluation of suspected pulmonary embolism. *Curr Prob Diagn Radiol* 1999;28:129-184.
50. Indik JH, Alpert JS. Detection of pulmonary embolism by D-dimer assay, spiral computed tomography, and magnetic resonance imaging. *Prog Cardiovasc Dis* 2000;42:261-272.
51. Johnson PR, Kanegoanker GS, Bates T. Indirect laryngoscopic evaluation of vocal cord function in patients undergoing transhiatal esophagectomy. *J Am Coll Surg* 1994;178:605-608.
52. Hulscher JB, van Sandick JW, Devriese PP, et al. Vocal cord paralysis after subtotal esophagectomy. *Br J Surg* 1999;86:1583-1587.
53. Tilanus HW, Hop WCJ, Langenhorst BLAM, van Lanschot JJB. Esophagectomy with or without thoracotomy. *J Thorac Cardiovasc Surg* 1993;105:898-903.
54. Gluch L, Smith RC, Bambach CP, et al. Comparison of outcomes following transhiatal or Ivor Lewis esophagectomy for esophageal carcinoma. *World J Surg* 1999;23:271-276.
55. Dia A, Valleix D, Dixneuf B, et al. The recurrent laryngeal nerve (RLN): Application to transhiatal oesophagectomy. *Surg Radiol Anat* 1998:20:31-34.
56. Liebermann-Meffert DM, Walbrun B, Hiebert CA, et al. Recurrent and superior laryngeal nerves: A new look with implications for the esophageal surgeon. *Ann Thorac Surg* 1999;67:217-223.
57. Pierie JP, Goedegebuure S, Schuerman FA, et al. Relation between functional dysphagia and vocal cord palsy after transhiatal oesophagectomy. *Eur J Surg* 2000;166:207-209.
58. Kraus DH, Ali MK, Ginsberg RJ, et al. Vocal cord medialization for unilateral paralysis associated with intrathoracic malignancies. *J Thorac Cardiovasc Surg* 1996;111:334-341.
59. Carew JF, Kraus DH, Ginsberg RJ. Early complications. Recurrent nerve palsy. *Chest Surg Clin N Am* 1999;9:597-608.
60. Zeitels SM. New procedures for paralytic dysphonia: Adduction arytenopexy, Goretex medialization laryngoplasty, and cricothyroid subluxation. *Otolaryngol Clin N Am* 2000;33:841-854.
61. Dougenis D, Walker WS, Cameron EW, et al. Management of chylothorax complicating extensive esophageal resection. *Surg Gynecol Obstet* 1992;174:501-506.
62. Alexiou C, Watson M, Beggs D, et al. Chylothorax following oesophagectomy for malignant disease. *Eur J Cardio-Thorac Surg* 1998;14:640-466.
63. Dugue L, Sauvanet A, Farges O, et al. Output of chyle as an indicator of treatment for chylothorax complicating oesophagectomy. *Br J Surg* 1998;85:1147-1149.
64. Merigliano S, Molena D, Ruol A, et al. Chylothorax complicating esophagectomy for cancer: A plea for early thoracic duct ligation. *J Thorac Cardiovasc Surg* 2000;119:453-457.
65. Ferguson MK. The anatomy and physiology of the thoracic duct. In Deslauriers J, Lacquet LK (eds): **Thoracic Surgery: Surgical Management of Pleural Diseases, Vol. 6**, "International Trends in General Thoracic Surgery," St. Louis, MO, C.V. Mosby Co., 1990, pp 353-356.
66. Miller JI. Diagnosis and management of chylothorax. *Chest Surg Clin N Am* 1996;6:139-148.

67. Ferguson MK. Thoracoscopy for empyema, bronchopleural fistula, and chylothorax. *Ann Thorac Surg* 1993;56:644-645.
68. Wurnig PN, Hollaus PH, Ohtsuka T, et al. Thoracoscopic direct clipping of the thoracic duct for chylopericardium and chylothorax. *Ann Thorac Surg* 2000;70:1662-1665.
69. van Sandick JW, Knegjens JL, van Lanschot JJ, et al. Diaphragmatic herniation following oesophagectomy. *Br J Surg* 1999;86:109-112.
70. Bains MS. Complications of abdominal right-thoracic (Ivor Lewis) esophagectomy. *Chest Surg Clin N Am* 1997;7:587-599.
71. Vecht J, Masclee AA, Lamers CB. The dumping syndrome. Current insights into pathophysiology, diagnosis and treatment. *Scand J Gastroenterol Suppl* 1997;223:21-27.
72. Sinha S, Padhy Ak, Chattopadhyay TK. Dumping syndrome in the intrathoracic stomach. *Trop Gastroenterol* 1997;18:131-133.
73. Scarpignato C. The place of octreotide in the medical management of the dumping syndrome. *Digestion* 1996;57 Suppl 1:114-118.
74. Vecht J, Gielkens HA, Frolich M, et al. Vasoactive substances in the early dumping syndrome: Effects of dumping provocation with and without octreotide. *Eur J Clin Invest* 1997;27:680-684.
75. Fok M, Cheng SW, Wong J. Pyloroplasty versus no drainage in gastric replacement of the esophagus. Am J Surg 1991;162:447-452.
76. Bemelman WA, Brummelkamp WH, Bartelsman JFWM. Endoscopic balloon dilation of the pylorus after esophagogastrostomy without a drainage procedure. *Surg Gynecol Obstet* 170:424-1990;426.
77. Mannell A, Epstein B. Exclusion of the oesophagus: Is this a dangerous maneuver? *Br J Surg* 1984;71:442-445.
78. Chambon JP, Robert Y, Remy J, et al. Mucoceles oesophagiennes compliquant la double exclusion de l'oesophage apres ingestion de caustique. *Ann Radiol* 1990;33:270-276.
79. Olsen CO, Hopkins RA, Postlethwait RW. Management of an infected mucocele occurring in a bypassed excluded esophageal segment. *Ann Thorac Surg* 1985;40:73-75.
80. Kamath MV, Ellison RG, Rubin JW, et al. Esophageal mucocele: A complication of blind loop esophagus. *Ann Thorac Surg* 1987;43:263-269.
81. Duranceau AC, Lafontaine ER, Archambault SC, et al. Motor function in the excluded esophagus and its implications in the management of patients with unresectable carcinoma of the esophagus. *Ann Surg* 1987;206:787-790.
82. Paramesh V, Rumisek JD, Chang FC. Spontaneous recanalization of the esophagus after exclusion using nonabsorbable staples. *Ann Thorac Surg* 1995;59:1214-1216.
83. Ramirez Schon G, Cebollero Marcucci J, Marquez Toro C. Distal-end esophagostomy of the excluded esophagus in the palliation of upper and mid-esophageal carcinoma. *Am J Surg* 1990;159:287-290.
84. Kron IL, Johnson AM, Morgan RF. Gastrotracheal fistula: A late complication after transhiatal esophagectomy. *Ann Thorac Surg* 1989;47:767-768.
85. Endredi J, Horvath OP. Late complications after pharyngogastrostomy. *Acta Chir Hung* 1997;36:76-78.

Index